Clinical echocardiography

DEVELOPMENTS IN
CARDIOVASCULAR MEDICINE

MASATSUGU IWASE and IWAO SOTOBATA
1st Department of Internal Medicine, Nagoya University School of Medicine, Nagoya, Japan

CLINICAL ECHOCARDIOGRAPHY

KLUWER ACADEMIC PUBLISHERS
DORDRECHT / BOSTON / LONDON

Library of Congress Cataloging in Publication Data

```
Iwase, Masatsugu, 1951-
    Clinical echocardiography / by Masatsugu Iwase and Iwao Sotobata.
        p.    cm. -- (Developments in cardiovascular medicine ; 95)
    Translated from Japanese.
    Bibliography: p.
    ISBN-13:978-94-010-6877-2    e-ISBN-13:978-94-009-0867-3
    DOI:10.1007/978-94-009-0867-3

    1. Echocardiography.  2. Cardiovascular system--Diseases-
-Diagnosis.   I. Sotobata, Iwao, 1932-   . II. Title.  III. Series:
Developments in cardiovascular medicine ; v. 95.
    [DNLM: 1. Cardiovascular Diseases--diagnosis.
2. Echocardiogrpahy.  3. Ultrasonic Diagnosis.   W1 DE997VME v. 95 /
WG 141.5.E2 I96c]
    RC683.5.U5I82 1989
    616.1'07543--dc19
    DNLM/DLC
    for Library of Congress                                    88-13665
                                                               CIP
```

ISBN-13: 978-94-010-6877-2   e-ISBN-13: 978-94-009-0867-3
DOI: 10.1007/978-94-009-0867-3

Published by Kluwer Academic Publishers,
P.O. Box 17, 3300 AA Dordrecht, The Netherlands.

Kluwer Academic Publishers incorporates
the publishing programmes of
D. Reidel, Martinus Nijhoff, Dr W. Junk and MTP Press.

Sold and distributed in the U.S.A. and Canada
by Kluwer Academic Publishers,
101 Philip Drive, Norwell, MA 02061, U.S.A.

In all other countries, sold and distributed
by Kluwer Academic Publishers Group,
P.O. Box 322, 3300 AH Dordrecht, The Netherlands.

This is the 3rd revised edition of *Clinical Echocardiography*.
The first edition and second revised edition appeared
in Japanese in 1984 and 1986 respectively.

Translated by Masatsugu Iwase and Mario A. Benavides G.

printed on acid free paper

Contents

Preface   IX
Foreword by Merrill P. Spencer   XI

1. *The basics of cardiac ultrasound*   1
    1. Physical properties of ultrasound   1
    2. Cardiac ultrasound imaging systems   2
    3. Doppler echocardiography   2

2. *Echocardiographic examination*   11
    1. Placement of the transducer   11
    2. Two-dimensional examination of the heart   11
      A. Left ventricular long axis view   11
      B. Left ventricular short axis view   12
      C. Four chamber view   12
    3. M-mode examination   14
    4. Contrast echocardiography   15
    5. Pulsed Doppler examination   17
      A. Left ventricular outflow   19
      B. Left ventricular inflow   21
      C. Right ventricular outflow   21
      D. Right ventricular inflow   21
    6. Continuous wave (CW) Doppler examination   21
    7. High PRF Doppler examination   25

3. *Acquired valvular heart disease*   28
    1. Mitral valve stenosis   28
    2. Giant left atrium   32
    3. Mitral valve regurgitation (rheumatic in origin)   32
    4. Mitral valve prolapse   33
    5. Ruptured chordae tendineae   37
    6. Aortic valve stenosis   37
    7. Aortic valve regurgitation   46
    8. Infective endocarditis   52
    9. Tricuspid valve stenosis   73

10. Tricuspid valve regurgitation   79
11. Pulmonary valve regurgitation   79
12. Prosthetic valve   80

4. *Congenital heart disease*   81
    1. Atrial septal defect   81
    2. Endocardial cushion defect   81
    3. Persistent left superior vena cava   82
    4. Ventricular septal defect   82
    5. Sinus of Valsalva aneurysm   84
    6. Patent ductus arteriosus   88
    7. Pulmonary stenosis   88
    8. Ebstein's anomaly   93
    9. Tetralogy of Fallot   93
   10. Double outlet of the right ventricle   99
   11. Single ventricle   99
   12. Corrected transposition of great arteries   99
   13. Tricuspid atresia   102
   14. Cor triatriatum   103
   15. Bicuspid aortic valve   105
   16. Supravalvular aortic stenosis   106
   17. Coronary artery fistula   106
   18. Anomalous origin of the left main coronary artery from the pulmonary
       trunk   121
   19. Marfan's syndrome   121

5. *Coronary artery disease*   122
    1. Wall motion abnormalities   122
    2. Wall thickening and echo intensity abnormalities   122
    3. Complications of myocardial infarction   123
       A. Ventricular aneurysm   123
       B. Mural thrombus of the left ventricle   123
       C. Rupture of the ventricular septum   136
       D. Mitral regurgitation   136
       E. Right ventricular myocardial infarction   136
    4. Ischemic cardiomyopathy   137
    5. Examination of coronary arteries   137

6. *Myocardial diseases*   138
    1. Hypertrophic cardiomyopathy   138
    2. Dilated cardiomyopathy   140
    3. Secondary cardiomyopathy   159
    4. Inflammatory process of the myocardium   159
    5. Myocardial abnormality due to toxic agents   159

7. *Other cardiac diseases*   160
    1. Left atrial myxoma   160
    2. Right atrial myxoma   160

3. Intracardiac rhabdomyoma — 160
4. Left ventricular fibroma — 168
5. Malignant primary cardiac tumor — 168
6. Secondary tumors of the heart — 168
7. Pericardial effusion — 168
8. Pleural effusion — 169
9. Constrictive pericarditis — 169
10. Pericardial defect — 169
11. False tendon — 169
12. Chiari network — 187
13. Atrial septal aneurysm — 187
14. Sigmoid septum — 188
15. Mitral anular calcification — 188
16. Aneurysm of the aorta — 188
17. Primary pulmonary hypertension — 188

8. *Evaluation of left ventricular function* — 189
1. M-mode echocardiography — 189
2. Two-dimensional echocardiography — 189
3. Doppler method — 192
   A. Evaluation of systolic function — 192
   B. Evaluation of diastolic behavior — 195
4. Age related changes in the left ventricular function — 213

9. *Pulmonary hypertension* — 214
1. M-mode echocardiographic evaluation — 214
2. Pulsed Doppler evaluation — 217

10. *Echocardiographic evaluation of arrhythmia* — 218
1. Bundle branch block — 218
2. Wall-Parkinson-White (WPW) syndrome — 218
3. Atrial fibrillation — 223
4. Atrial flutter — 223
5. Ectopic atrial rhythm — 237
6. Supraventricular premature contraction — 237
7. Ventricular premature contraction — 239
8. Abnormal atrio-ventricular conduction — 248
9. Cardiac pacing — 248

11. *Color coded Doppler flow mapping* — 250

References — 282

Additional references — 296

Index of subjects — 299

Preface

Recently, much progress has been made with echocardiography and Doppler techniques and these ultrasound methods have grown in importance and reliability as non-invasive diagnostic procedures for many cardiovascular disorders. The objective of this textbook is to offer a detailed yet concise overview of the echocardiographic diagnosis of the various cardiovascular diseases. The book focuses upon the practical echocardiographic (including Doppler) examination. Accordingly, the fundamental principles of echocardiography and the Doppler techniques (pulsed and continuous wave and color flow mapping are covered briefly but comprehensively). A copious amount of representative figures and illustrations is included so that the reader is able to understand the clinical application of each modality in the various cardiovascular pathologies and the echocardiographic diagnosis. In keeping with the concept of an integrated echocardiographic examination, the two-dimensional, M-mode and Doppler echocardiographic findings are included in many of the diseases.

Usually, the echocardiographic examination is approached first by two-dimensional imaging to give an understanding of the anatomical correlations, if necessary adding M-mode to clarify the time course of intracardiac movements, and secondly by each Doppler technique to evaluate the hemodynamic conditions. When familiar with these approaches, one can make not only the diagnosis of many cardiovascular diseases with echocardiography alone, but also the rational and expeditious management of patients. Today, some of the cardiac diseases (Atrial Myxoma, Atrial Septal Defect, Infective endocarditis and so forth) have been operated based only on echocardiographic findings. Echocardiographic examination before catheterization also allows the procedure to be carried out more safely and within a shorter time. With the increasing importance of echocardiography in clinical cardiology, it is necessary for clinicians to understand the many aspects of this diagnostic approach as well as possible. I hope that this textbook will help fulfil this need.

Thanks are due to Dr. Mario A. Benavides G. from Mexico and Mr. Jim Chapman for their assistance with the translation and editing of the work.

MASATSUGU IWASE

Foreword

Recent progress in cardiac Doppler represents a great success story in the recent history of echocardiography. After the early beginnings with pulse Doppler, followed by the vision of color M-mode provided by Brandestini and practical demonstrations of continuous-wave Doppler capabilities by Hatle, the combination of modalities of continuous-wave spectral analysis and 2-D color display brought us to a powerful capability in noninvasive diagnostic techniques. Dr. Iwase early grasped the meaning of these trends and has, through excellent performance, led us into the future. This book is a superb state-of-the-art example brought together in a format which is well illustrated and clearly explained. It represents a benchmark in cardiac ultrasound from which we can move forward to higher levels of patient care.

MERRILL P. SPENCER
Founding President
International Cardiac Doppler Society and
Medical Director, Institute of Applied
Physiology and Medicine
Seattle, U.S.A.

The basics of cardiac ultrasound

1. Physical properties of ultrasound

Ultrasound is sound that has a frequency above the audible range (20–20 000 Hz). The velocity is equal to the frequency multiplied by the wavelength, i.e. $C = f \times \lambda$, where C is the velocity, f is the frequency of the sound, and λ is the wavelength. The wavelength and frequency, and hence the velocity, vary according to the medium in which the sound travels. Also, wavelength and frequency are related to each other – the higher the frequency, the shorter the wavelength. Ultrasound used for imaging applications is formed into a beam and has the physical properties of both a beam and sound, such as (1) attenuation, (2) reflection, (3) refraction, (4) characteristic velocity in each medium, (5) straight propagation through homogeneous medium and (6) Doppler effect.

When ultrasound propagates through a medium, its energy is attenuated depending on the distance traveled and on its frequency. The longer the distance, the greater the attenuation. The higher the frequency, the greater the attenuation. In the 'near field', ultrasound propagates as a beam in a straight line from the transmitting element through the homogeneous medium. It diverges in the 'far field' as uncontrolled sound energy. The boundary between the near field and the far field is the transition point. The distance from the transition point to the transmitting element is assumed to be $P = D^2/4\lambda$, where P is the distance from the transmitting element to the transition point, D is the diameter of the transmitting element and λ is the wavelength. The larger the diameter of the transmitting element, the longer the distance to the transition point. In a commercially available transducer, the typical transition point is about 24 cm. For higher frequencies (shorter wavelengths), the distance is longer. As the ultrasound propagates through a medium, it undergoes reflections and refractions at interfaces between two media. The magnitude of the reflection is dependent on differences in acoustic impedance and on the degree of refraction. By definition, the acoustic impedance is the density of the medium times the velocity that sound travels through that medium. Refraction is related to the difference of the velocities in the two media. When the ultrasound beam strikes an interface with a large acoustic mismatch, such as the interface between liquid and gaseous media, most of the ultrasound is reflected. The amount of reflection to the transducer is also affected by the angle of incidence to the interface. The closer the incident angle is to 90 degrees, the greater the amount of reflection. Each medium through which the ultrasound beam passes has a characteristic acoustic velocity . When the ultrasound beam travels through a homogeneous medium, it moves with its characteristic velocity and undergoes no reflection or refraction. A frequency range of 1 MHz through 10 MHz is used for imaging ultrasound systems. In cardiac diagnosis, a frequency range of 2.25–7.5 MHz is implemented.

2. Cardiac ultrasound imaging systems

Echoes (reflected or back-scattered signals) in the ultrasound beam are mainly generated from the interfaces between structures or tissues inside the body. The propagation velocity (about 1540 meters per second) is assumed to be the same through all kind of soft tissues. The depth at which the echo is generated is then calculated as half of the round-trip time divided by the propagation velocity, or $d = (t/2)/C$, where d is the depth generating the echo, t is the elapsed time from transmitting to receiving the echo, and C is the propagation velocity. The magnitude of the echo depends on the types of interfaces between tissues or structures causing it. For example, posterior pericardial echoes are most strong since they originate between the heart and lung.

Displaying the magnitude of the echoes as amplitude on a cathode ray tube (CRT) is called 'A-mode' (amplitude mode). Usually, the magnitude is used to modulate the intensity (brightness) on the CRT image, which is called B-mode (brightness mode). When a B-mode image is swept over an area, it is called two-dimensional mode (Figure 1.1). A cross-section of the heart is obtained by this two-dimensional imaging mode. For scanning the heart, the sector format is usually employed. Another format, the rectangular format (linear scan) is not usually used to view the heart because of the strong echoes from the ribs. However, a linear scanner is often applied to the neonate and children because their ribs are not yet ossified. To produce sector images, either a mechanical scanner or a phased array can be used. The popular mechanical scanner creates the sector image by mechanically oscillating or rotating between one and three transducer elements. The phased array uses varying electrical delay lines, without any mechanical motion.

Cardiac ultrasound imaging systems usually produce images at the rate of about 30–60 frames/sec. This depends on the depth setting and sector angles as well as the number of acoustic vectors used to construct each image. The operator can see the cardiac images in real time, permitting a spatially accurate representation of the anatomy. Fewer acoustic data have been obtained far from the transducer than in the near field due to attenuation. The area very close to the apex of the sector (1 to 2 cm) is often difficult to observe clearly, because of the reverberation of the echoes and difficulty in focusing. Sweeping a B-mode line from left to right on a CRT as a function of time is called the M-mode (time motion mode). M-mode echocardiography has been used to evaluate cardiac wall and valve motion because of its rapid sampling rate and high degree of temporal resolution.

3. Doppler echocardiography

The Doppler effect is well known as the change in pitch of a train whistle or of an ambulance siren moving past a stationary observer. When the sound source moves toward the stationary observer, the wavelength of the sound is compressed and it is perceived as a higher pitched sound. The sound becomes lower in pitch when it moves away from the listener (Figure 1.2). Doppler echocardiography is based on this effect.

When a transducer transmits a known frequency of sound into the heart or blood vessels, the sound waves reflect off the moving red blood cells, creating frequency shifts. The

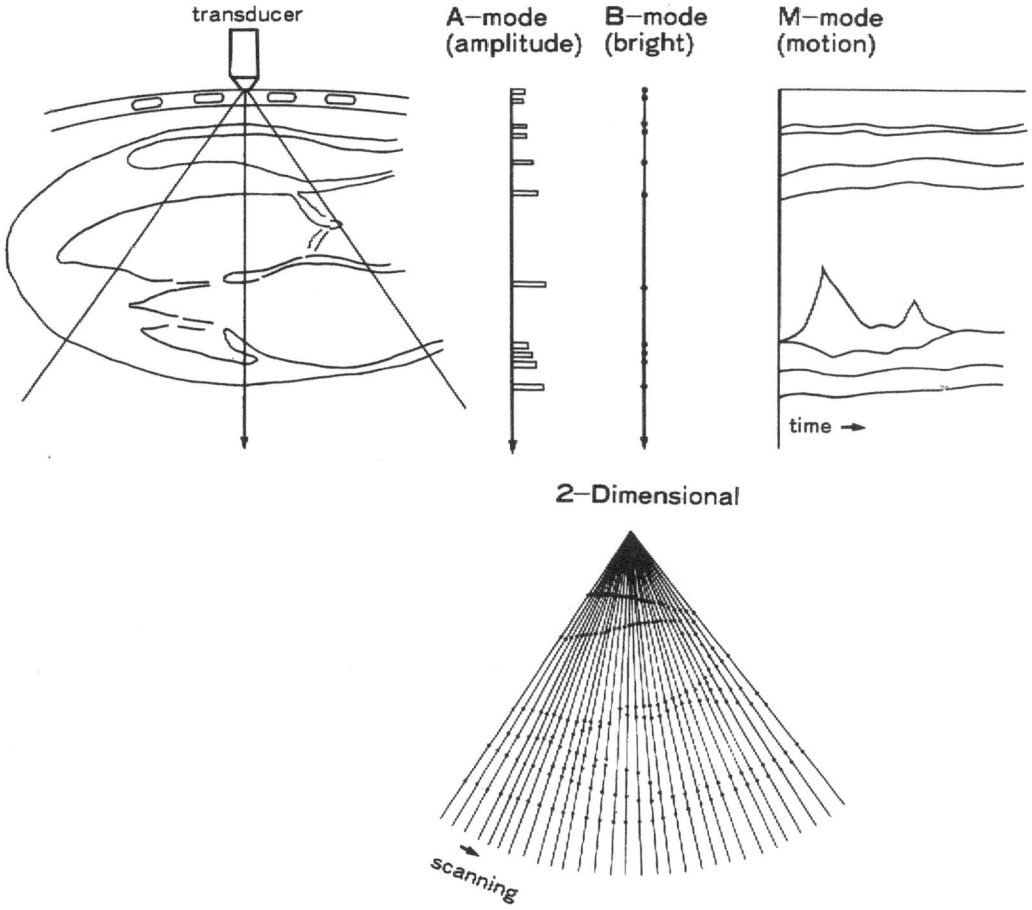

Figure 1.1. Diagrams illustrating the principles of echocardiographic imaging using pulsed, reflected ultrasound. (See text for details.)

transducer receives this returning sound. The transmitted frequency is compared with the returning frequency, and the frequency shifts created by the moving blood cells are determined as the vector component of the blood flow velocity along the beam line (Figure 1.3). The Doppler equation can be used to calculate blood flow velocity from the shifted frequency if the speed of sound in tissue is known as well as the angle between blood flow and the ultrasound beam (Figure 1.4). This Doppler frequency is within the audible range, so it can be heard as sound from a loudspeaker. Ultrasound fetal monitors and Doppler stethoscopes simply employ this sound. However, this audio sound alone is not enough to analyze blood flow dynamics, since not all blood cells move at the same velocity and in the same direction. Real blood flows often produce complex shifted frequencies that contain information about the motion of all blood cells moving at a variety of velocities within the ultrasound beam. This complex signal must be then processed through a computer that does a calculation of the discreet Fourier transform using an FFT (Fast Fourier Transformation or chirp Z algorithm). This process results in the breakdown of the complex composite signal into its individual frequency elements and amplitudes (spectral analysis). In order to display the spectral

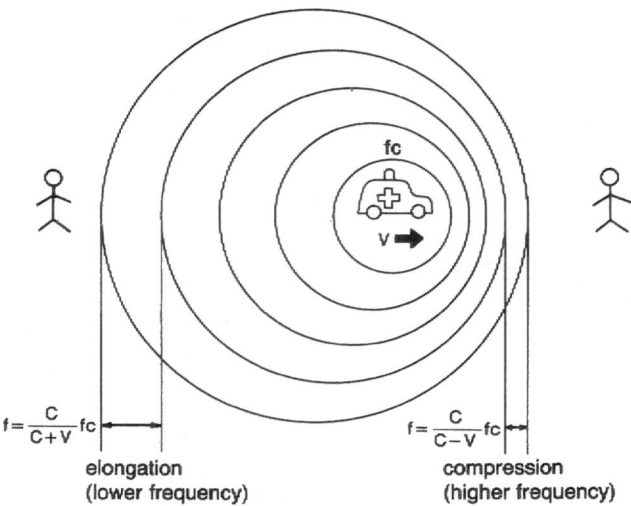

$$f = \frac{C}{C+V} \, fc$$

elongation
(lower frequency)

$$f = \frac{C}{C-V} \, fc$$

compression
(higher frequency)

Figure 1.2. Doppler effect. When an ambulance moves at a speed of V with its siren wailing, the wavelengths are compressed in front of the ambulance and the frequency of the waves, or the pitch, is increased for the stationary listener. Likewise, it is heard as a low pitch sound as it moves away because the wavelength is elongated. fc: frequency of the siren. C: sound velocity. V: speed of the ambulance.

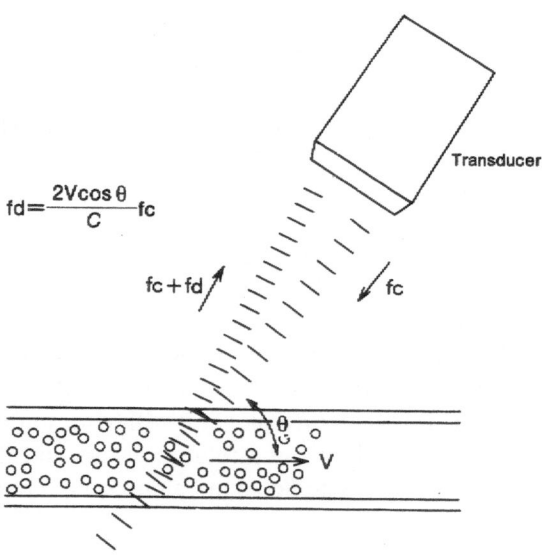

$$fd = \frac{2V \cos \theta}{C} \, fc$$

Figure 1.3. Blood flow measurement by Doppler effect. The transmitted frequency (fc) is shifted to $fc + fd$ by the reflection of moving blood cells according to Doppler effect. The Doppler shifted frequency is calculated into the blood flow velocity by the Doppler equation. C: propagation velocity through a body. fc: transmitting frequency. fd: Doppler shifted frequency. θ: angle between the flow and ultrasonic beam direction.

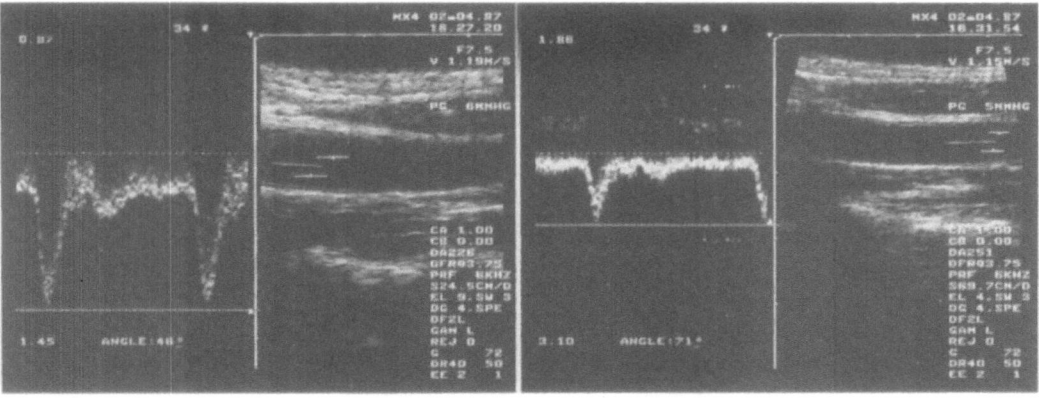

Figure 1.4. Measurement of carotid arterial flow velocity calculated by inserting different angle correction factors. Right, with a larger angle between the blood flow and the ultrasound beam (Doppler angle; *DA*), a lower frequency shift is sampled. However, both calculated velocities (arrow) are similar, by the Doppler equation, when the angle is corrected for.

analysis, a small range of velocities is deposited into a 'bin' of information and plotted over time. At a given point in time, more blood cells are moving at the velocity represented by the most intense (bright) bin than are moving at other velocities. Usually, blood flow toward the transducer is displayed above the zero line (base line), while flow away from the transducer is displayed below the zero line (Figure 1.5). The greater the distance from the zero line, the more the Doppler shift and hence the higher the velocity. In normal conditions the blood flow is laminar, which means that most of the blood cells move in a uniform direction with a smooth variation in velocity. However, abnormal flow such as regurgitant, stenotic or shunt flow may become turbulent, so that blood cells move in a variety of directions at various velocities. The laminar flow displays narrow band spectra, while the turbulence shows wide band spectra (Figure 1.6).

Cardiac Doppler systems are fundamentally of two types, pulsed and continuous wave, both taking advantage of the Doppler effect. In the pulsed wave (PW) Doppler system, a transducer transmits the short burst of the ultrasound and only functions as a receiver for a limited period or 'window' of time (time gate or range gate). This time period is proportional to the interval required for the sound reflecting from a specific area (sample volume) to be received. Therefore, the pulsed Doppler instrument receives information corresponding to the location of the sample volume and ignores echoes returning from other areas (Figure 1.7A). The sample volume may be located anywhere within the heart or great vessels using a two-dimensional image for spatial orientation. Pulsed Doppler systems have two limitations due to the use of a pulsed wave. One is the maximum measurable Doppler shifted frequency (Fd_{max}) and the other is the maximum measurable depth. The Nyquist limit (Fd_{max}) is the theoretical maximum frequency that a sampling system can accurately measure. For example, if pulses are transmitted every 250 μsec, then the pulse repetition frequency (PRF) is calculated to be 4 kHz. The Fd_{max} is half of the PRF, by the sampling theorem, or 2 kHz. The maximum measurable depth is limited by the turnaround time of the pulses. For example, if it is 250 μsec, the maximum measurable depth is half of the propagation velocity (1540 m/sec × 250 × 10^{-6} sec), or about 19 cm. This is the reason why there are limitations in measuring high blood flow velocities in deep areas (Figure 1.8). When the Doppler shifted frequency exceeds

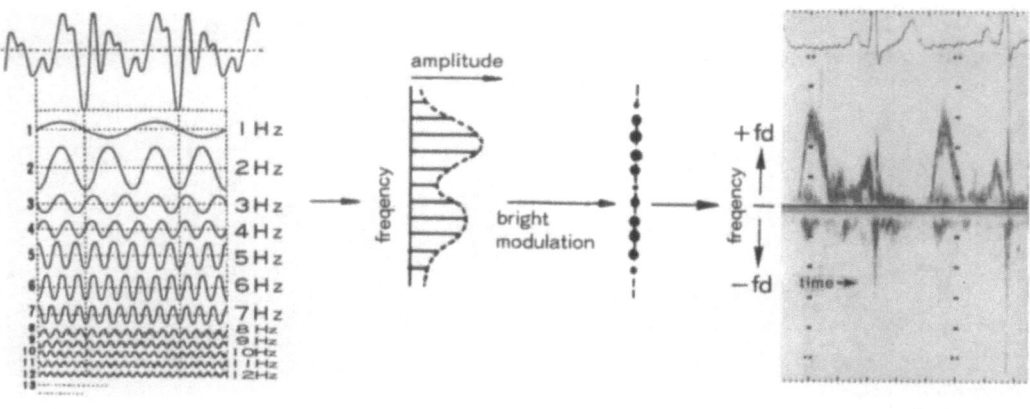

spectrum display

Figure 1.5. Frequency analysis and display of Doppler echocardiography. The complex frequency-shifted signal is a sum of various sinusoidal frequency components on which a discrete Fourier transform may be performed. The spectral tracing demonstrates the Doppler-shifted frequency of the vertical axis and time on the horizontal axis. The flow toward the transducer is presented above the baseline (zero line), and the flow away from the transducer appears below the baseline (by convention). The greater the distance from the baseline on the vertical axis, the greater the frequency shift (or velocity).

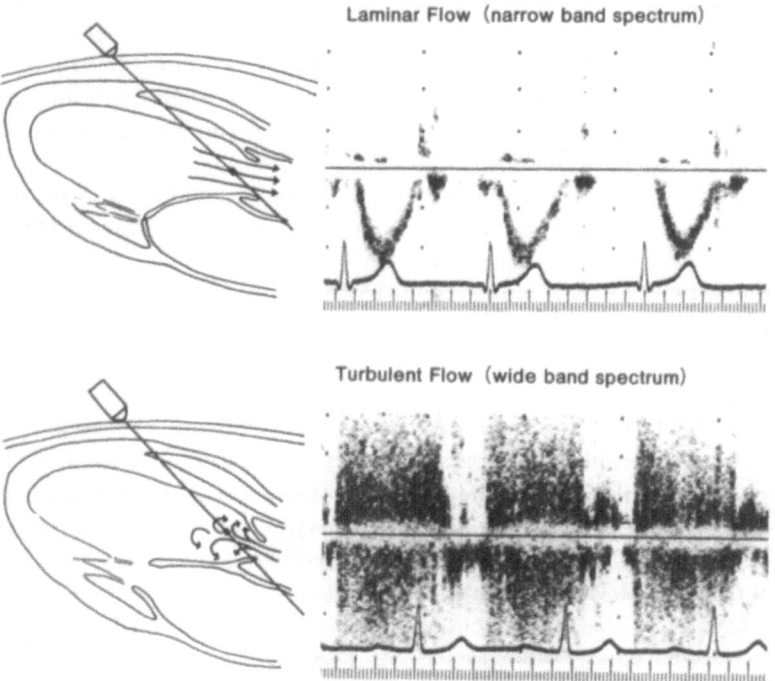

Figure 1.6. Spectral patterns of normal and abnormal flow velocity tracings by pulsed Doppler echocardiography. The normal blood flow is laminar, which implies the red blood cells move in the same direction with a fairly uniform velocity. The abnormal flow shows turbulence, indicating that the red blood cells move in different directions with a variety of velocities. This abnormal flow regime appears to be bi-directional, and it is difficult to identify the direction of blood flow.

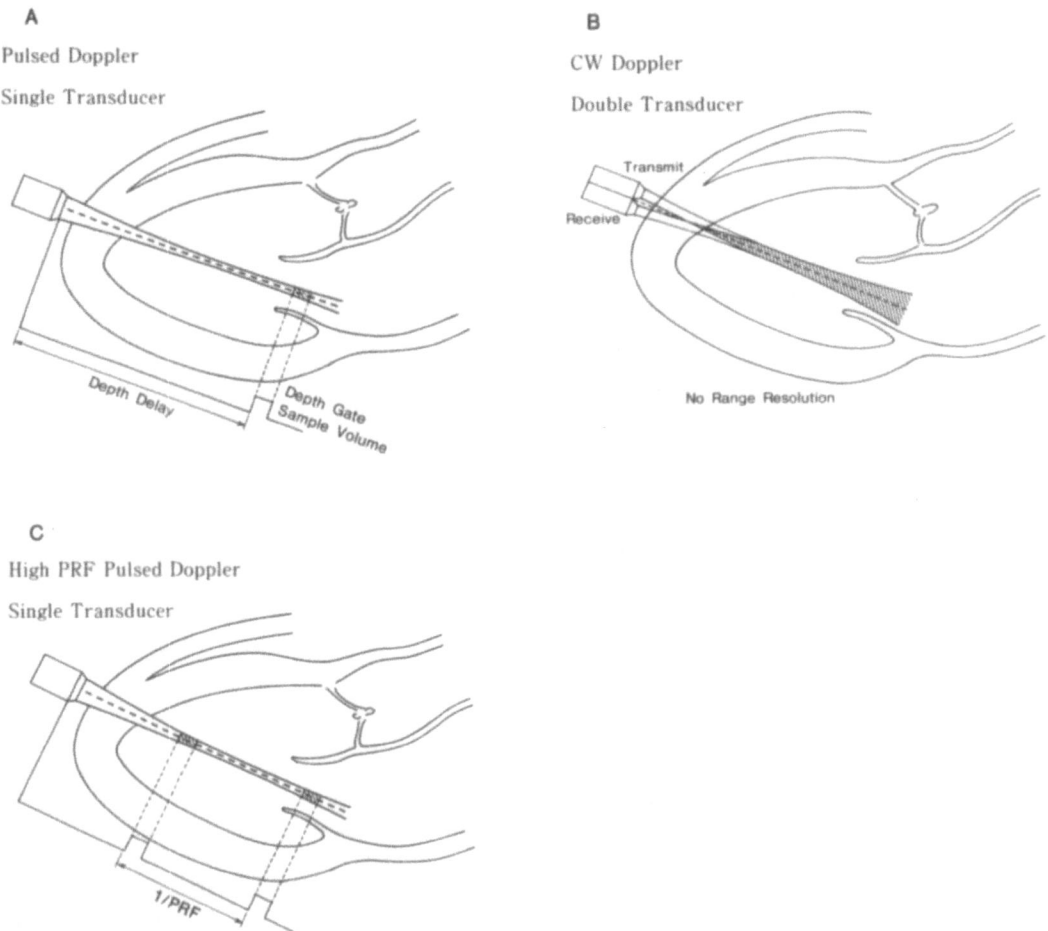

A

Pulsed Doppler

Single Transducer

Depth Delay Depth Gate Sample Volume

B

CW Doppler

Double Transducer

Transmit

Receive

No Range Resolution

C

High PRF Pulsed Doppler

Single Transducer

1/PRF

Figure 1.7. Three different modes of Doppler echocardiography. (A) Pulsed Doppler Mode: The time-gated echoes from the specific depth are sampled and analyzed to the blood flow spectra. (B) CW Doppler Mode: All of the echoes along with the beam direction are sampled and analyzed. (C) High pulse repetition frequency (PRF) Doppler Mode: The gated echoes are received not only from the specific depth but also from the ambiguous sampling points. The ambiguous sampling points are located every 1/PRF (sec). The PRF can be increased independently of the depth setting.

Fd_{max}, aliasing occurs and the spectra come up from $-Fd_{max}$. It is possible to deal with aliasing by merely adding the top portion of the flow velocity signal (which had 'rolled over' and been displayed at the bottom of the record) to the truncated portion of the flow velocity record (Figure 1.9). Recently introduced equipment can shift the zero line (zero shift) and display double the normal scale ($2Fd_{max}$) in one direction (Figure 1.10). To measure velocities which exceed $2Fd_{max}$, continuous wave (CW) or high pulse repetition frequency (high PRF) Doppler methods are mandatory.

The CW Doppler transducer has two elements mounted close to each other. One transmits the ultrasound wave continuously, and the other receives the returning sound continuously (Figure 1.7B). Therefore, there are no limitations in the measurable Doppler shifted frequency and the measurable depth. Since the receiver obtains all of the echoes along the beam line, it is not possible to identify the echoes from specific depth, and is difficult to separate

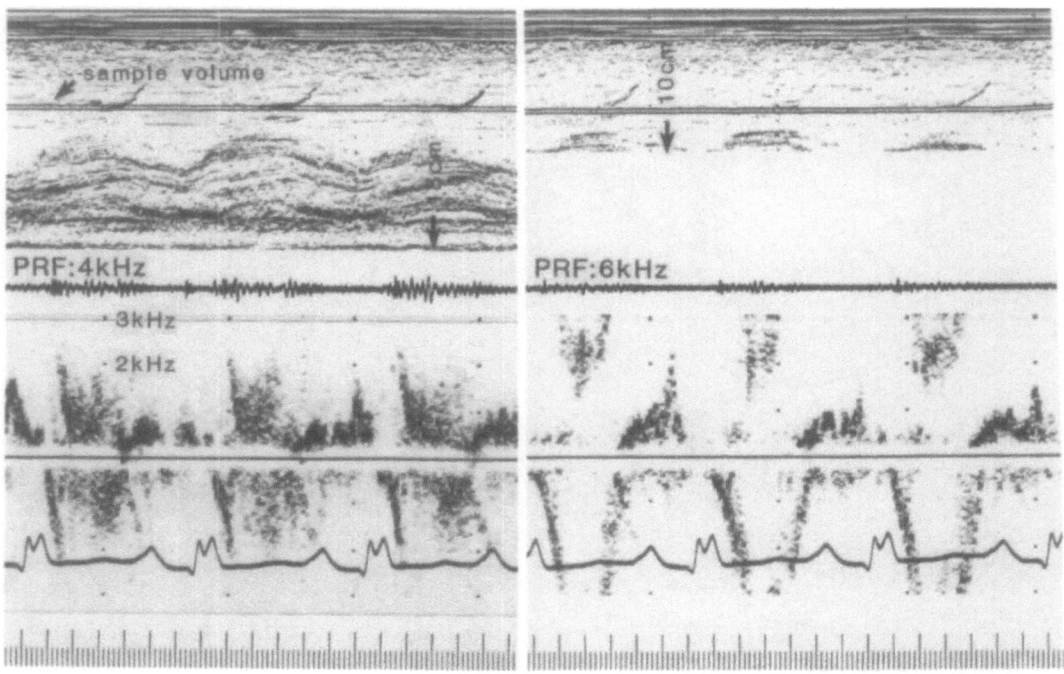

Figure 1.8. Changes in the spectral display of tricuspid regurgitant flow with different PRF. When the PRF is set to 4 KHz, the maximum measurable Doppler shifted frequency is ± 2 KHz and identification of the blood flow direction is rather difficult due to bi-directional appearance (left). When the PRF is increased to 6 KHz, the maximum measurable Doppler-shifted frequency becomes ± 3 KHz, and the direction of tricuspid regurgitant flow is recognized as being away from the transducer with the aliasing being clearly identified (right). In the M-mode trace, the maximum depth is limited to 10 cm by the PRF of 6 KHz, while at 18 cm depth the maximum applicable PRF is 4 KHz.

different signals from two or more flows. Therefore, the specific beam direction must be aligned with only one flow. In clinical practice, one should choose between these two methods, as necessary, to meet specific needs. For example, to localize a sample volume to specify the area for cardiac output measurement one uses pulsed Doppler and to measure high velocities, CW Doppler is implemented. High pulse repetition frequency (PRF) Doppler systems which implement the range ambiguity phenomenon have been developed to measure high velocities in a specific sample volume. In these systems, a higher repetition rate than conventional pulsed Doppler systems allows an increase in Fd_{max}, but they can also pick up ambiguous signals. These arise from the simultaneous reception of ultrasonic signals from earlier pulses at greater depths than the intended sample depth (Figure 1.7C). Accordingly, the high PRF Doppler method permits assessment of the higher velocities and provides some localization capability using a conventional two-dimensional transducer. Another recent development in echocardiographic equipment is the multi-gated pulsed Doppler system. In this system, one can obtain a simultaneous display of three Doppler signals at different sampling points on the same beam line (Figure 1.11). By virtue of having three different gate circuits which process the receiving signals of different time gates (different depths), these different channels can emit separate Doppler signals from each depth. Three different Doppler signals are run through the same FFT circuit. The samples are analyzed in a time-sharing mode, analyzed signals coming from the three channels are read out of the

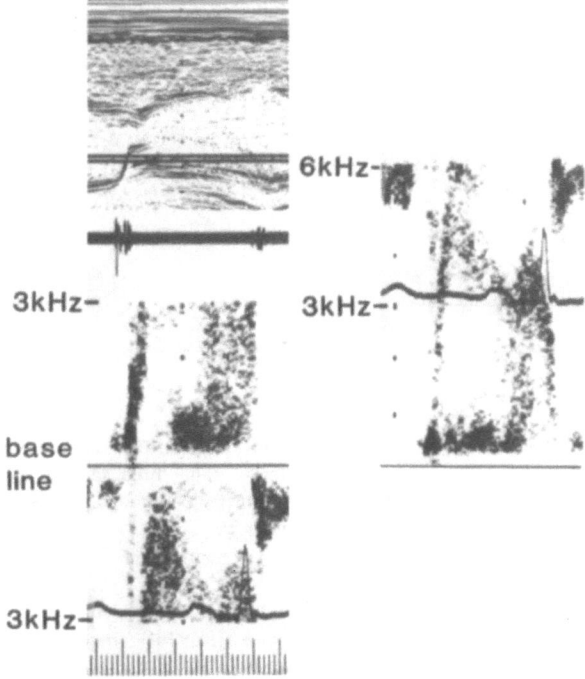

Figure 1.9. Pulsed Doppler recording of stenotic mitral flow with aliasing, and an illustration of a manual stacking technique. The left panel shows a stenotic transmitral flow, which has aliased. The signal has 'wrapped around' so that the peak velocity appears at the bottom of the spectral display. The right panel shows the same waveform with the aliased portion summed with the unaliased segment.

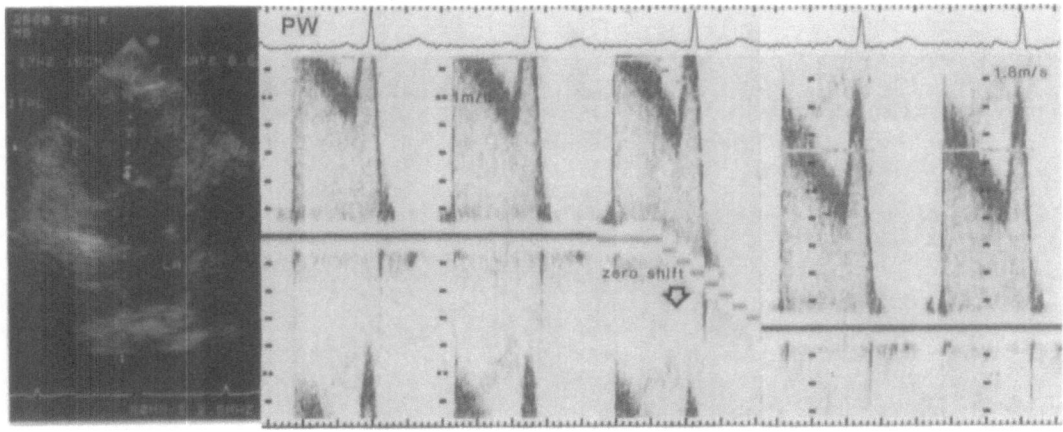

Figure 1.10. Pulsed Doppler recording of stenotic mitral flow with aliasing and zero shift. The trace on the left demonstrates a stenotic transmitral flow, whose velocity is high enough to cause the aliasing. Therefore, it is rather difficult to evaluate the flow profile in this trace. When the zero line is shifted downwards, the flow profile becomes acceptable. The zero shift allows one to display velocities exceeding the Nyquist limit to twice Fd_{max} in one direction.

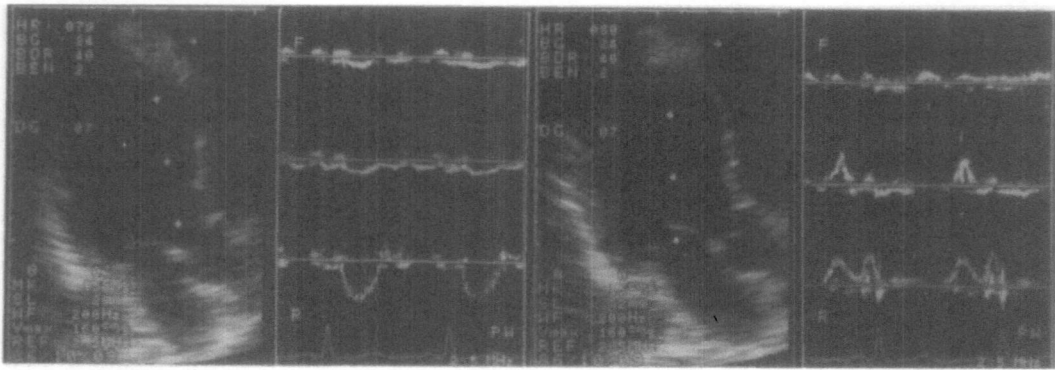

Figure 1.11. Multi-gated Doppler recordings of left ventricular outflow and inflow in three different sample volumes of a patient with an old myocardial infarction. The three sample volume locations in the left ventricular outflow and inflow tracts are shown in the two-dimensional image and each velocity trace is presented simultaneously.

output memory at the same time and can be displayed simultaneously. When three different Doppler signals are displayed simultaneously, the time lag among these three signals is not more than 3 msec, which is believed to be negligible in clinical practice.

Another new method is color coded flow mapping, which can display blood flow information on two-dimensional images. Details of this method are addressed in Chapter 11.

CHAPTER 2

Echocardiographic examination

1. Placement of the transducer

Ultrasound waves do not travel well through gaseous or calcified media, such as lung or bone. Thus, the sites at which a transducer may be located in order to obtain cardiac ultrasound images are limited. These limited areas, so-called 'acoustic-windows', lie on the left sternal border (parasternal), over the apex (apical), below the xiphoid (subcostal), and in the suprasternal notch (suprasternal). Because the heart lies at a variable depth within the thorax, parasternal cardiac imaging is often facilitated by positioning the patient on his left side so that the heart falls against the left anterior chest wall. These transducer locations have been named by the American Society of Echocardiography (A.S.E.) for standardization.

2. Two-dimensional examination of the heart

The major cross-sectional images used for observing the various structures of the heart are the long axis, short axis, and four chamber views. The long axis images present a major axis of the left ventricle, and can be obtained by positioning the transducer either parasternally or apically. The short axis images present the minor axis of the left ventricle, and can be obtained by either parasternal or subcostal positioning. The four chamber images present the major axis of the left ventricle with maximum right-side heart, and can be obtained by either apical or subcostal positioning. The suprasternal long axis presents the aortic arch, while the short axis presents the transverse image of the aortic arch. The above is a summary of usage; however, modified approaches and cross-sections are sometimes necessary to obtain specific information depending on the disease conditions.

A. Left ventricular long axis view

The parasternal long axis view is obtained by placing the transducer on the left sternal border between the second and fifth intercostal space and directing the index mark of the transducer toward the patient's right shoulder. Usually, the transducer is placed on the third or fourth intercostal space, and the sector plane is aligned parallel to the longitudinal axis of the left ventricle. Careful control of the transducer is required to avoid improper angulation of the scan plane tangentially through the ventricle and to scan both the aortic and mitral valves (Figure 2.1). In cases of cardiac enlargement, sliding the transducer slightly away from the

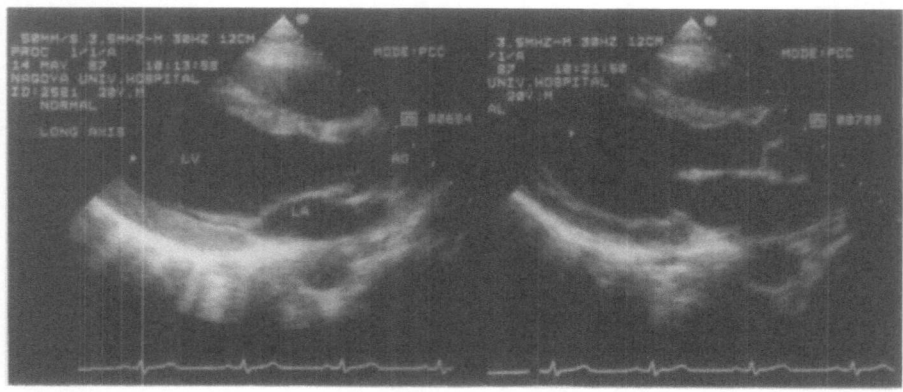

Figure 2.1. Left ventricular long axis view.

sternal border often produces better images than the ordinary way. The parasternal long axis is commonly used to evaluate the left ventricle, the left atrium, the aortic root and aortic and mitral valves. M-mode tracing is performed using the parasternal long axis view (details are described below).

The left ventricular long axis images are also obtained by the apical approach using the apical long axis view, which is suitable for left-sided Doppler recordings.

B. Left ventricular short axis view

Serial short axis views of the left ventricle are obtained by orienting the sector plane perpendicular to the long axis of the left ventricle from a standard parasternal long axis transducer placement on the chest wall. The short axis sweep is performed by maintaining the transducer in a fixed location on the chest wall and slowly angling the image plane from aorta (cephalad) to apex (caudad) to obtain the various parts of the short axis view such as aortic valve, mitral valve and papillary muscle level (Figure 2.2). The image at the aortic valve level demonstrates the cusps of the aortic valve and the sinuses of Valsalva. It is important to assess the morphology as well as the valve opening and closure. Often, at this level, left and right coronary arteries are observed. Images at the mitral valve level demonstrate the movements of anterior and posterior leaflets. At this level, the mitral valve orifice is evaluated, especially for mitral stenosis. At the papillary muscle level, the contraction and relaxation of the left ventricle are observed. In the case of right ventricular pressure or volume overload, the interventricular septum inclines to the left ventricle, so-called processing of the 'D-shaped' interventricular septum.

C. Four chamber view

The four chamber view is obtained by placing the transducer over the cardiac apex (apical four chamber view) or locating the transducer below the xiphoid (subcostal four chamber view) and the tomographic plane directed perpendicular to the ventricular and atrial septa and through the plane of the mitral and tricuspid orifices to permit simultaneous display of both atria and ventricles, atrioventricular valves and cardiac septa (Figure 2.3). In the apical four chamber view, a dropout of interatrial septal echoes as produced by an atrial septal defect is

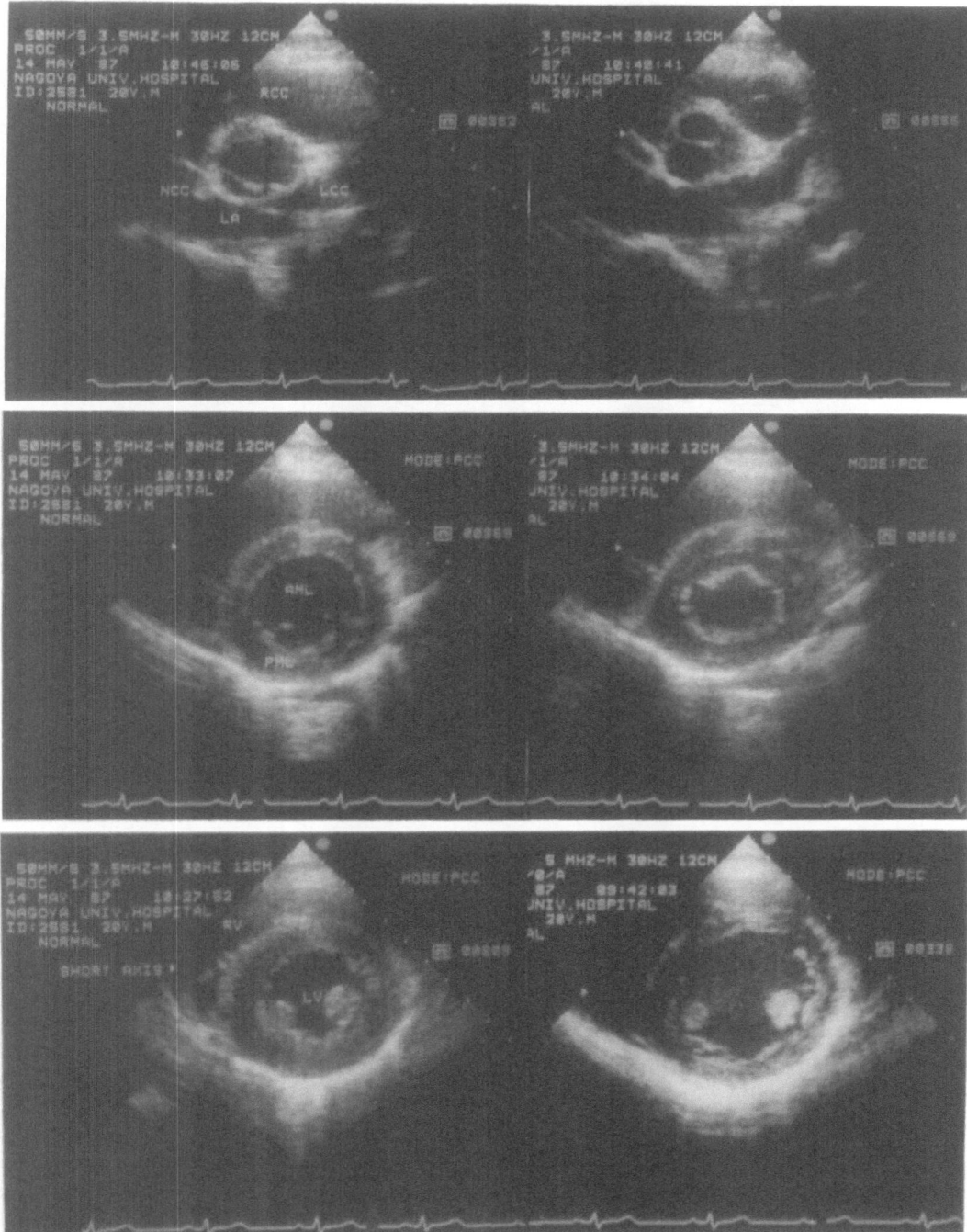

Figure 2.2. Left ventricular short axis view. Upper: aortic valve level, middle illustrates mitral valve level, and lower: left ventricular level.

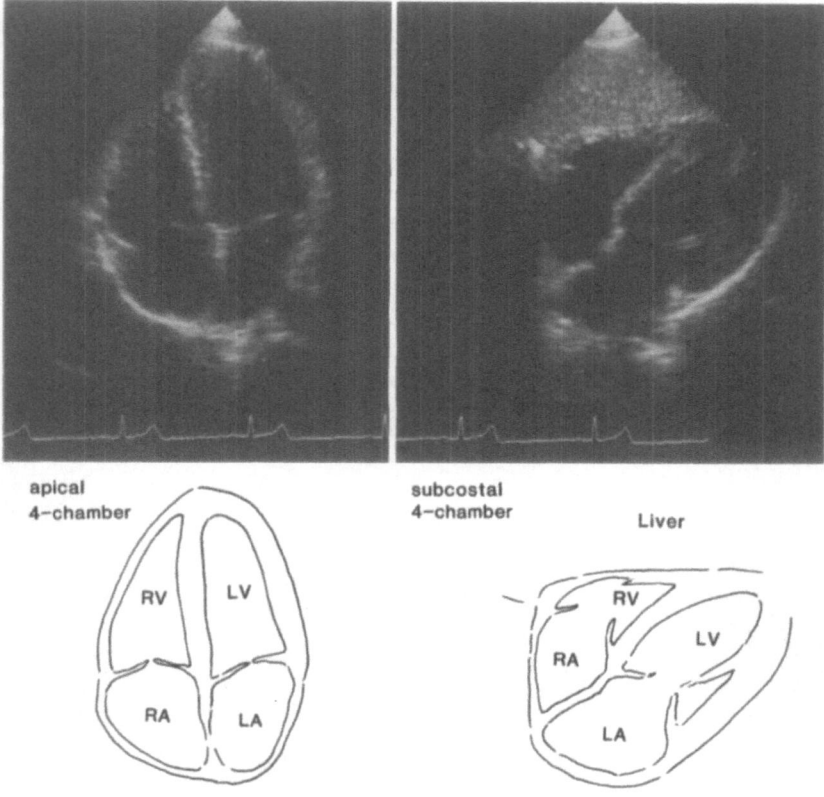

Figure 2.3. Four chamber view.

frequently observed in normal subjects, because the interatrial septum lies on the ultrasonic beam direction, so that fewer echoes are received. To evaluate the defect of the atrial septum, the subcostal four chamber view is prefered.

3. M-mode examination

M-mode tracings of the left heart are obtained using the parasternal long axis view. When the beam is directed to the aortic valve, the aortic valve motion and the left atrium are demonstrated. The mitral valve motion is recorded when the beam is directed so as to obtain the maximum opening of the anterior leaflet. M-mode tracing of the left ventricle is recorded when the beam is steered between the mitral valve and the papillary muscle where the left ventricular cavity presents its maximum diameter. This level demonstrates the contraction and relaxation of the left ventricle (Figure 2.4). It is necessary to direct the beam perpendicularly to both the interventricular septum and the posterior wall of the left ventricle for these measurements. However, it is sometimes difficult to direct the beam perpendicularly to the interventricular septum in cases of aged or obese patients. The steering of the M-mode beam from the aortic valve to the left ventricle is known as the 'M-mode scan', which exposes the motion and the anatomical relationships of the cardiac structures (Figure 2.5). M-mode measurements of the left side of the heart are referred to in Figure 2.6. Calculations of the cardiac functions are addressed in Chapter 8.

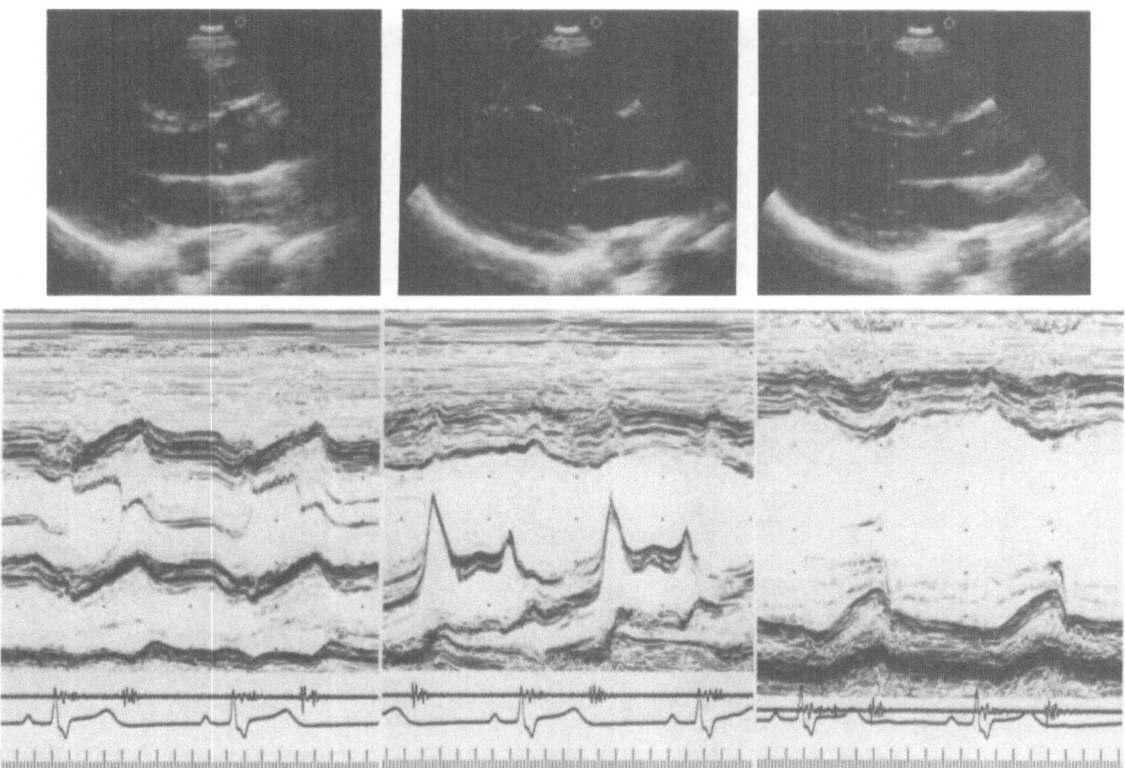

Figure 2.4. M-mode traces of the left side heart.

M-mode tracing of the pulmonary valve is recorded with the right ventricular outflow view which is obtained by placing the transducer on the second or the third intercostal space and the sector plane parellel to the sternum. The tricuspid valve is recorded with the right ventricular inflow view that is obtained by placing the transducer lower than the parasternal long axis view, rotating it counterclockwise and then tilting the plane up or down to obtain the best image (Figure 2.7). In normal subjects, it is usually difficult to record the pulmonary or the tricuspid valve motion through the entire cardiac cycle. However, it is often possible to record the valve motion entirely in the case of right ventricular enlargement.

4. Contrast echocardiography

Contrast echocardiography can present a cloud of echoes in the area of the echocardiogram caused by blood flow using the rapid injection of a medium such as indocyanine green, saline solution, dextrose in water or a carbon dioxide gas mixture of such solutions. The rapid injection from the peripheral vein through a needle or cardiac catheter produces micro-bubbles. The strong echo is processed by the difference in acoustic impedance between blood and microbubbles. This technique is useful to detect abnormal flow such as shunt or regurgi-tant flow and also to diagnose congenital abnormalities through the blood flow. For example, the contrasted flow from the right ventricle to the right atrium through the tricuspid valve is visible during systole in the case of tricuspid valve insufficiency (Figure 2.8). More recently,

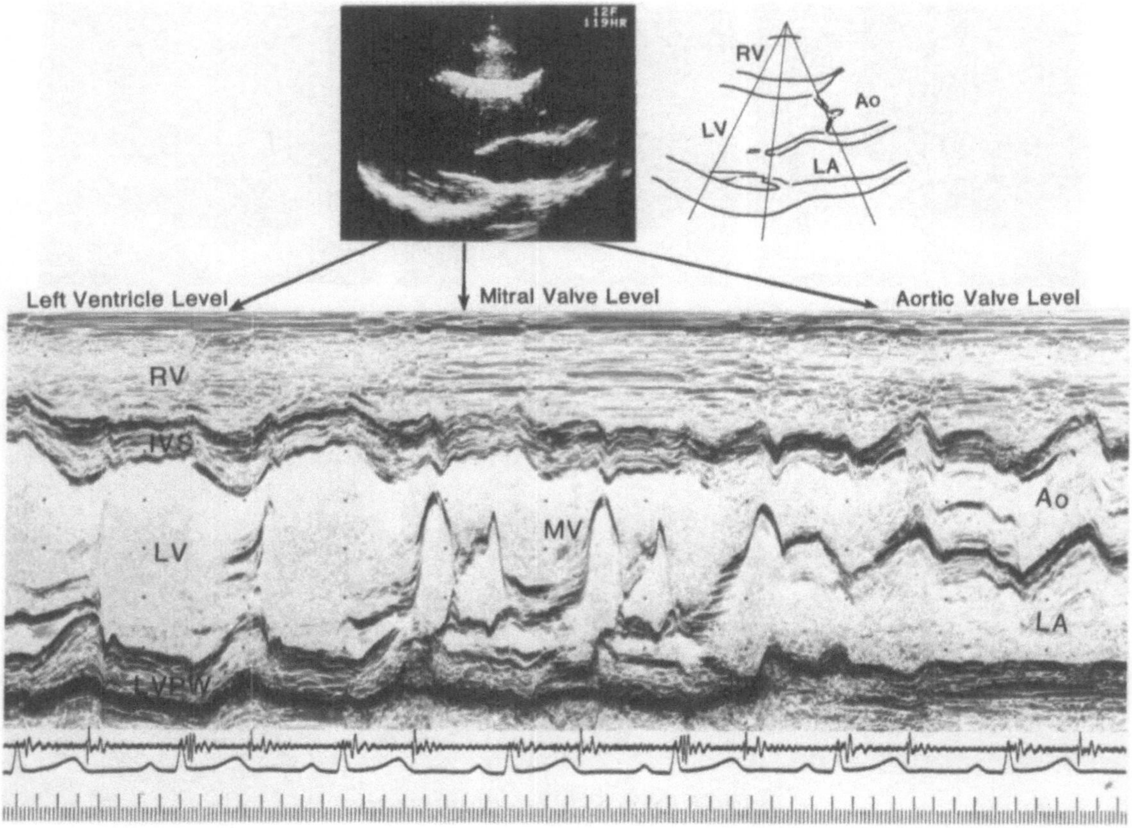

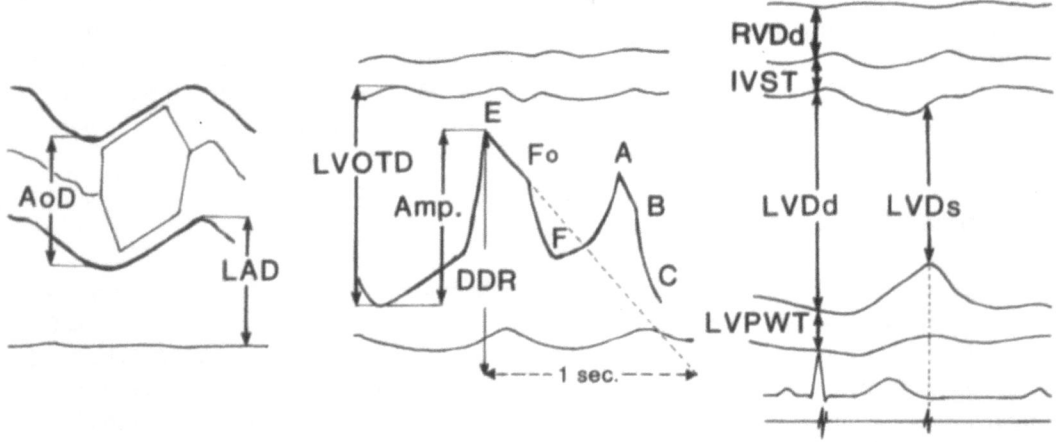

Figure 2.5.   M-mode scan of left side heart.

Figure 2.6.   M-mode measurement of left side heart. The measurements are performed between the leading edges of the traces. The end-systole is land-marked by the second heart sound, and end-diastole by the peak of R-wave of ECG.

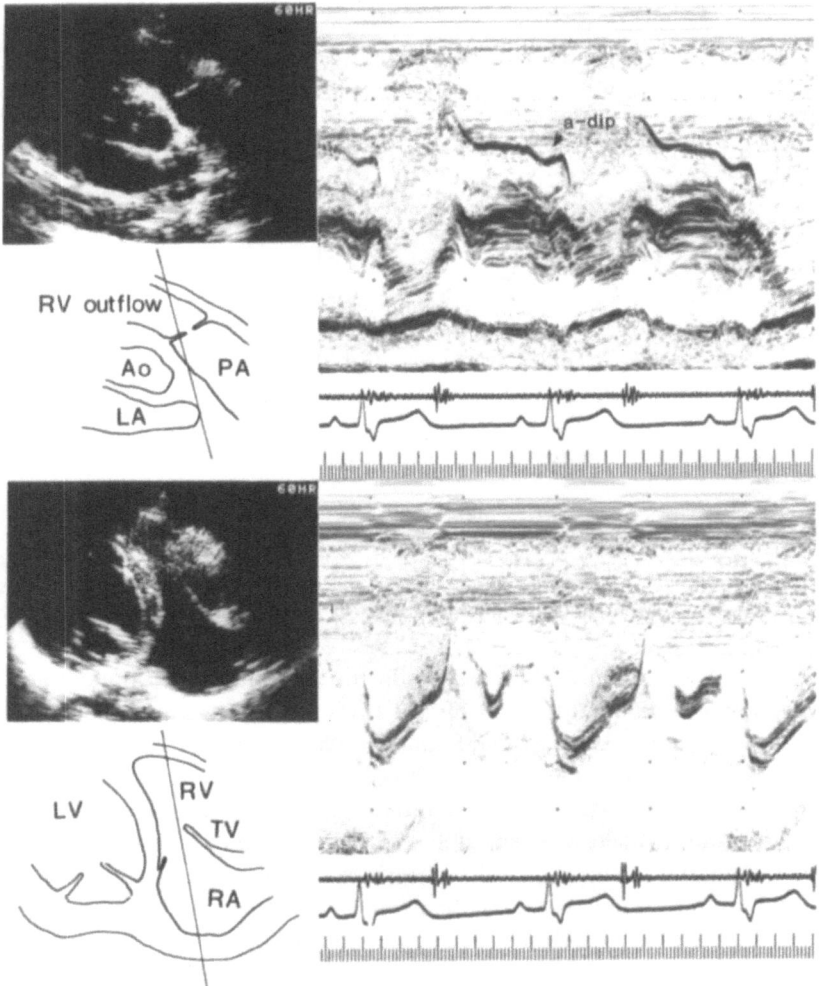

Figure 2.7. M-mode traces of pulmonary and tricuspid valve. Normally, the pulmonic valve is usually recorded only in diastole and missed in systole. The tricuspid valve is only recorded during systole and early diastole in normal conditions.

the cardiac Doppler technique has been substituted for contrast echocardiography in detecting shunt or regurgitant flow. An obvious advantage is that the cardiac Doppler examination is a noninvasive method while contrast echocardiography is somewhat invasive. However, contrast echocardiography is still an important method for identifying the venous chamber or pulmonary artery in complex malformations (see Figure 4.41).

5. Pulsed Doppler examination

In order to reduce the Doppler angle to zero, and to measure blood flow velocity accurately, the transducer must be directed so as to orient the ultrasound beam as nearly parallel to the blood flow as possible. A narrow band signal will yield the least spectral dispersion. The apical approach is frequently applied to detect the flow through the left chambers. Because two-

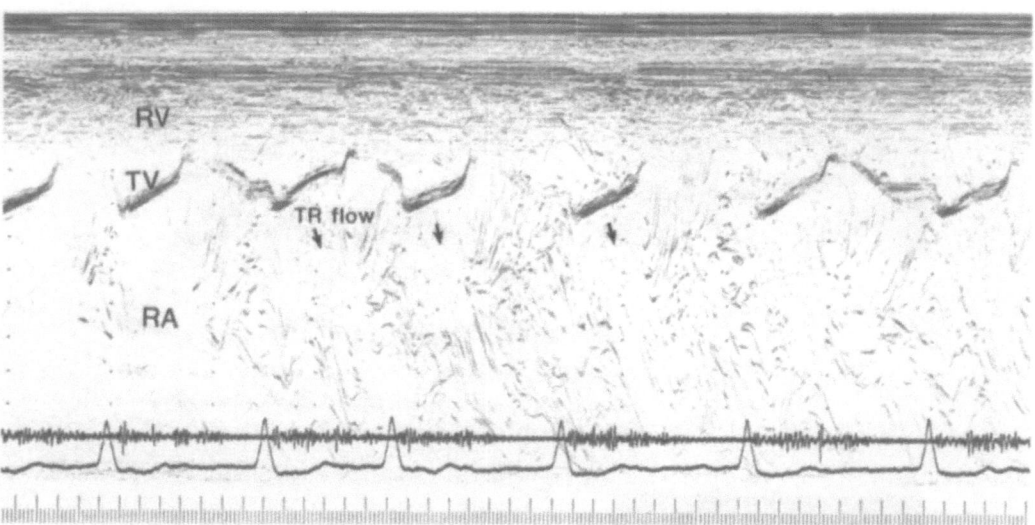

Figure 2.8. Contrast M-mode echocardiogram of the tricuspid regurgitation. The contrast echoes (marked as arrows) are visible in systole as they pass from the right ventricle to the right atrium through the tricuspid valve.

dimensional guidance does not always provide the direction of Doppler sampling in the azimuth plane, further slight adjustments in the transducer's angulation may be necessary to obtain a clear-cut spectral display of the highest modal velocities. The audio signal can also help to orient the transducer and is in fact the only means of ascertaining that a parallel alignment to flow has been obtained. An optimum audio signal will accompany a spectral trace which contains a narrow band high velocity component when good alignment is achieved. The regurgitant flow is turbulent, so proper beam alignment is not so essential for detection, but it is important to evaluate the peak velocity (see Figures 3.21, 22). Proper gain adjustment is required to detect the best Doppler signal (Figure 2.9). A wall motion filter is used to reject the frequency range from 100 Hz to 1600 Hz, eliminating the artifact caused by valve or wall motion. These Doppler signals are low frequency and are very strong. They can

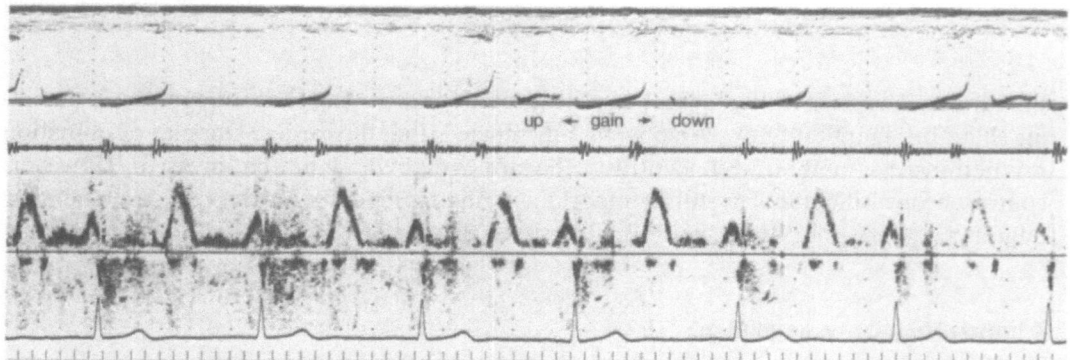

Figure 2.9. Pulsed Doppler spectral change under various gain controls. Excessive gain (left side) produces the noise in the background, and the mirror image in the opposite side of the base line. In this condition, the verification of the regurgitant flow is difficult. The lower gain spectrum (right side) does not present a proper velocity profile.

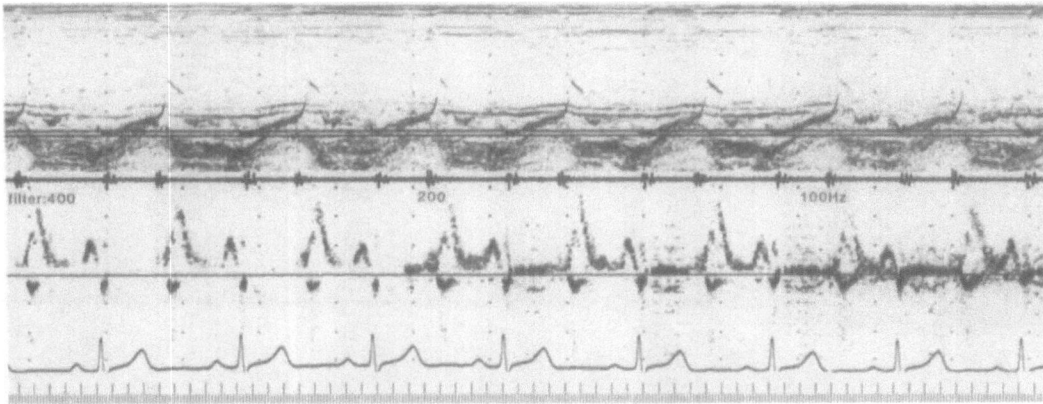

Figure 2.10. Pulsed Doppler spectral change under various wall filters. The FFT spectra are well recorded by setting the wall filter to 400 Hz; however, the rise time is rather damped. Under a 200 Hz wall filter, the appropriate spectra with proper rise time and acceptable noise level are obtained. The spectra under a 100 Hz wall filter demonstrate the noisy trace and is difficult to identify the blood flow information, because the cardiac wall or valve motions overlie on the blood flow spectra.

often saturate the amplifier. A wall motion filter of 400 Hz is commonly used for pulsed Doppler examination. If a lower frequency filter is used, it is usually impossible to separate the blood flow signals from the artifacts. According to the locations of the sample volume and anatomical conditions, however, a lower frequency filter is sometimes acceptable and lower velocity information is available (Figure 2.10). The volume length of a sample is variable and usually the smallest size is adequate in most clinical situations, for integrating both normal and abnormal flows. When measuring flows in the heart or the great vessels, it may sometimes be necessary to increase the sample volume length in order to obtain the most clinically relevant information.

A. Left ventricular outflow (Figure 2.11)

The sample volume is located in the center of the left ventricular outflow tract just below the aortic valve when monitoring the apical long axis or apical five chamber view (modified apical four chamber view that is obtained with somewhat superior angulation of the transducer to visualize the aortic root as it appears like the fifth chamber). The spectrum is normally a narrow band and its peak is in early systole.

B. Left ventricular inflow (Figure 2.11)

The sample volume is located in the center of the mitral annulus when monitoring the apical long axis view. It usually has two peaks caused by rapid filling in early diastole and atrial contraction in late diastole. Sometimes, with higher heart rate, these peaks are merged into a single peak.

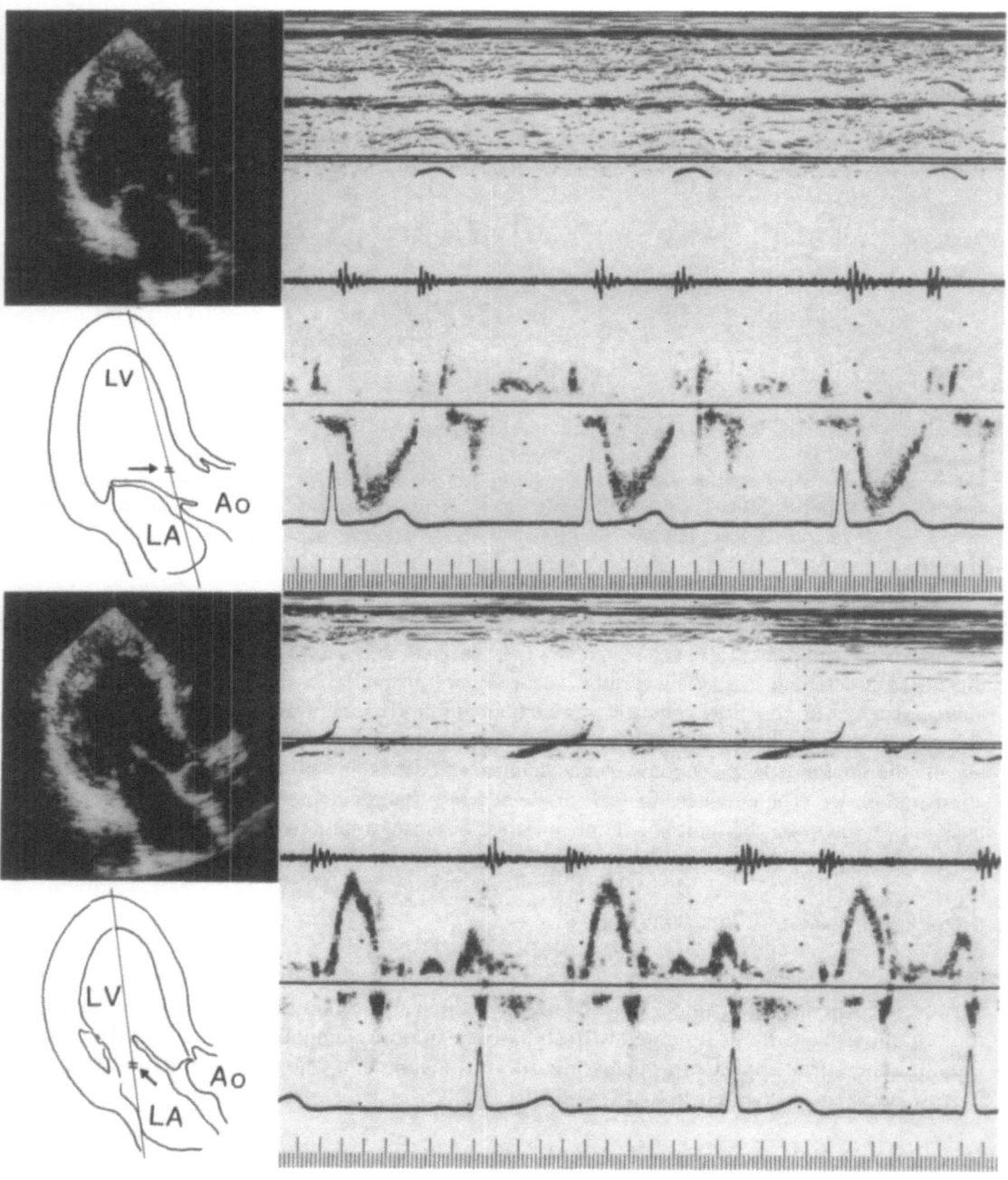

Figure 2.11. Pulsed Doppler examinations of the normal left ventricular outflow and inflow tracts. In the left ventricular outflow tract, the spectra are narrow band with a single peak point in early systole. In the left ventricular inflow tract, the narrow band spectra have two peaks in one cardiac cycle. The first higher peak demonstrates the left ventricular rapid filling and the second is the left ventricular inflow due to the atrial contraction.

C. Right ventricular outflow (Figure 2.12)

The sample volume is located just above the annulus of the pulmonic valve when monitoring the long axis view of the right ventricular outflow tract. The normal spectrum has a peak in mid systole that rises as a slow, dome-like trace with low acceleration. The spectrum of pulmonary hypertension presents rapid rising and it becomes similar to the normal left ventricular outflow velocity. One may frequently note a diastolic leakage of the normal pulmonary valve. This flow has a characteristic low velocity wide band signal, which is often more intense in late diastole (see Figure 3.84).

D. Right ventricular inflow (Figure 2.12)

The sample volume is located in the center of the tricuspid annulus when monitoring the right ventricular inflow view from the apex of the right ventricle. The right ventricular inflow (tricuspid flow) has two peaks similar to those of left ventricular inflow. In many cases, it is difficult to record good right ventricular inflow because of difficulty in aligning the beam parallel to the flow in the azimuthal plane. The right ventricular inflow is often affected by the respiratory cycle. The presence of a small leakage in the normal tricuspid valve is a frequent finding. While the flow itself is of little hemodynamic importance, the ability to measure the peak systolic gradient for estimation of right ventricular pressure is quite useful.

6. Continuous wave (CW) Doppler examination

Two types of transducer are used to perform CW Doppler echocardiography examinations. One is a hybrid imaging transducer and the other is a non-imaging, dedicated transducer. Using the hybrid imaging transducer, CW Doppler echocardiographic examination is easily performed by locating the Doppler beam direction on the two-dimensional image, but approaches are rather limited. A dedicated smaller transducer allows a wider degree of angulation from various acoustic windows. This independent Doppler transducer often operates at a lower frequency than an imaging probe and may be designed to optimize the Doppler signal. Thus, technically adequate signals can be obtained in subjects with normal and abnormal flows that are anatomically difficult to insonicate with a Doppler angle near zero. The angulation of the non-imaging transducer is guided by listening to the audio signal, and observing the spectral pattern, to discern beam location within the heart and great vessels. In the case of higher velocity flow, the highest pitch audio indicates that angulation of the ultrasound beam to the jet is optimal.

The transducer approach when dealing with normal flow is similar to that of pulsed Doppler echocardiography. The envelope of the spectrum is almost the same as with broadened spectra (Figures 2.13, 14). Since the range of the normal blood flow velocity is within the measurable velocity range of pulsed Doppler echocardiography, the CW Doppler echocardiographic examination is not usually necessary for normal flow recordings. However, abnormal flow such as stenotic or regurgitant flow usually has a high velocity and exceeds the measurable maximum velocity range (Fd_{max}) of pulsed Doppler echocardiography. These abnormal flows often cause multiple aliasing due to the high peak velocity, the spectral recording demonstrates bi-directional wide band with signals in this severely aliased pulsed Doppler tracing. In these situations, the CW Doppler examination replaces pulsed Doppler echocardiography, and it is possible to measure even the highest velocities that will be encountered in a physiological state.

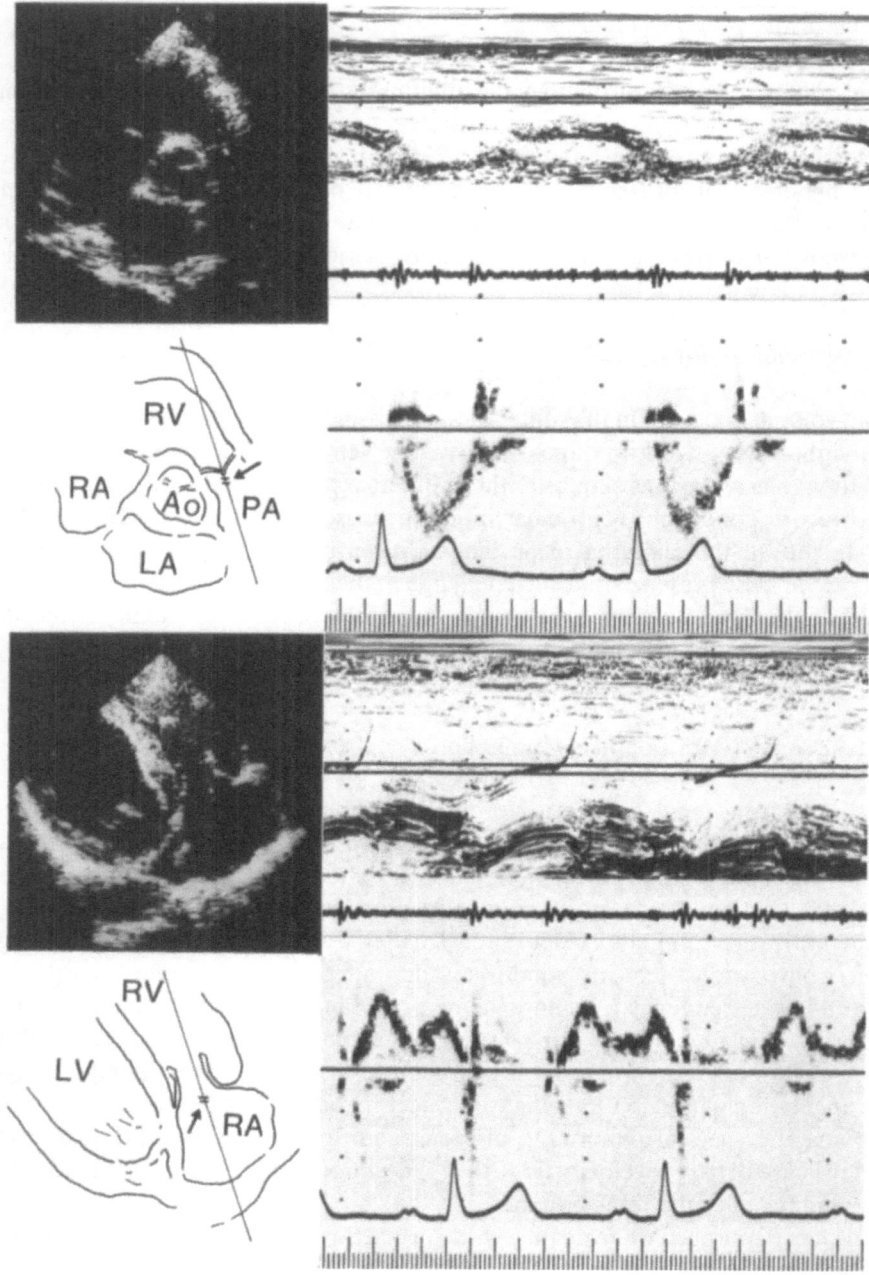

Figure 2.12. Pulsed Doppler examinations of right ventricular outflow and inflow tracts. In the right ventricular outflow tract, the narrow band, and damped single peak appears in mid-systole as the ejection flow. In the right ventricular inflow tract, the narrow band dual peaks appear in one cardiac cycle as with the left ventricular inflow tract.

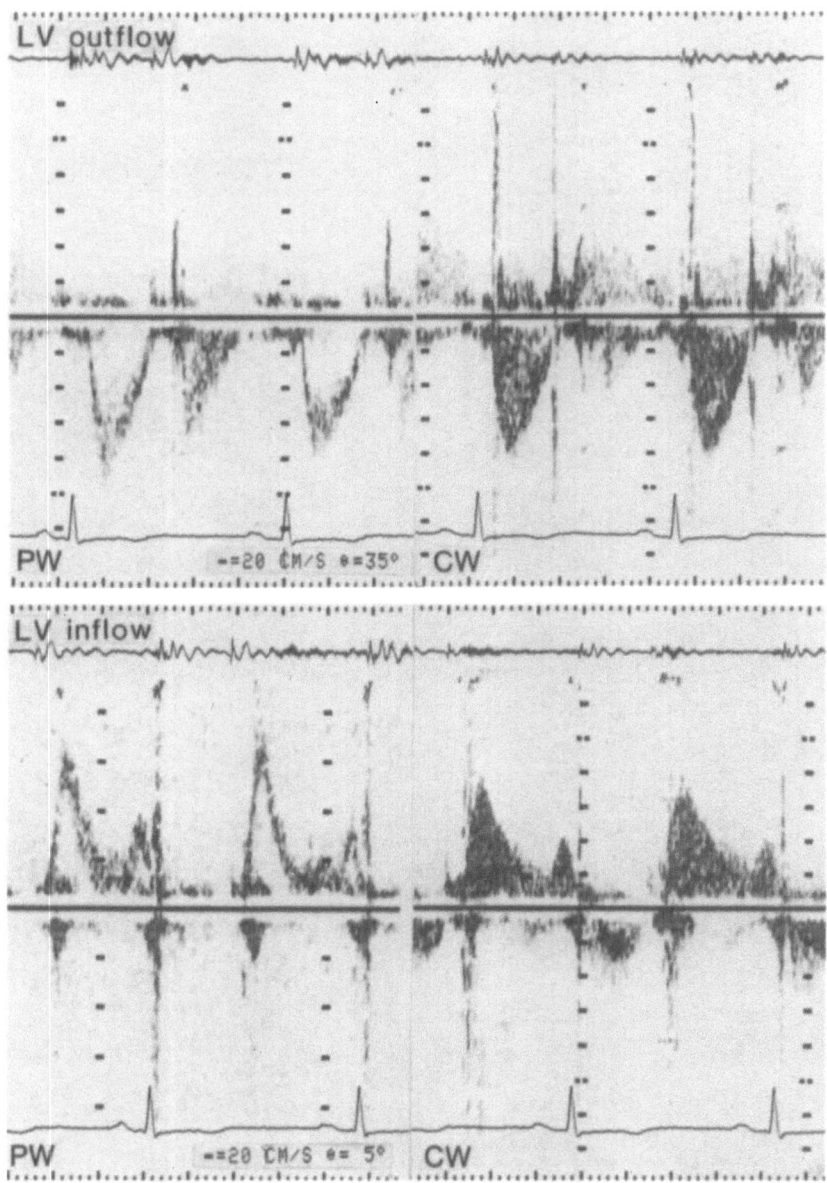

Figure 2.13. Comparisons of the normal left ventricular outflow and inflow velocity tracings by pulsed versus CW Doppler technique. These recordings are performed by both the pulsed and continuous methods by placing the different transducers at different places, to obtain the maximum velocity from the dedicated CW Doppler transducer, and monitoring the clear two-dimensional images for the Doppler beam direction as parallel as possible by pulsed Doppler method. The maximum velocity obtained properly by the continuous method is the same as that obtained by the pulsed method with angle correction. The patterns are also similar to each other. However, the CW Doppler spectra include the artifact due to the processing of all the echoes along the beam direction.

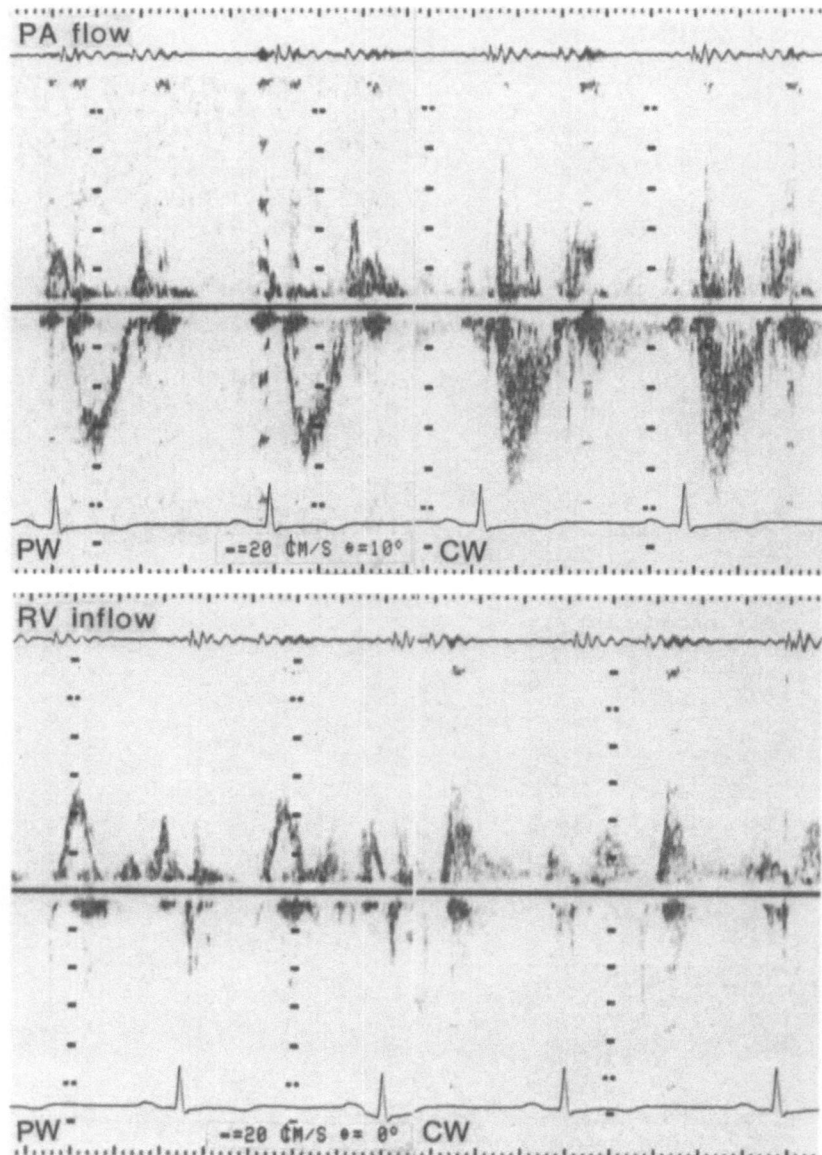

Figure 2.14. Comparisons of the normal right ventricular outflow and inflow velocity tracings by pulsed versus CW Doppler technique.

In recent years, the non-invasive assessment of the cardiac pressure measurements has become widely accepted. The simplified Bernoulli equation is commonly used for the calculation of the pressure gradient, as the pressure gradient $(PG) = 4V^2$ where PG is a pressure difference in mm Hg across the stenotic valve, and V is the peak velocity of the transvalvular flow in m/sec.

Some investigators have implemented the angle between the blood flow and the beam direction to correct for the angle, by using color flow mapping when CW Doppler echocardiography is performed. This permits one to obtain the angle corrected maximum velocity quantitatively (see Figure 11.9). It must be pointed out that color flow mapping guided placement of the CW Doppler is a rough approximation of a parallel alignment. The flow volume being sampled is three dimensional, the Doppler sample volumes are three dimensional, and the CW Doppler beam must be implemented simultaneously with the color flow study while the angle is being corrected. It should also be stated that if the angle is over-estimated by color flow mapping, the error is squared when the pressure is calculated and can lead to significant overestimation of the severity of the lesions. For these reasons it is suggested that the color flow mapping be used to rapidly position the CW Doppler, then the audio signal be used for the final alignment.

The value of the CW Doppler echocardiographic examination is for measuring high flow velocities rather than observing flow characteristics such as laminar or turbulent flow. This evaluation should be done by pulsed Doppler echocardiography, because CW Doppler echocardiogram includes all the blood flow information along the beam direction.

7. High PRF Doppler examination

The implementation of high pulse repetition frequency (PRF) Doppler examination is basically the same technique as with conventional pulsed Doppler. When one locates the sample volume (main sampling) on the two-dimensional image, the ambiguous sample volumes are marked in the display (Figure 2.15). When there are two or more high velocity flows along the beam line, one should take care that measurements are not being based on the ambiguous signal contribution. Figure 2.16 demonstrates the spectra of the mitral regurgitation at several pulse repetition frequencies. The spectra vary according to the pulse repetition frequency. If the maximum measurable velocity is 1.2 m/sec, one can only read bi-directional aliased signals. However, it is possible to recognize the higher peak velocity and its direction, away from the transducer (even if aliasing occurs), when the range of 3.2 m/sec is employed (PRF:

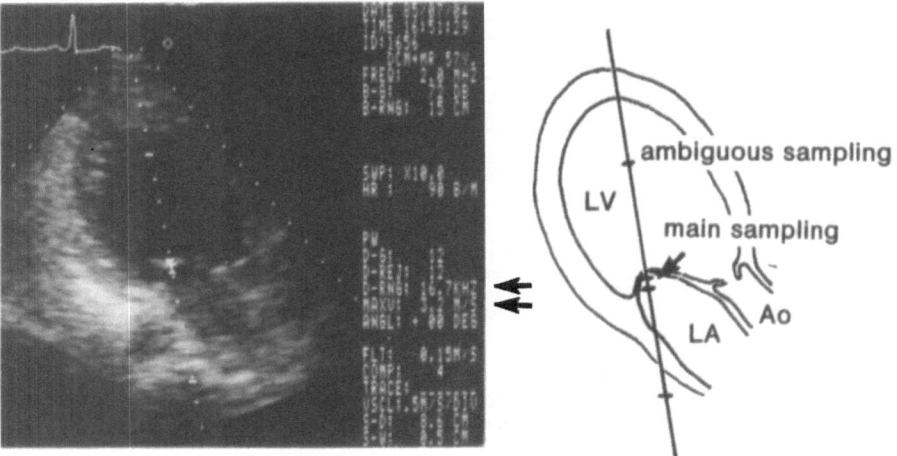

Figure 2.15. Ambiguous sampling points in the two-dimensional image by high PRF Doppler echocardiography. With this method, the main sampling point that is the place of interest, and the ambiguous sampling points where the unexpected echoes are received from, are displayed in the two-dimensional image. The pulse repetition frequency, which is referred to as D-RNG (16.7 KHz), and the measurable maximum velocity, that is referred to as MAX *V* (3.2 m/sec) are noted in the display (arrow).

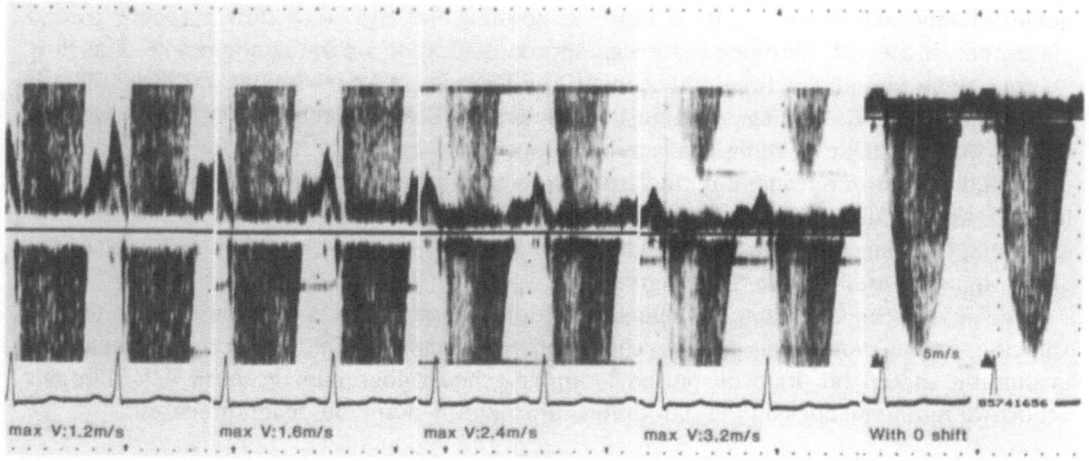

max V:1.2m/s max V:1.6m/s max V:2.4m/s max V:3.2m/s With 0 shift

Figure 2.16. The spectral change of the mitral regurgitant flow by the various pulse repetition frequencies. By increasing the pulse repetition frequency with zero shift, it becomes possible to identify the entire spectral profile of the mitral regurgitant flow. The above examples demonstrate the changes in the spectral display with each measurable maximum velocity. When the lower PRF is employed to perform the examination, multiple aliasing occurs and it looks like the bi-directional flow without identification of flow direction.

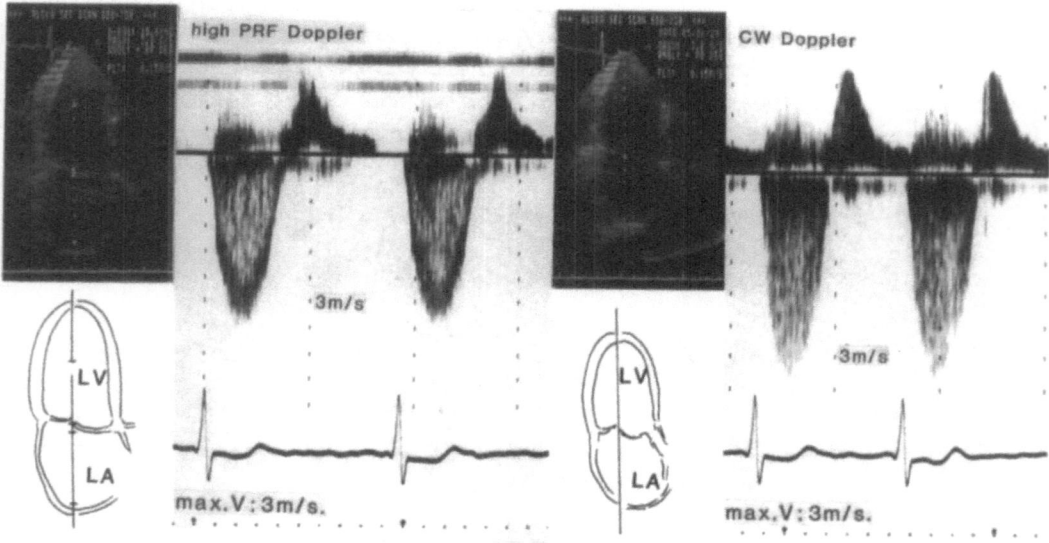

Figure 2.17. Comparison of the mitral regurgitant flow by high PRF versus CW Doppler methods. Using the same transducer with imaging and placing it at the same place, the mitral regurgitant flow is recorded by the high PRF method and CW method. The envelope of the spectra is more clearly visible by the high PRF method than CW method due to limited sample volume.

16.7 KHz). When the zero line is shifted, the maximum velocity of regurgitant flow that can be measured is 5 m/sec. When the left ventricular inflow, which has a maximum velocity of 1 m/sec, is recorded using this setting, the spectrum is depressed and not suitable for evaluation. A careful control of PRF is therefore required, depending on the purpose. In this mode, simultaneous presentation of the spectra and M-mode is impossible. The high PRF Doppler method produces velocity tracings with less broadening of the spectra than that of conventional CW Doppler echocardiography (Figure 2.17). This is a useful technique for measuring high velocity with some range resolution.

Acquired valvular heart disease

1. Mitral valve stenosis

Mitral stenosis is one of the most common acquired valvular heart diseases. Doppler ultra-sound and echocardiography are the most useful method for such evaluation. Two-dimensional echocardiography provides anatomical findings that include: doming of the anterior mitral leaflet in the long axis view, and stenotic mitral orifice like the appearance of a fish mouth in the short axis view (Figure 3.1). The assessment of the mitral valve area can be obtained using parasternal short axis view by planimetry. Depending on the mitral valve area (MVA), the severity is divided into three classes: (1) Mild MVA > 2 cm², (2) Moderate MVA 1–2 cm², and (3) Severe MVA < 1 cm². However, clinical symptoms do not always correspond to this assessment. Sometimes they are related to a low cardiac output state, severe mitral valve calcification and the presence of aortic regurgitation. In these patients, it is also necessary to evaluate the characteristics of the mitral valve leaflets and subvalvular apparatus. The presence of calcification and chordal shortening or fusion should be determined, because these factors have an important role in determining the surgical procedure (commissurotomy or valve replacement). In this entity, an enlarged left atrium, a small left ventricle and a small aortic root dimension are present in severe cases (Figures 3.3, 4). These findings reflect the disturbance of the transmitral flow. M-mode echocardiography provides qualitative rather than quantitative information about mitral stenosis, such as decreased E–F slope and excursion of anterior leaflet with diastolic anterior motion of posterior leaflet (Figures 3.2, 4).

In the presence of mitral stenosis, the transmitral flow becomes accelerated and turbulent with prolonged deceleration of rapid filling due to a persistent pressure gradient between left ventricle and atrium. When the flow is accelerated, an additional pressure drop is required for convective acceleration.

$$P_1 - P_2 = \frac{1}{2}\varrho(V_2^2 - V_1^2).$$

1 and 2 indicate two different positions across the stenotic valve, P indicates pressure (mm Hg), ϱ is the constant for mass density of blood and V is the flow velocity (m/sec). Since the flow velocity proximal to the stenosis (V_1) is usually much smaller than the maximum velocity in the post-stenotic jet (V_2) (Figure 3.5), one can usually neglect V_1 and obtain a simplified Bernoulli equation to calculate the pressure drop.

$$P_1 - P_2 = 4V_2^2.$$

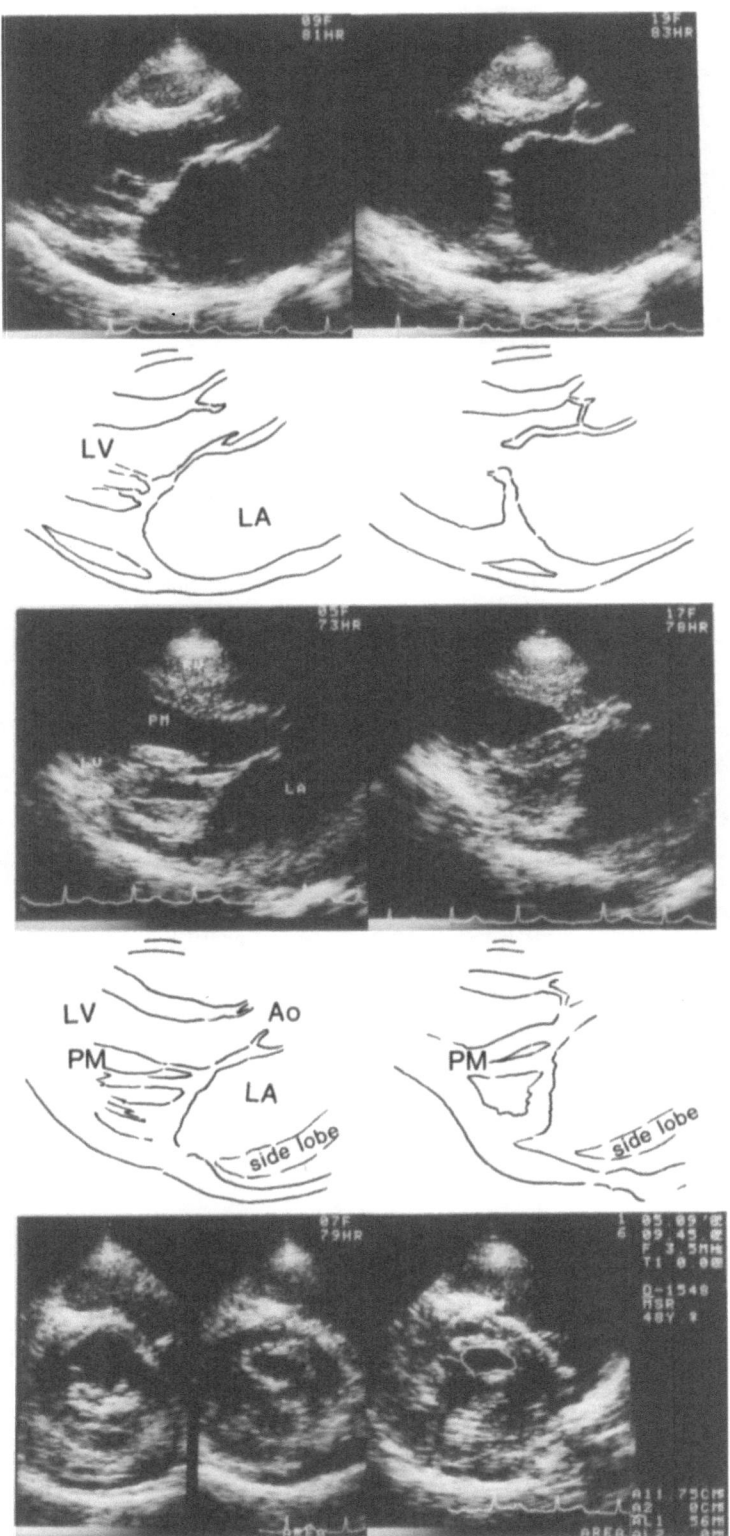

Figure 3.1 Parasternal long and short axis view from a patient with mitral stenosis. The upper figure shows a doming of anterior leaflet and left atrial enlargement. The middle figure shows a subvalvular fusion. The lower figure shows the stenotic mitral valve orifice and its planimetric measurement.

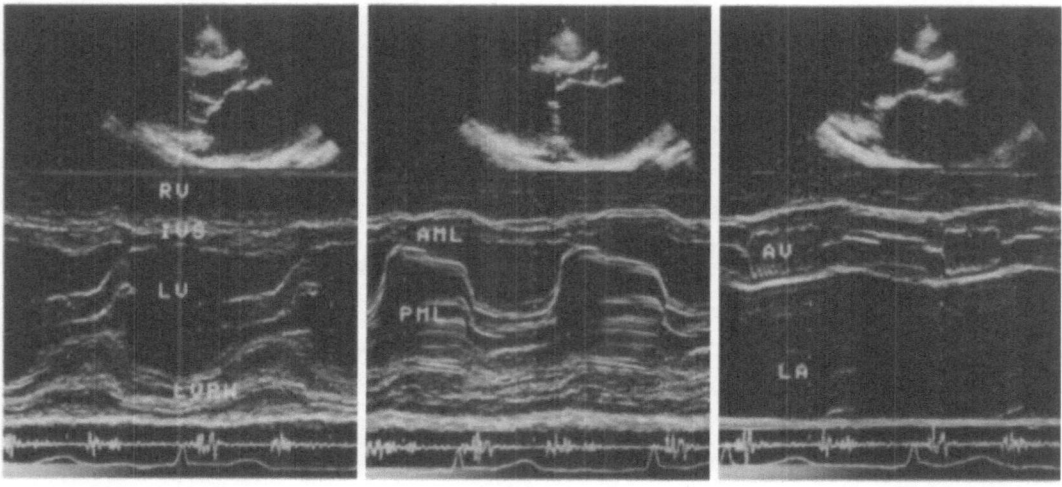

Figure 3.2. Two-dimensional and M-mode echocardiograms from a patient with mitral stenosis. The M-mode illustrates a decreased E–F slope of the anterior mitral leaflet. One also notes a diastolic anterior motion of the posterior mitral leaflet and an enlarged left atrium.

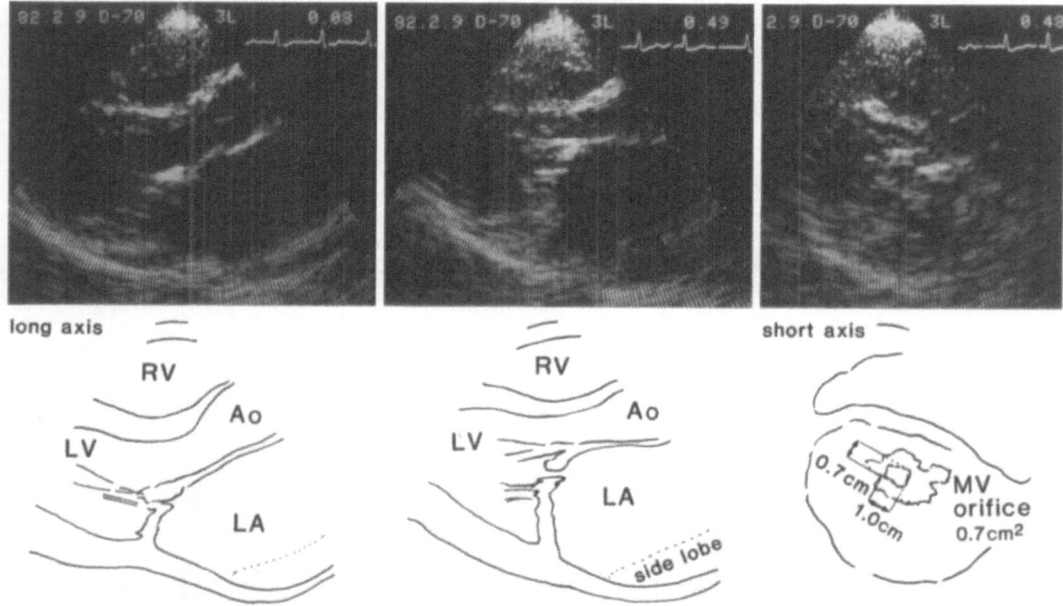

Figure 3.3. Parasternal long and short axis views from a patient with severe mitral stenosis. A calcified mitral valve with an area of less than 1 cm² is observed. Left atrial enlargement and small left ventricle can also be seen.

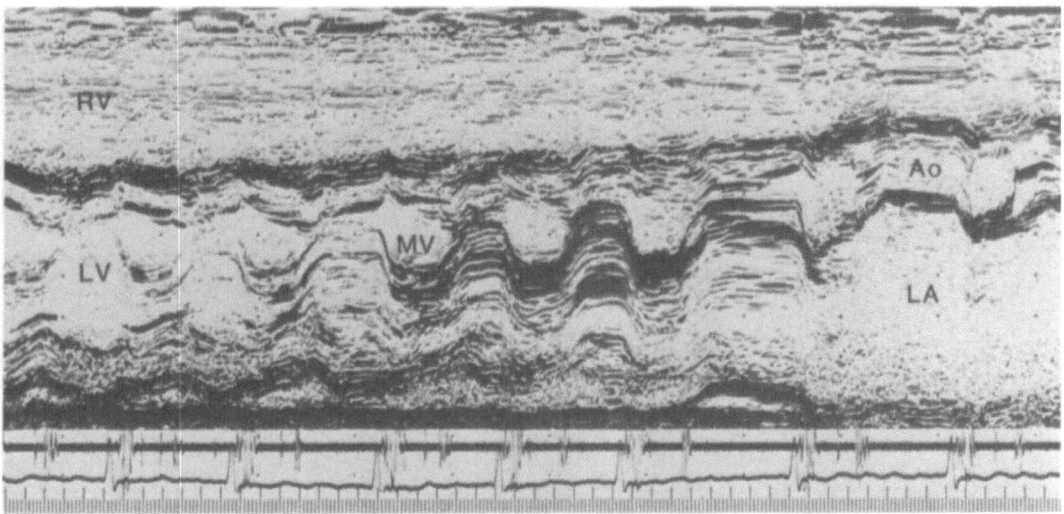

Figure 3.4 M-mode scan demonstrating a severely calcified and stenotic mitral valve.

Using Doppler echocardiography, it is possible to obtain the transmitral pressure gradient (Figure 3.6) which correlates well with cardiac catheterization. The time course of the pressure gradient can be expressed as pressure half-time, which is obtained by dividing the peak velocity by $\sqrt{2}$ and by measuring the time from peak velocity to the point where this decrease in velocity is found (Figure 3.7). In severe mitral stenosis, the pressure half-time becomes over 300 msec (Figure 3.8). When mild obstruction is present, the pressure half-time shows below 100 msec (Figure 3.9). The pressure half time is well correlated with mitral valve area (MVA) and Hatle *et al.* have described the following formula to calculate the MVA from the estimated pressure half time.

$$MVA \; (cm^2) = \frac{220}{\text{pressure half time (ms)}}$$

These Doppler measurements are easily obtained by an echocardiographic equipment interfaced with a micro-computer system (Figure 3.10).

In patients with mitral stenosis, the enlargement of left atrium and the presence of atrial fibrillation can produce intracavitary left atrial thrombus. Usually, the presence and location of large thrombi are easily detected by echocardiography (Figures 3.11, 12, 13). But, in cases with small and/or multiple thrombi, one should be careful during the examination and use several views (Figures 3.14, 15). Left atrial thrombi are usually attached to the posterior wall, but in rare cases, floating thrombi are present and can protrude into the mitral orifice (Figure 3.16).

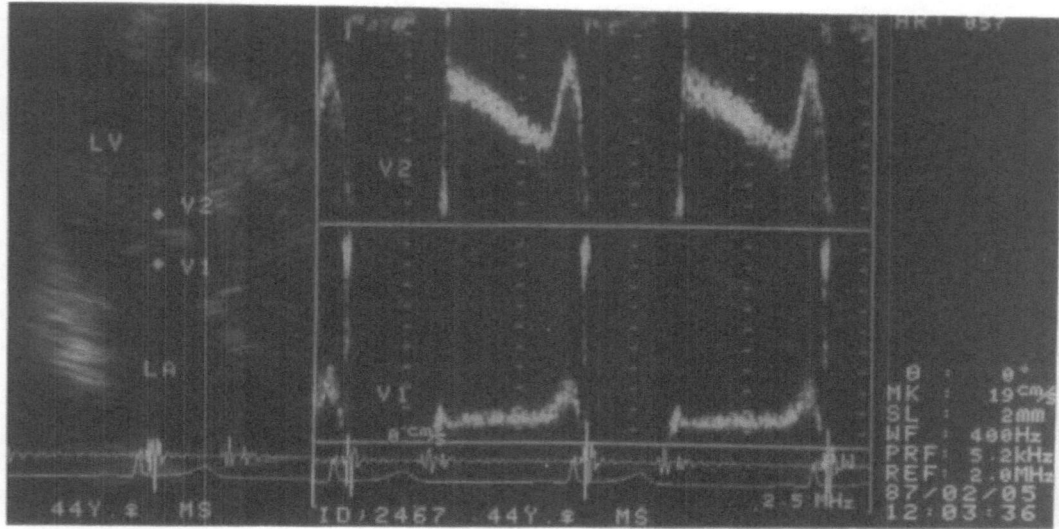

Figure 3.5. Multi-gated pulsed Doppler echocardiogram from a patient with mitral stenosis. Simultaneous recordings of pre (*V*1) and post (*V*2) stenotic valve flow demonstrating accelerated flow in *V*2.

2. Giant left atrium

In chronic rheumatic mitral valve disease, a giant left atrium is sometimes found. In this condition, the blood flow stasis in the left atrium may become echogenic and can then be seen (smoky echo appearance) using two-dimensional and M-mode echocardiography (Figures 3.17, 18).

3. Mitral valve regurgitation (rheumatic in origin)

Mitral regurgitation (MR) is detected by Doppler techniques and two-dimensional echocardiography, which not only identifies its origin but also indicates the hemodynamic repercussion (left ventricular and atrial dilatation) secondary to volume overload. The echocardiographic findings of rheumatic mitral regurgitation consist of valve thickening along with some degree of stenosis and left atrial and ventricular enlargement (Figure 3.19). In M-mode, the mitral valve echoes commonly show a slightly decreased E–F slope with a good excursion, but these findings are nonspecific (Figure 3.20). Pulsed Doppler demonstrates the systolic turbulent flow within the left atrium. Because the regurgitant flow will have non-laminar elements, it can be recorded not only from the apical approach but also from the parasternal views, where the ultrasound beam is relatively perpendicular to the regurgitant jet (Figure 3.21). When the distance between the probe and the regurgitant flow is decreased, the regurgitant flow signal will usually be stronger than that recorded from the apex. The velocity of mitral regurgitant flow is so high that aliasing occurs with pulsed Doppler or CFM. CW or high PRF Doppler must be implemented to assess the direction and peak velocity in these cases (Figure 3.22). Usually, the 'flow mapping technique' is the method of choice to evaluate the severity of valvular regurgitation. This method utilizes a grading criterion similar to that applied in cardiac catheterization even though the observed parameters are quite different.

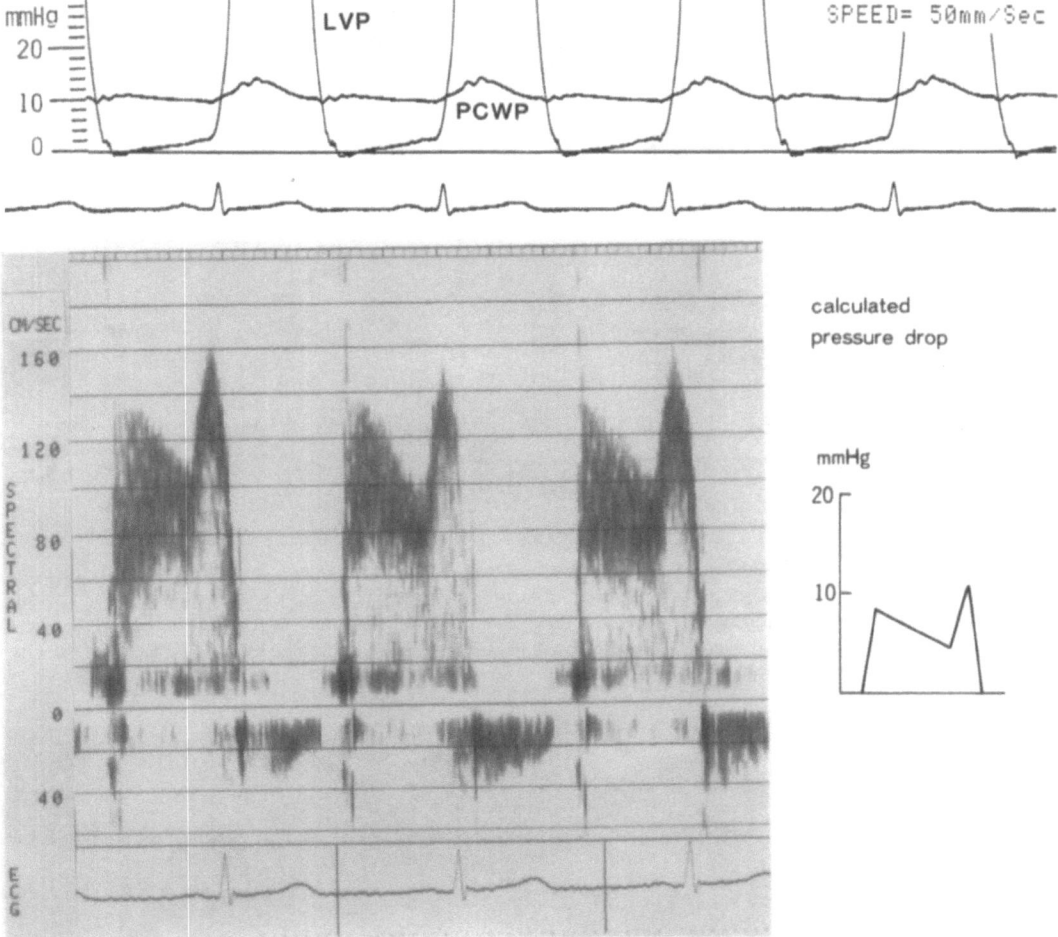

Figure 3.6 Pulsed Doppler echocardiogram and simultaneous recording of left ventricular pressure (LVP) and pulmonary capillary wedge pressure (PCWP) of a patient with mitral stenosis. The figure on the left illustrates the increased peak velocity of the transmitral flow. The right-hand figure shows a measurement of the transmitral pressure gradient by a simplified Bernoulli equation. This Doppler pressure gradient is very similar to pressure recordings.

The severity of mitral regurgitation is graded to delineate the spatial extent of the regurgitant flow in the left atrium (Figure 3.23). This method can correlate well with left ventriculography (Figure 3.24).

4. Mitral valve prolapse

Echocardiography is playing an important role in our understanding of mitral valve prolapse (MVP), but it has introduced some controversial problems concerning its diagnosis. In mitral valve prolapse, the valvular abnormality is principally a displacement or bulging of one or both mitral leaflets into the left atrium. Two-dimensional echocardiography provides useful information about the spatial orientation of prolapse; by angulating the transducer, it is possible to demonstrate the anterolateral, middle and posteromedial commissure (Figure

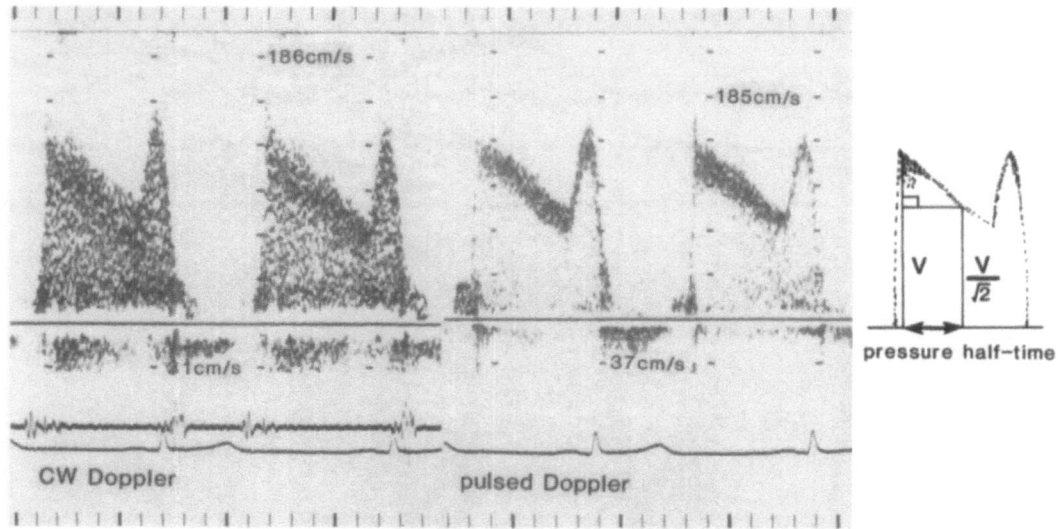

Figure 3.7. CW and pulsed Doppler echocardiogram from a stenotic mitral valve flow and the measurement of pressure half-time. The pulsed mode recording of a stenotic mitral flow generally has a narrower spectral bandwidth than the corresponding continuous wave (CW) recording. The pressure half-time is calculated as the time interval required for the peak velocity to decrease to the pressure half-velocity which is obtained by dividing the peak velocity by $\sqrt{2}$.

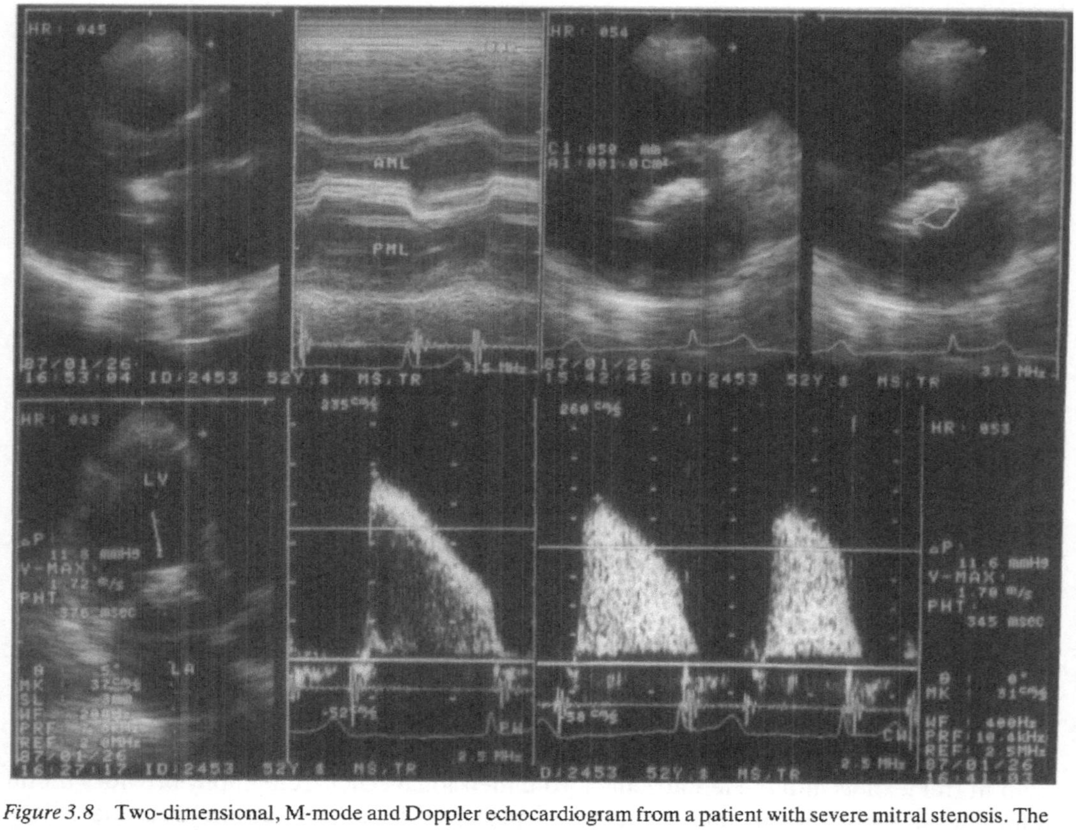

Figure 3.8 Two-dimensional, M-mode and Doppler echocardiogram from a patient with severe mitral stenosis. The parasternal short axis view reveals severely obstructed mitral valve area (1 cm²). Pulsed and continuous wave Doppler show the almost similar prolonged pressure half-time (376 and 345 msec). The horizontal line shows the pressure half-velocity.

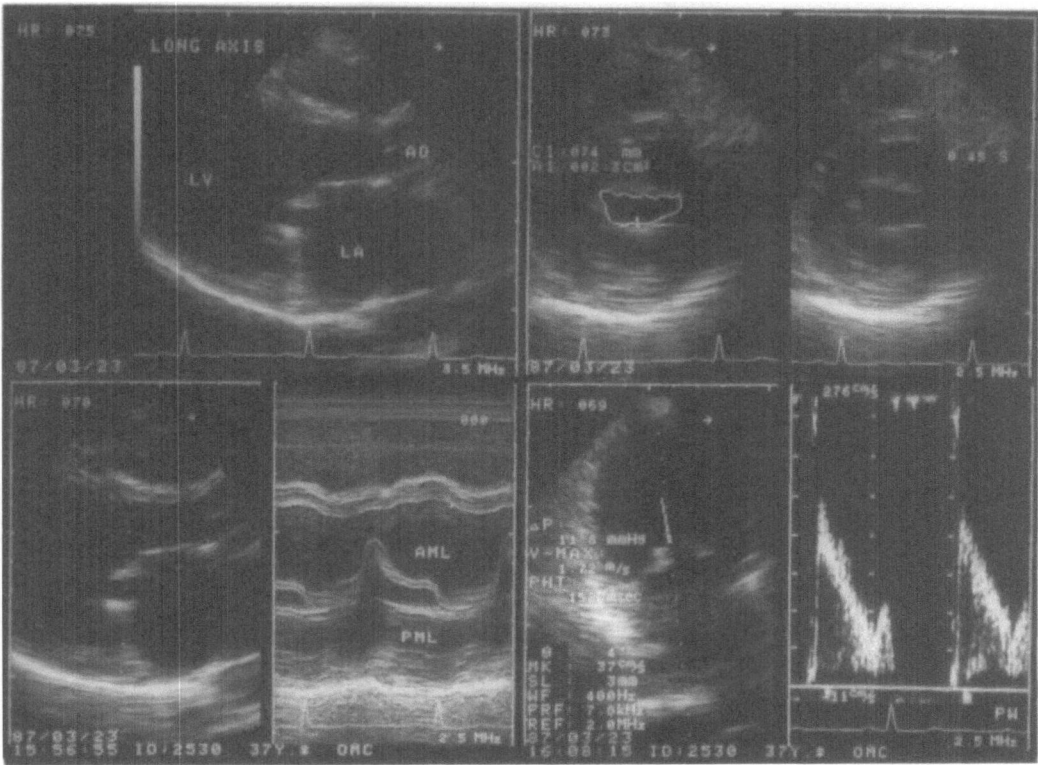

Figure 3.9. Two-dimensional, M-mode and pulsed Doppler echocardiogram from a patient with mild mitral stenosis after open mitral commisurotomy (OMC). The parasternal long and short axis view reveal a mildly obstructed mitral valve area (2.3 cm²). The M-mode echocardiogram shows slightly decreased E–F slope with increased echo intensity. The pulsed Doppler echocardiogram recorded from an apical approach shows the mildly prolonged pressure half-time (152 msec).

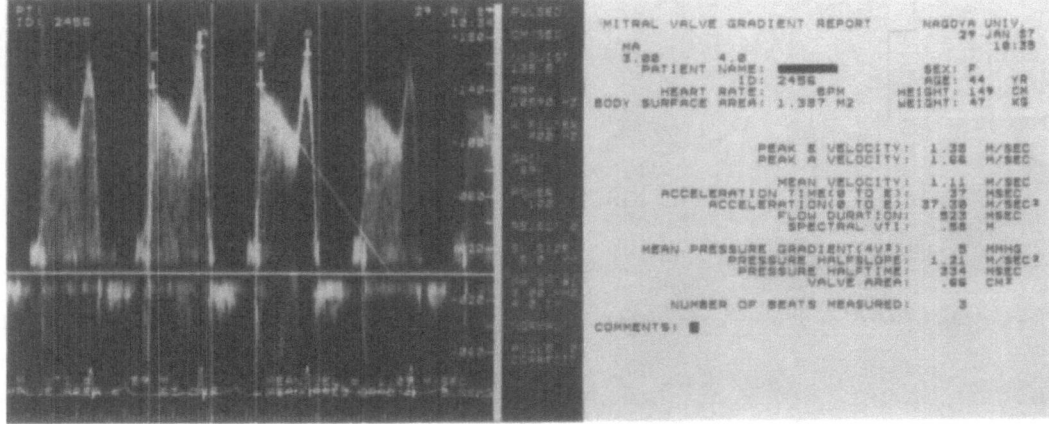

Figure 3.10. Measurement of mean peak velocity, pressure gradient and pressure half-time in the setting of mitral stenosis by an echocardiographic equipment interfaced with a microcomputer system.

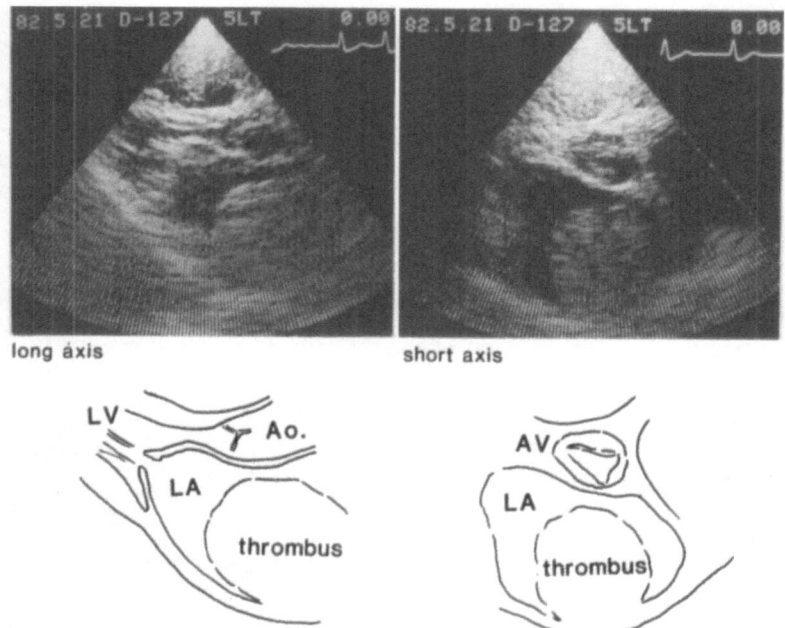

long axis   short axis

Figure 3.11.   Parasternal long and short axis views demonstrating a large left atrial thrombus.

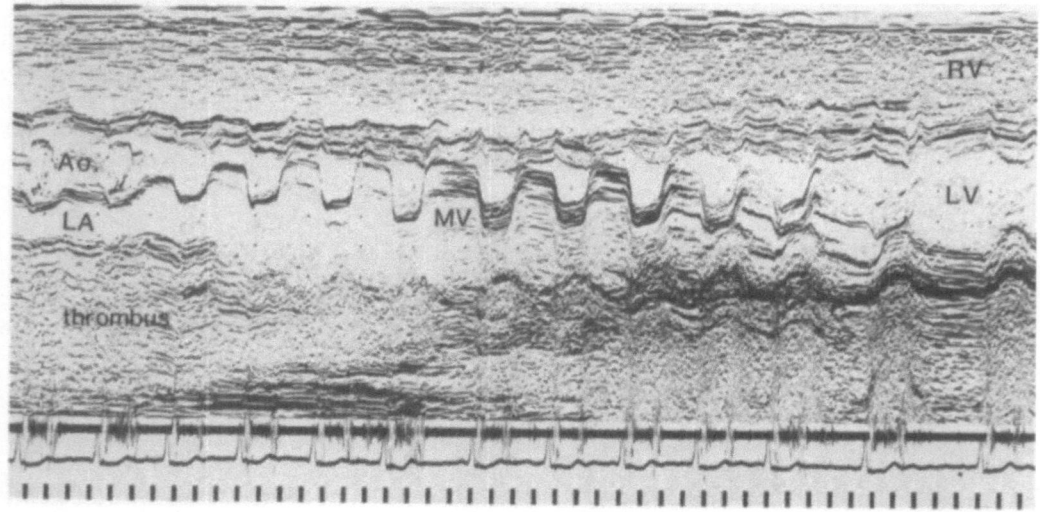

Figure 3.12.   M-mode scan illustrating an abnormally large cloud of echo due to thrombus on the posterior wall of the left atrium.

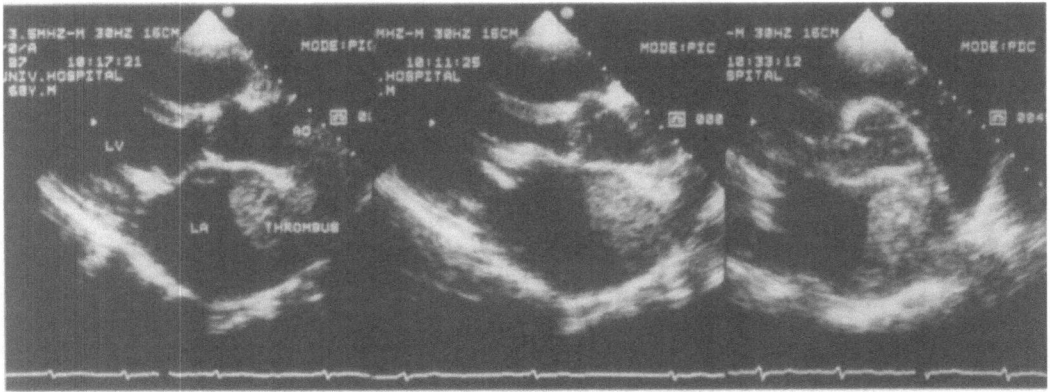

Figure 3.13. Parasternal long and short axis view demonstrating a left atrial thrombus attached to the antero-lateral side of the left atrium.

3.25). M-mode echocardiography shows the characteristic findings of the valvular motion such as systolic buckling or bowing (Figures 3.26, 27), but these findings are not always present, or they may escape observation, because of the limited spatial resolution obtained with this method (Figures 3.28, 29). Mitral valve prolapse is frequently accompanied by regurgitation and Doppler techniques can detect the presence and direction, and can estimate the severity of the mitral regurgitation. In those cases of mitral regurgitation due to anterior mitral valve prolapse, the regurgitant flow is usually directed to the posterior wall of the left atrium (Figure 3.27). In patients with mitral regurgitation, secondary to posterior mitral valve prolapse, the regurgitant jet is frequently directded toward the anterior wall (Figure 3.26).

Mitral valve prolapse is sometimes accompanied by abnormal motion of a papillary muscle and/or chordae tendineae (Figures 3.30, 31, 32) or a mixomatous degeneration of the leaflets (Figure 3.33). Tricuspid valve prolapse may also be present in this entity, and the pulsed Doppler method is useful in this situation since the differentiation of which valve is incompetent is easily made (Figure 3.34).

5. Ruptured chordae tendineae

Chordae tendineae can be ruptured due to inflammatory or ischemic process, but there are also idiopathic origins. Ruptured chordae tendineae can be identified using two-dimensional echocardiography, especially in patients with endocarditis (Figures 3.35, 36). This entity usually produces a flailing mitral valve with severe mitral regurgitation (Figures 3.37, 38, 39).

6. Aortic valve stenosis

Acquired aortic stenosis (AS) is secondary to rheumatic or atherosclerotic changes. Using two-dimensional echocardiography, one can evaluate the morphology of the aortic valve, the presence of calcification and LV hypertrophy. Until now, the application of the aortic valve area assessment has had many limitations, in comparison with the mitral valve area (Figures 3.40, 42). M-mode echocardiography can demonstrate the reduced opening of the aortic valve (Figure 3.41), but this finding is not always representative of the severity of the stenosis. In

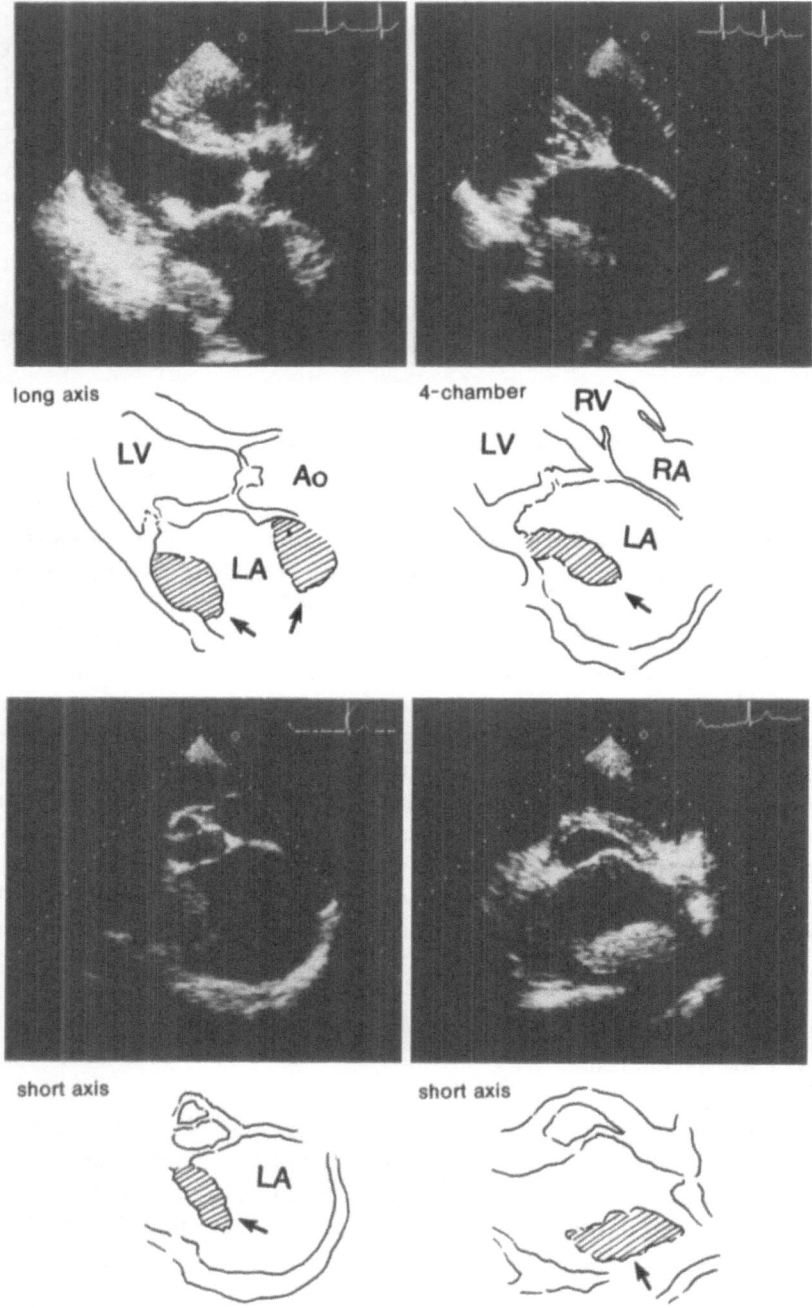

Figure 3.14. Two-dimensional echocardiogram demonstrating thrombi in the left atrium (arrow). In this patient, the long axis view permits identification of two different thrombi.

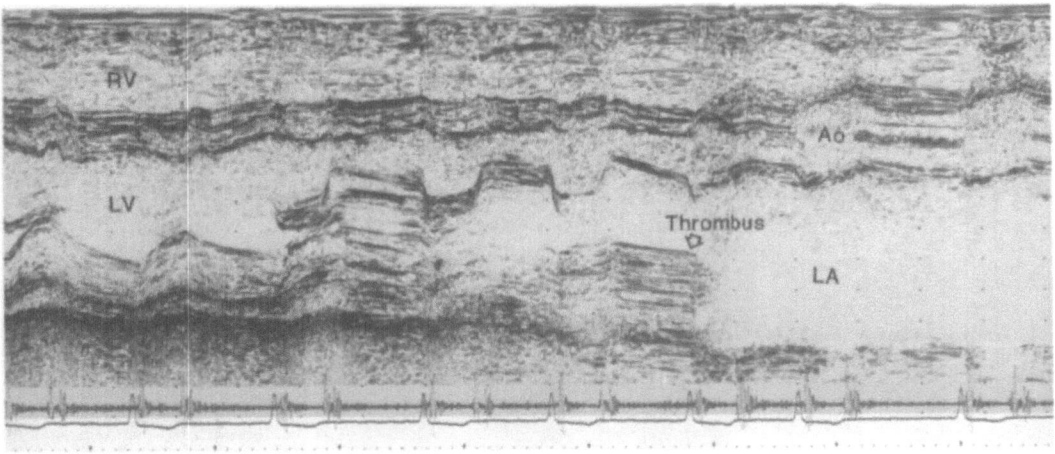

Figure 3.15. M-mode scan of the same patient (Figure 3.14). One can see only one thrombus on the posterior wall, which indicates one of the possible limitations of this method for evaluating the thrombus.

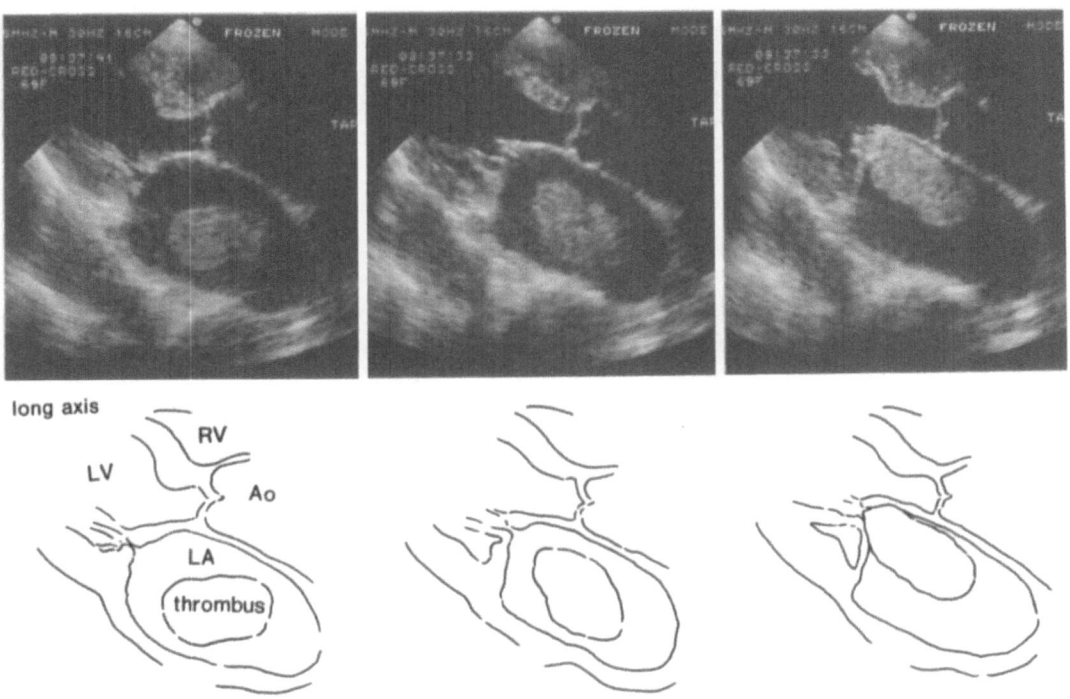

Figure 3.16. Two-dimensional long axis view of a patient with mitral stenosis and floating LA thrombus. The free motion and the protrusion into the mitral orifice (right panel) may be clearly seen.

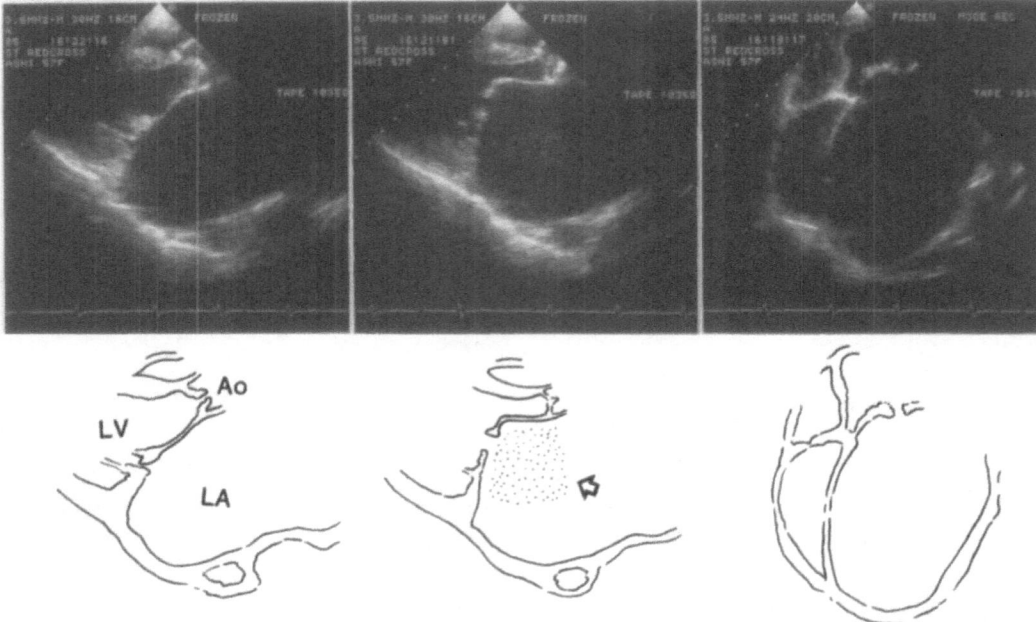

Figure 3.17. Parasternal long axis and apical four chamber view of a patient with rheumatic mitral stenosis and regurgitation accompanied with giant left atrium. Intra-atrial smoke-like echoes are noted, due to flow stasis (arrow).

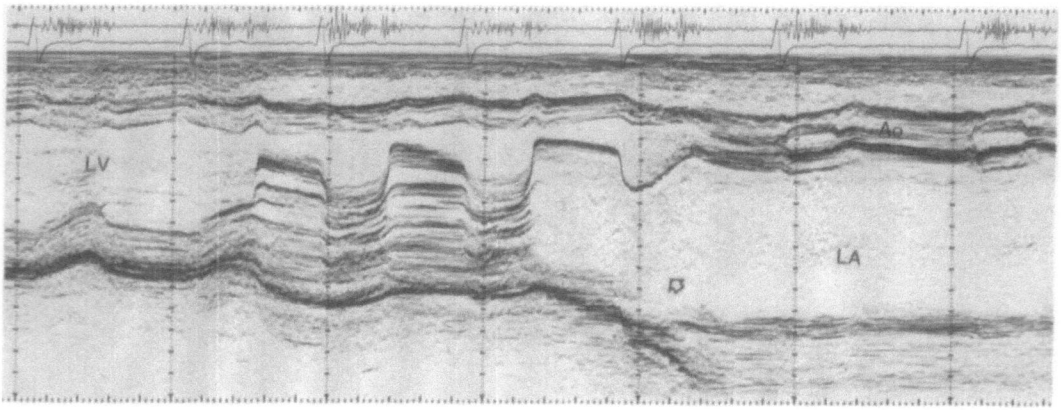

Figure 3.18. An M-mode scan illustrating mitral stenosis with giant left atrium. The blood stasis is evident in the left atrium (arrow).

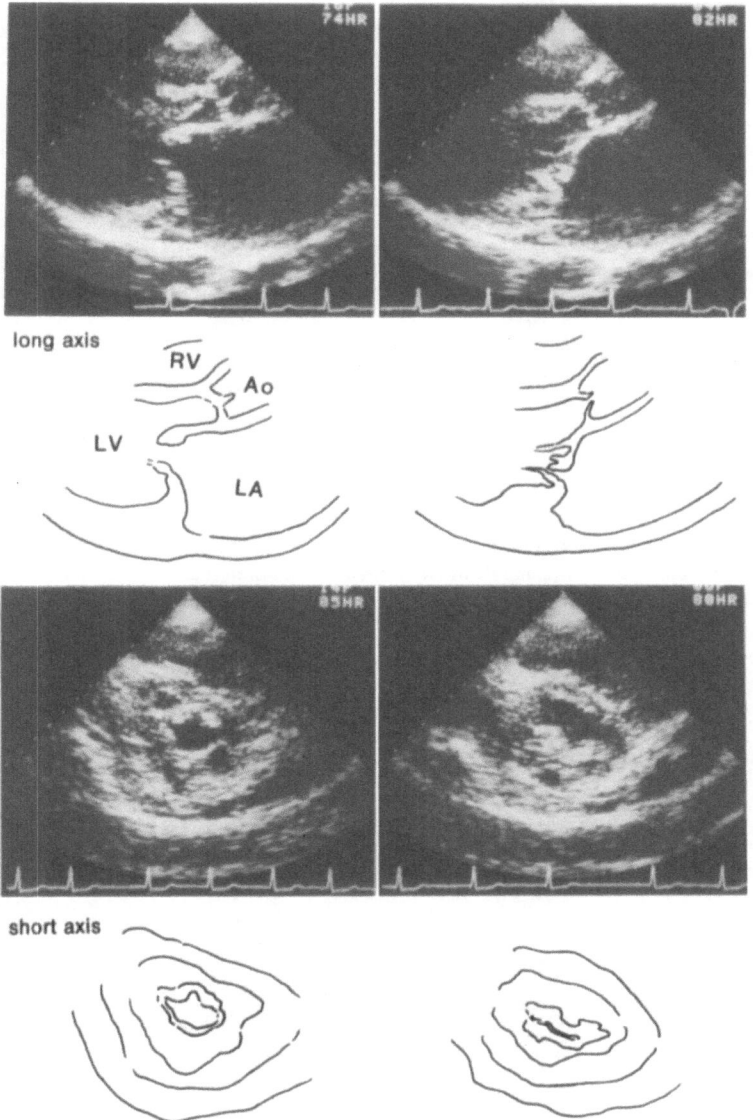

Figure 3.19. A long and short axis view of a patient with predominant rheumatic mitral regurgitation. Mitral valve thickening with a mild degree of stenosis and incomplete systolic closure are illustrated.

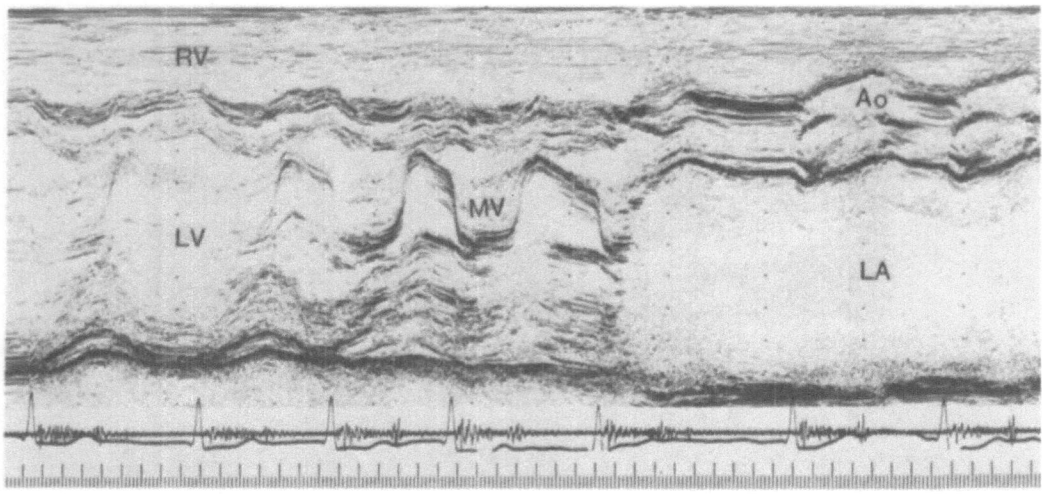

Figure 3.20.   An M-mode scan demonstrating mitral valve thickening, decreased E–F slope and good excursion of the anterior leaflet. Left atrial and ventricular dilatation is noted secondary to volume overload.

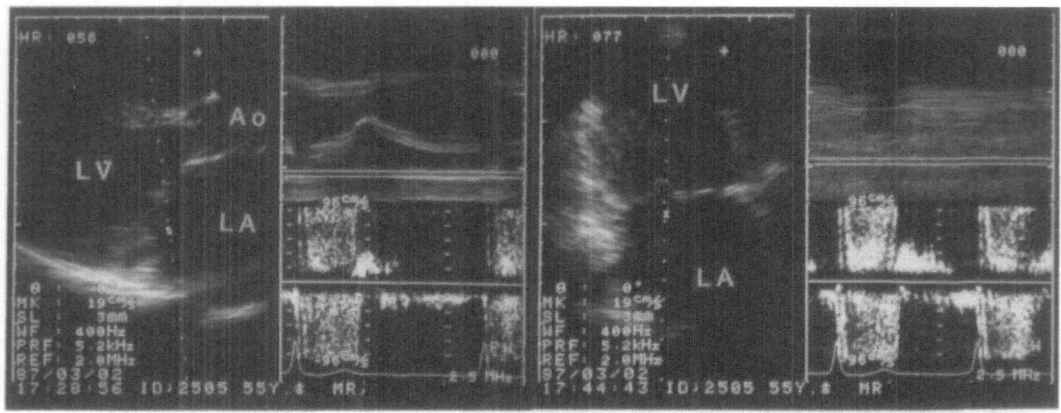

Figure 3.21.   A pulsed Doppler echocardiogram of mitral regurgitation from apical and parasternal windows. The sample volume can be positioned in the left atrium from both the parasternal approach (left) and apical approach (right). The systolic regurgitant signal is similarly demonstrated from both approaches. These regurgitant signals are due to non-laminar elements and the high velocity, which exceeds the Nyquist limits for pulsed Doppler, resulting in aliasing.

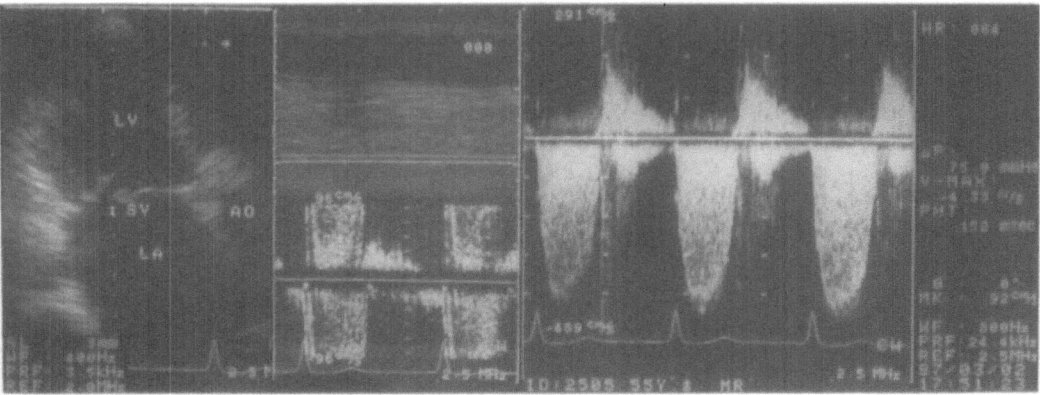

Figure 3.22. A pulsed and CW Doppler echocardiogram of mitral regurgitation recorded from apical window. The pulsed Doppler echocardiogram shows an aliased and turbulent flow signal (mitral regurgitation), which results in directional ambiguity and limitations on peak velocity measurements. CW Doppler does show the direction and peak velocity of the regurgitant flow in the same patient.

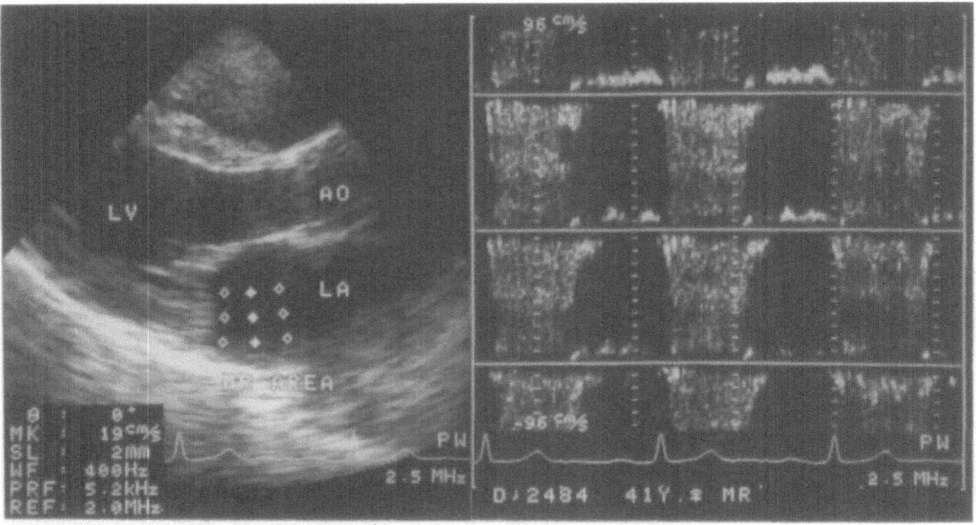

Figure 3.23. Flow mapping evaluation of mitral regurgitation using multi-gated pulsed Doppler echocardiography. Left: the location of the regurgitant flow (indicated area). *Right:* the mitral regurgitant flows in athree different sample volume simultaneously.

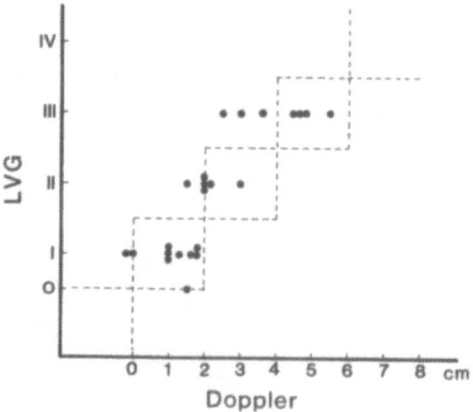

Figure 3.24. Correlation between pulsed Doppler flow mapping and left ventriculography, in grading the severity of mitral regurgitation (by modified Sellers). A very good correlation of the maximal distance of regurgitant flow and the degree of mitral regurgitation is demonstrated.

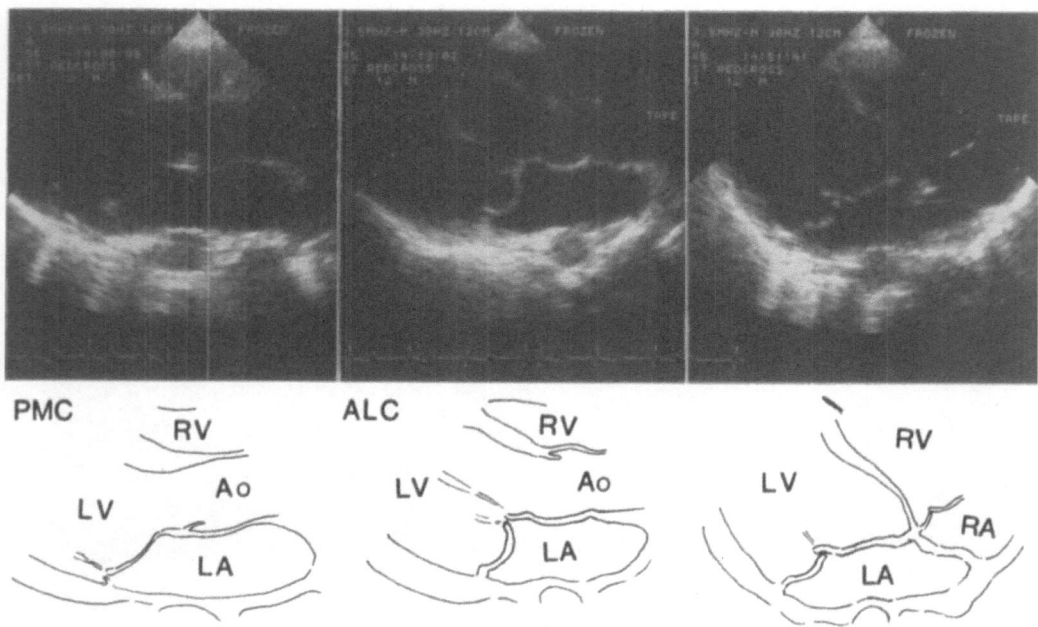

Figure 3.25. Parasternal long axis and apical-four chamber views of a patient with posterior mitral valve prolapse. The left panel does not show the mitral valve prolapse on postero-medial commisural (PMC) side. The middle panel clearly shows the significant posterior mitral valve displacement on antero-lateral commisural (ALC) side. The right panel also demonstrates the prolapse of the posterior leaflet.

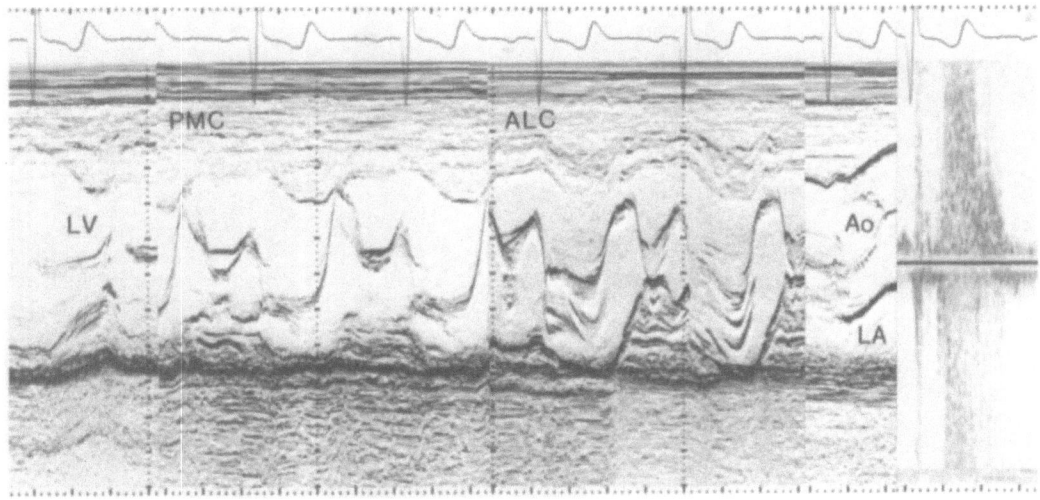

Figure 3.26. An M-mode echocardiogram of a patient with posterior mitral valve prolapse. The mitral valve echo of postero-medial commisural (PMC) side does not demonstrate abnormal findings. Antero-lateral commisural (ALC) side demonstrates the characteristic late systolic and posterior buckling of the mitral valve. The pulsed Doppler echoacardiogram shows a systolic and turbulent flow in the left atrium, which is mainly directed toward the anterior wall due to posterior mitral valve prolapse.

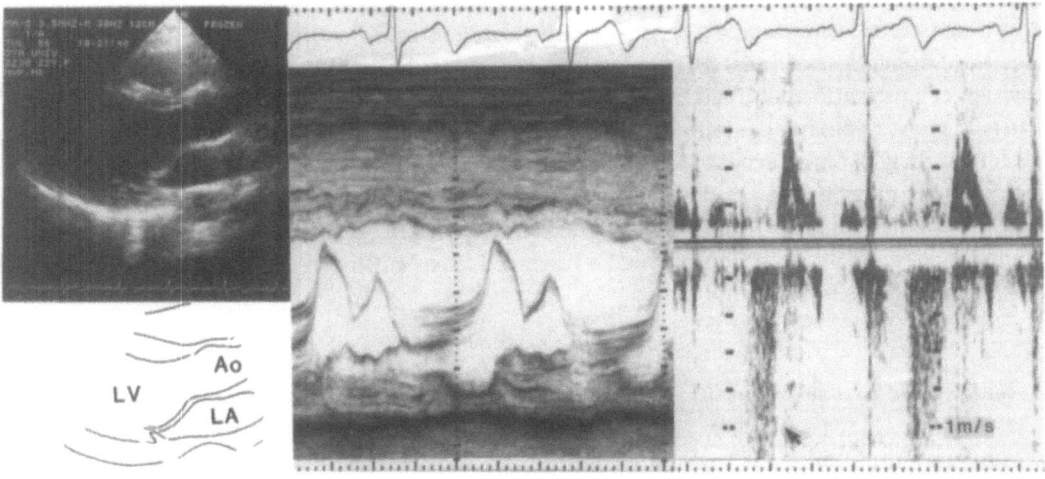

Figure 3.27. Parasternal along axis view, M-mode and pulsed Doppler echocardiogram from a patient with anterior mitral valve prolapse. A late systolic regurgitant signal is demonstrated by the pulsed Doppler echocardiogram.

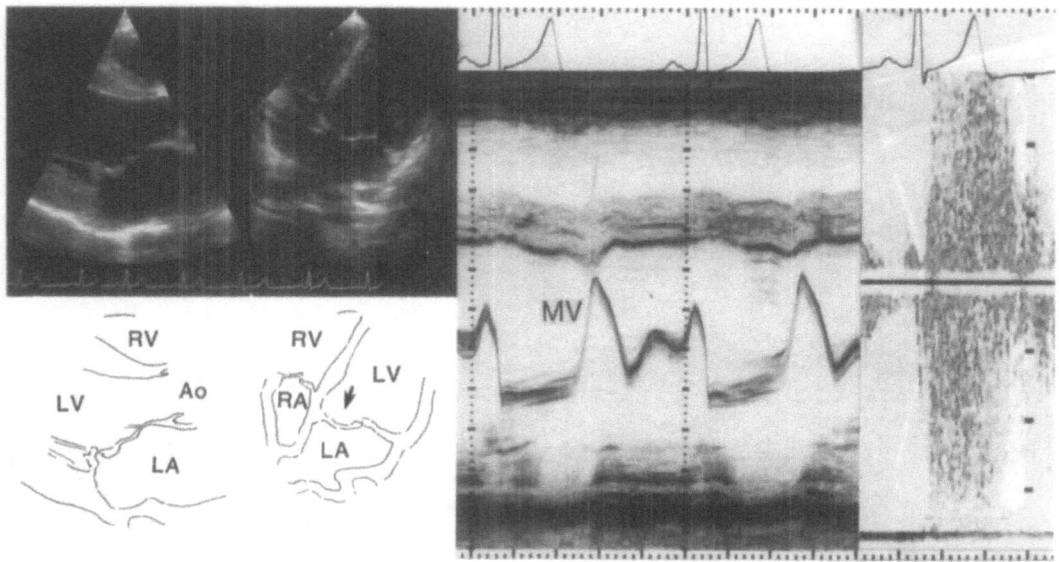

Figure 3.28. Parasternal and apical long axis views, M-mode and pulsed Doppler echocardiogram from a patient with anterior mitral valve prolapse. The two-dimensional echocardiogram illustrates an abnormal coaptation of the anterior leaflet (arrow). Holosystolic prominent echoes of mitral valve are evident, without typical buckling or bowing changes. Pulsed Doppler shows a systolic turbulent flow in the left atrium (mitral regurgitation).

severe cases, one cannot appreciate accurately the degree of aortic stenosis using M-mode and two-dimensional echocardiography, due to prominent calcification (Figure 3.42, 43). Usually, the application of pulsed Doppler echocardiography to the evaluation of the stenotic flow is very limited, and CW Doppler is preferable for its quantitative evaluation (Figure 3.44). The peak velocity of stenotic flow should be assessed using several approaches, such as the left and right parasternal, apical, subcostal and suprasternal windows since the highest peak velocity may be measured more accurately from one window than another (Figures 3.45, 46). For the assessment of the transaortic systolic pressure gradient, a simplified Bernoulli equation ($p = 4V^2$) can be employed. This method is well correlated with cardiac catheterization (Figure 3.47).

7. Aortic valve regurgitation

Aortic regurgitation (AR) has many aetiologies such as: rheumatic, atherosclerotic, inflammatory, annuloaortic dilatation and valve prolapse. Usually, two-dimensional echocardiography cannot visualize the abnormalities of the aortic valve in aortic regurgitation (Figures 3.48, 50). In severe cases, it is accompanied by LV dilatation due to volume overload. In M-mode echocardiography, sometimes double or multiple diastolic echoes of the aortic valve with mitral valve fluttering can be observed (Figure 3.49). Fluttering of the anterior mitral leaflet may be recorded if the regurgitant jet is oriented toward the mitral leaflet (Figure 3.51). The presence of a diastolic mitral valve flutter is a specific but not sensitive finding in aortic regurgitation, and provides no indication of severity. Aortic regurgitation is sometimes secondary to the aortitis syndrome (Figures 3.52, 53), aortic valve prolapse due to idiopathic origin (Figures 3.54, 55) or related to a membranous VSD (see

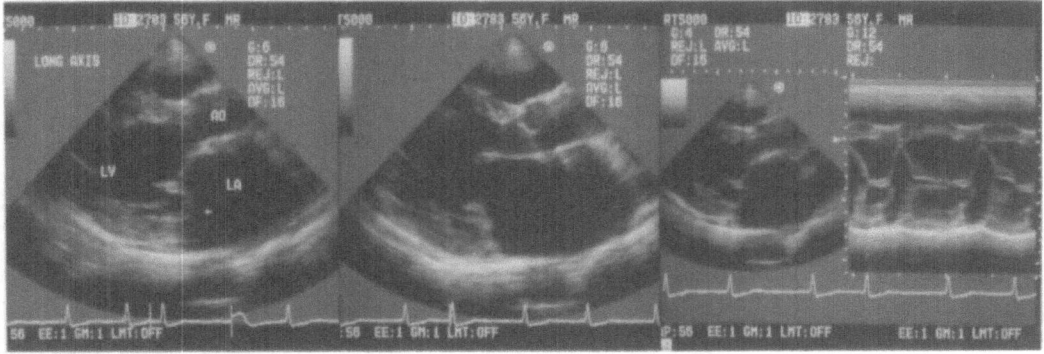

Figure 3.29. Parasternal and M-mode echocardiogram of a patient with posterior mitral valve prolapse. The two-dimensional echocardiogram illustrates an abnormal prolapsing of posterior leaflet (arrow), whereas the M-mode cannot reveal any abnormal findings (buckling or bowing).

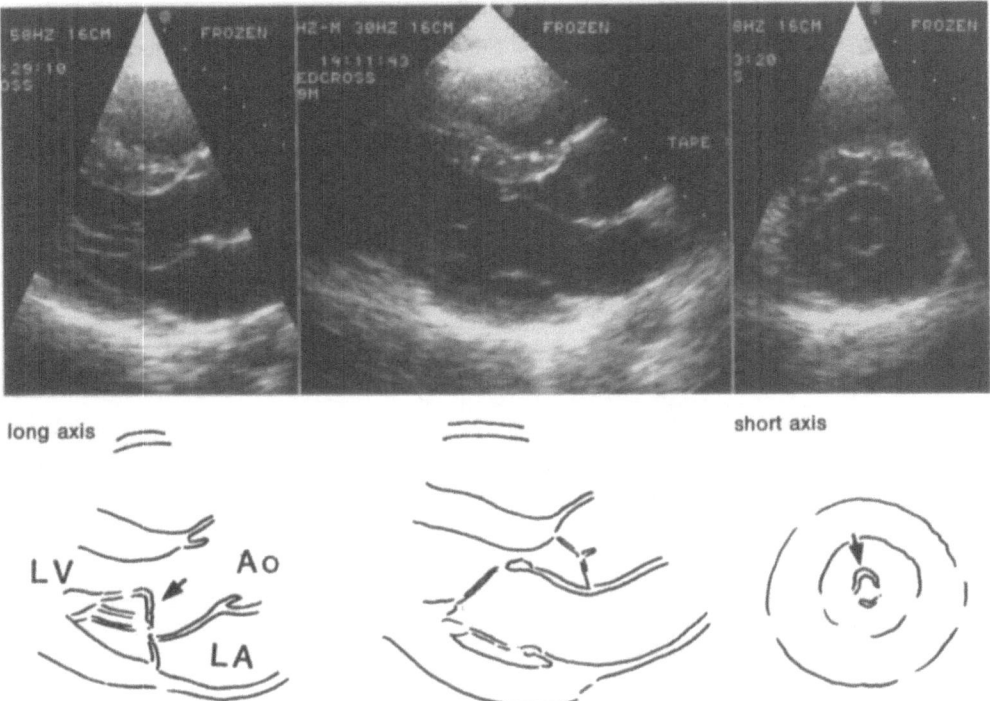

Figure 3.30. Parasternal long and short axis view demonstrating systolic anterior movement (SAM) of the chordae tendineae (arrow), and mitral valve prolapse.

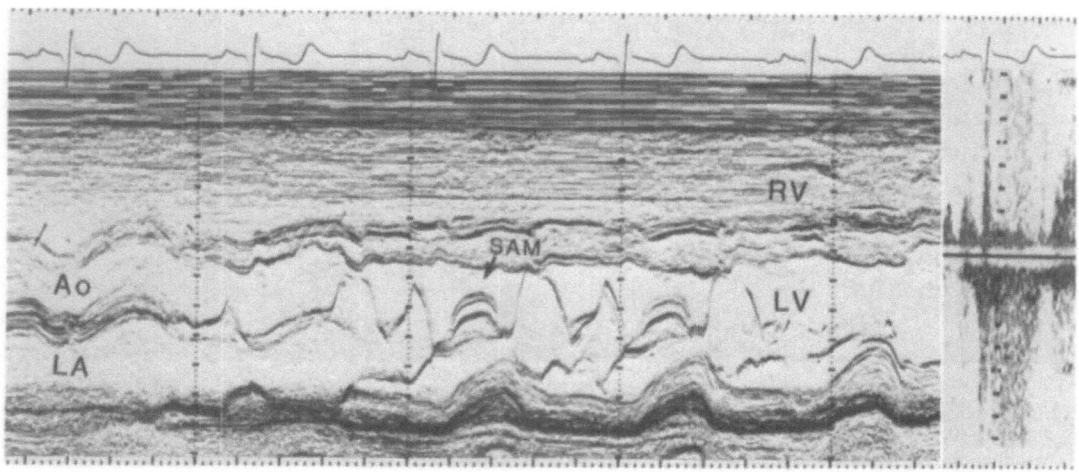

Figure 3.31. M-mode scan shows a prominent SAM of the chordae tendineae and pulsed Doppler evidences the mitral regurgitant flow.

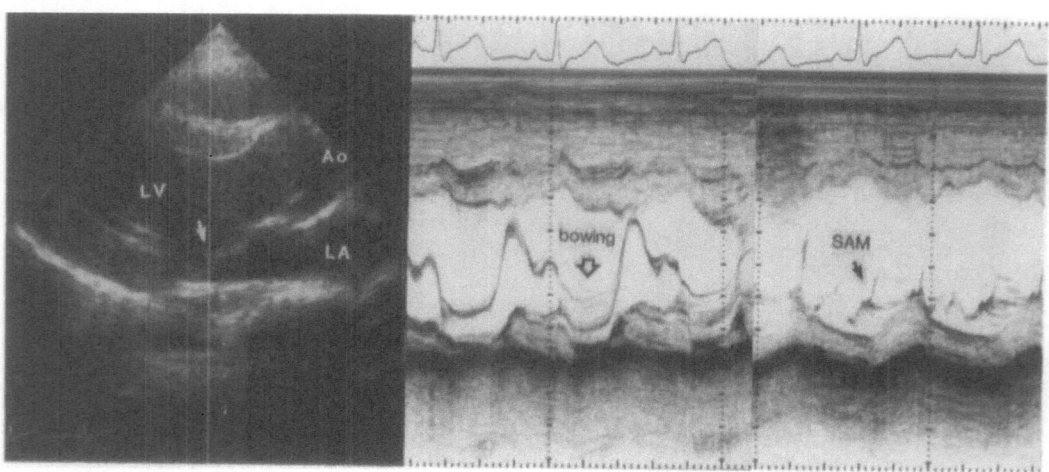

Figure 3.32. Parasternal long axis and M-mode echocardiogram of a patient with anterior mitral valve prolapse and SAM. The M-mode echocardiogram recorded from the mitral valve level shows prominent holosystolic bowing. The M-mode echocardiogram recorded from the left ventricular level demonstrates systolic anterior movement (SAM) of the chordae tendineae.

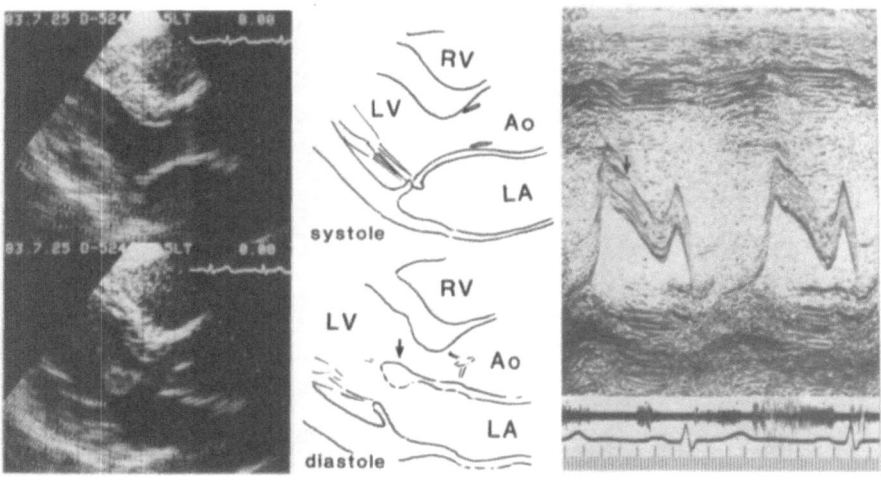

Figure 3.33. Parasternal long axis view and M-mode echocardiogram of a patient with mixomatous degeneration of anterior mitral valve leaflet (arrow).

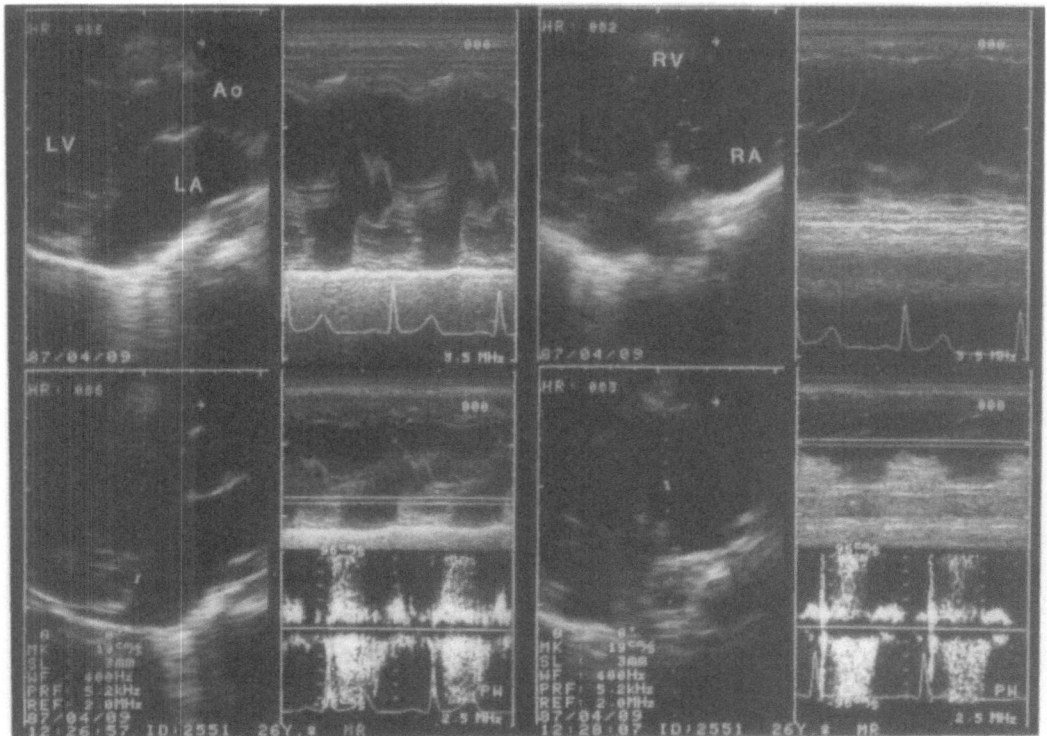

Figure 3.34. Two-dimensional, M-mode and pulsed Doppler echocardiogram of a patient with prolapse of the anterior mitral leaflet and the anterior tricuspid leaflet. The left panel shows an anterior mitral valve prolapse and holosystolic bowing with mitral regurgitation. The right panel shows an anterior tricuspid valve prolapse, systolic bowing and pulsed Doppler demonstrates the tricuspid regurgitation.

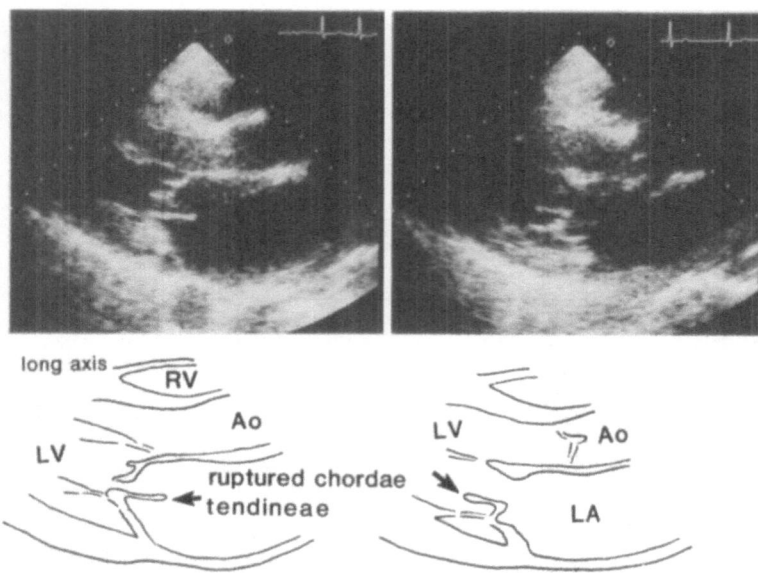

Figure 3.35. Parasternal long axis view of a patient with endocarditis and ruptured chordae tendineae. During systole (left) the chordae tendineae protrudes into the left atrium (arrow) and during diastole, the chordae is located in the left ventricle (arrow). Only minimal abnormality during the systolic coaptation of the mitral leaflets in this patient can be seen.

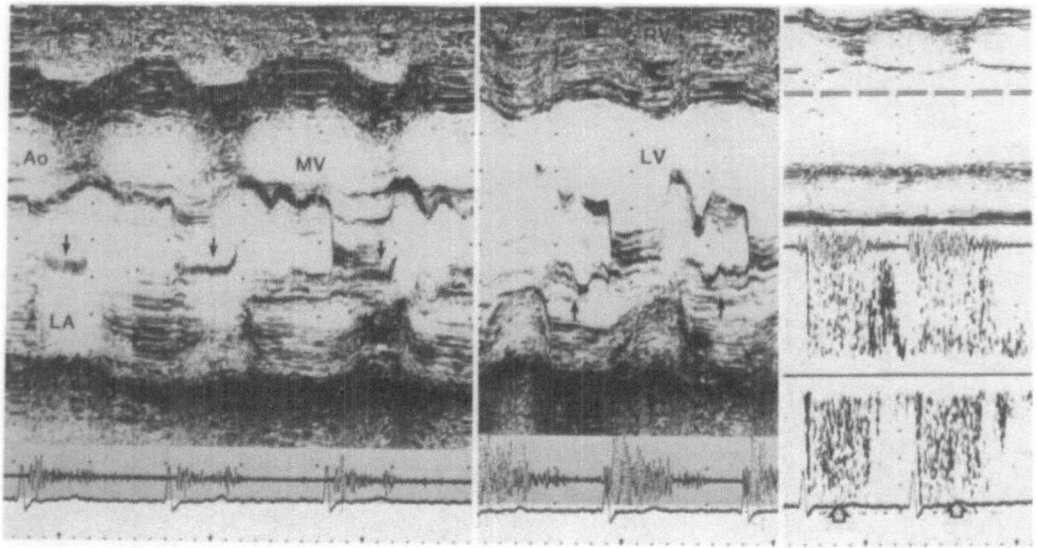

Figure 3.36. An M-mode and pulsed Doppler echocardiogram demonstrating the presence of chordae tendineae in the left atrium during systole (small arrow) and mitral regurgitant flow (large arrow).

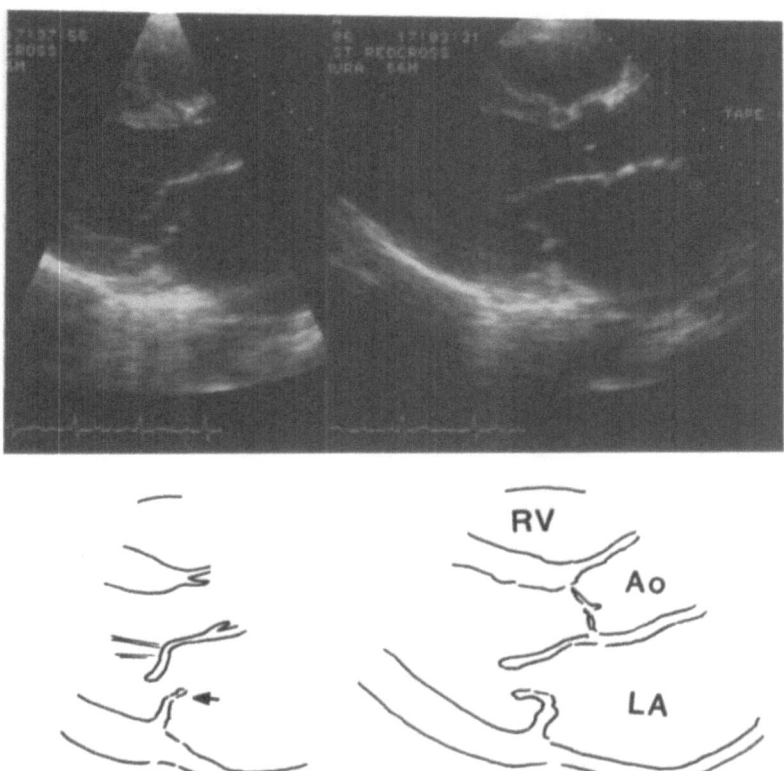

Figure 3.37. Parasternal long axis view of a patient with ruptured chordae tendineae demonstrating the flail posterior mitral valve (arrow).

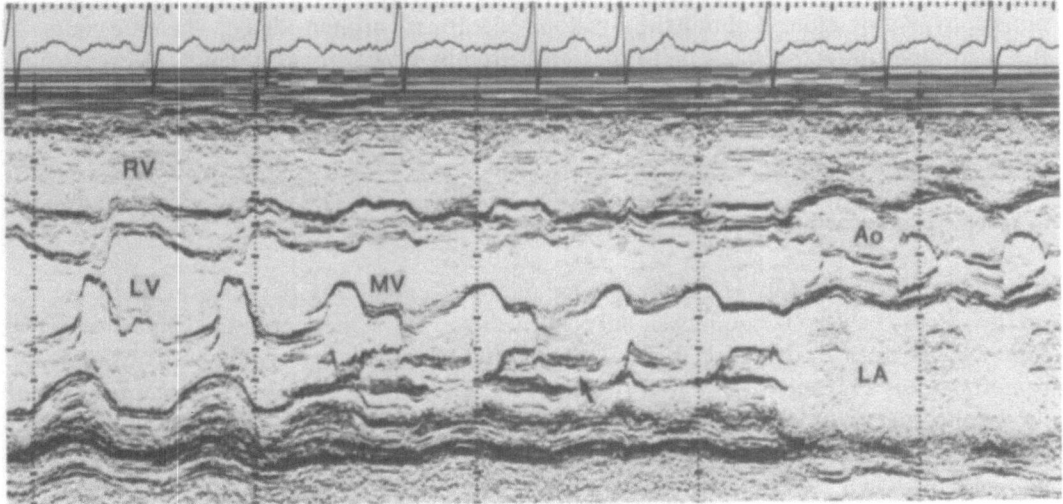

Figure 3.38. An M-mode scan illustrating a systolic bowing (arrow) of the mitral valve due to ruptured chordea tendineae.

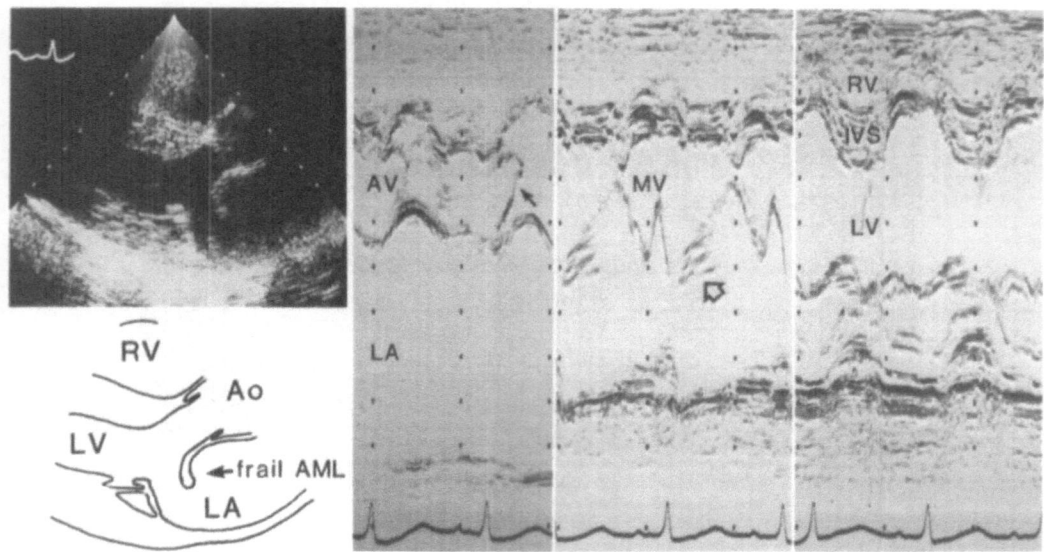

Figure 3.39.   Parasternal long axis view and M-mode echocardiogram of a patient with ruptured chordae tendineae and flail anterior mitral leaflet. M-mode shows a premature closure of aortic valve, with hyperdynamic LV wall motion due to severe mitral regurgitation.

Figures 4.22, 23). The diagnosis and hemodynamic evaluation of aortic regurgitation can be carried out by Doppler techniques. Pulsed Doppler echocardiography provides information about the location and severity of the regurgitant flow in the left ventricle (Figure 3.56). The 'flow mapping technique' provides the semi-quantitative evaluation of aortic regurgitation that is well correlated with aortography (Figure 3.57). When the sample volume is located in the ascending or descending aorta, aortic regurgitant flow is recorded as a lower velocity retrograde flow due to a lower pressure gradient (Figure 3.58). Using CW Doppler echocardiography, it is possible to obtain the envelope of aortic regurgitant signal. The time course of the regurgitant flow (pressure half-time) measured by CW Doppler tends to decrease with increasing severity of aortic regurgitation. Hatle *et al.* found that a pressure half-time less than 250 msec indicated the presence of severe aortic regurgitation (Figure 3.59).

8. Infective endocarditis

Infective endocarditis (IE) is usually accompanied by vegetations that are principally located on the cardiac valves. Two-dimensional echocardiography is the method of choice for detection. Ordinarily, the vegetation is mobile with increased echo intensity (Figure 3.60, 62), and sometimes it is attached to a previously diseased valve (Figure 3.64). Using M-mode echocardiography, one can appreciate the characteristically 'shaggy' echoes on the involved structures (Figures 3.61, 63, 65). During the acute phase, infective endocarditis is commonly accompanied by valvular regurgitation and sometimes with valvular perforation (Figures 3.66, 67, 68) or abscess formation (Figures 3.69, 70, 71). Two-dimensional echocardiography provides sufficient information for the correct medical management and surgical procedure. Vegetation formations in the right side on the heart usually occur due to congenital abnormalities such as VSD or PDA (Figures 3.72, 73, 74).

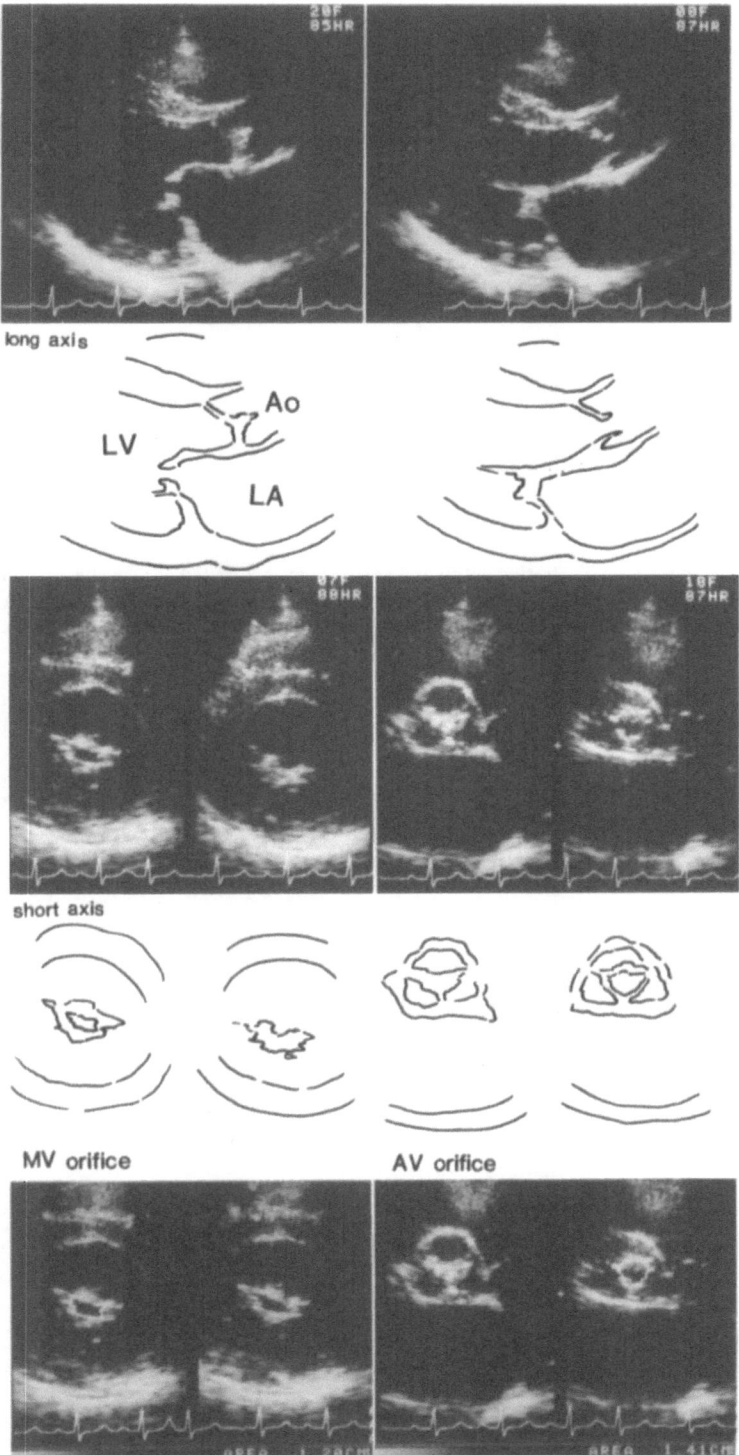

Figure 3.40. Parasternal long and short axis view of a patient with mitral and aortic stenosis. The increased echo intensity of the aortic and mitral valves with limited opening can be seen. In this patient, in particular, it is possible to evaluate the mitral and aortic valve area by the planimetric method.

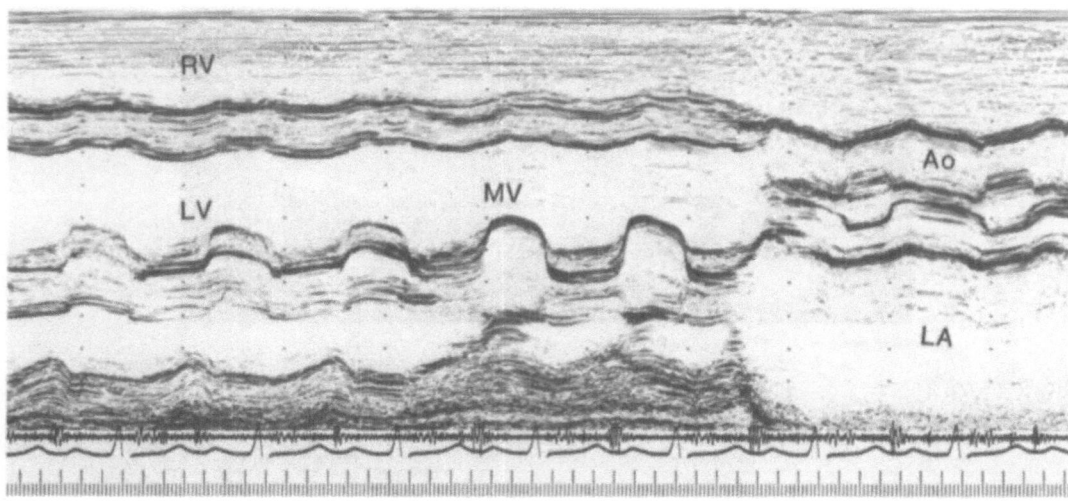

Figure 3.41.   An M-mode scan illustrating mitral and aortic stenosis. Limited aortic valve opening with prominent diastolic echoes can be seen. Mitral valve echoes show decreased E–F slope due to stenosis.

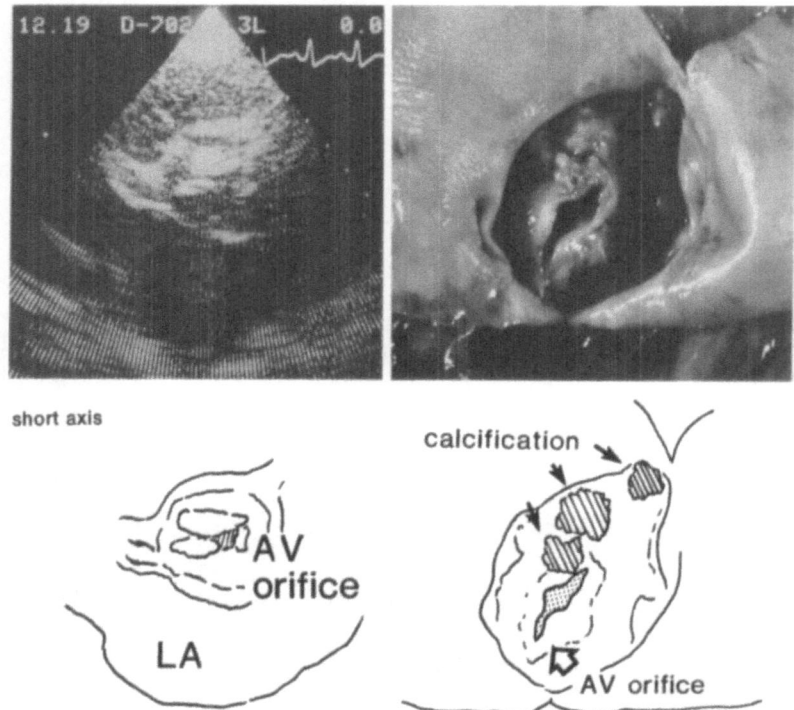

Figure 3.42.   Parasternal short axis view of a patient with severe aortic stenosis and an autopsy specimen from the same patient. Two-dimensional echocardiographic assessment of aortic valve area is almost impossible due to severe calcification, in comparison with autopsy findings.

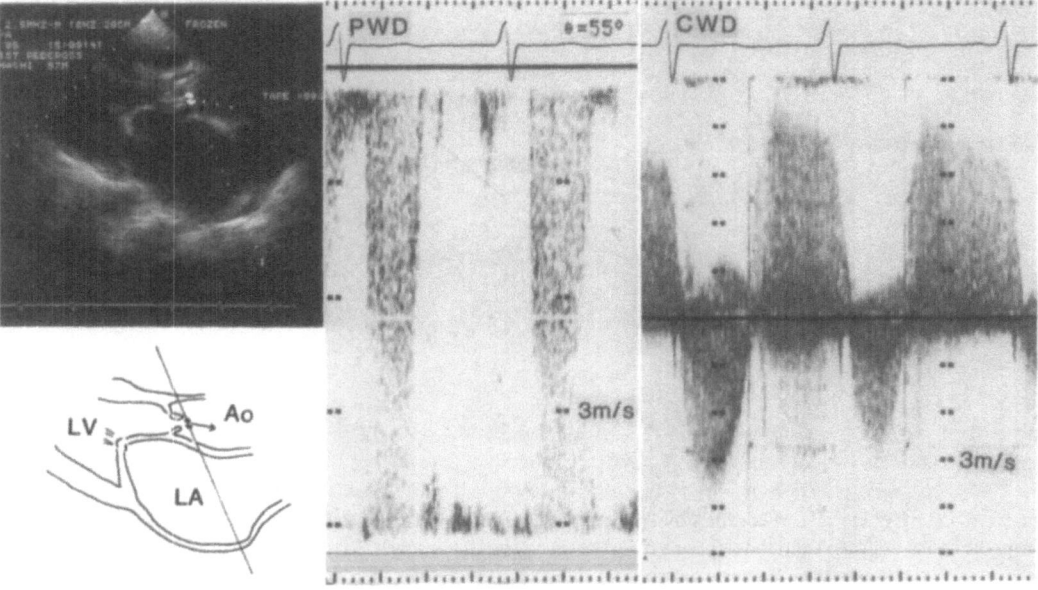

Figure 3.43. M-mode echocardiogram of a patient with severe aortic stenosis. The left panel shows a cloud of echo in the aortic root and the aortic valve motion can not be identified due to severe calcification. The middle and right panels show a poor mitral valve motion and LV hypokinesis due to depressed cardiac function.

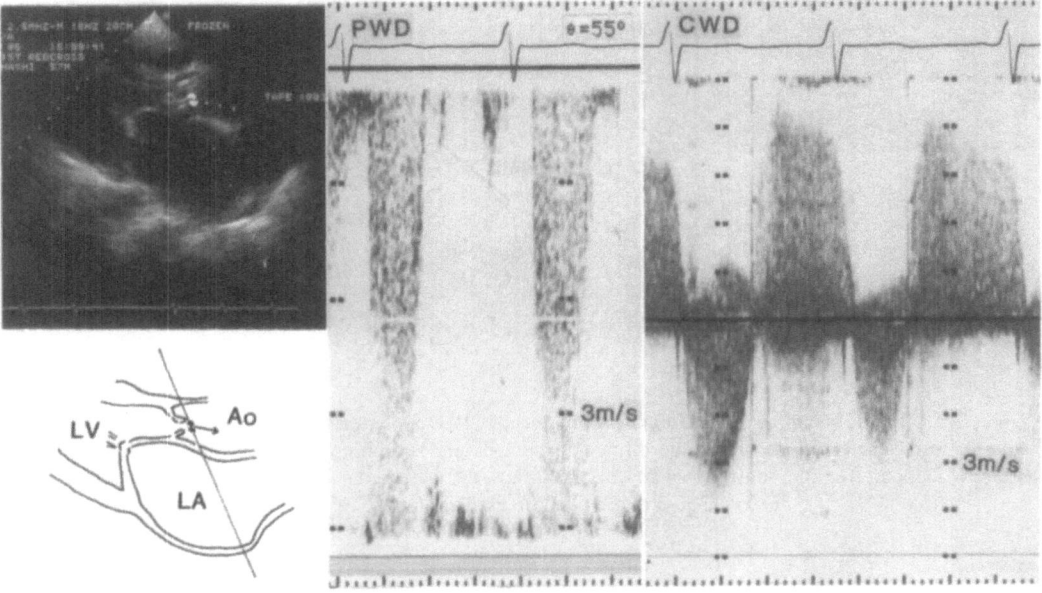

Figure 3.44. Pulsed and CW Doppler echocardiogram of a patient with aortic stenosis. In the parasternal long axis view, pulsed Doppler with angle correction shows turbulent flow with increased peak velocities (about 3 m/sec). The large angle correction (55 degrees) may introduce some errors in quantification. CW Doppler illustrates the peak velocity more clearly and also demonstrates an aortic regurgitant flow in the apical approach.

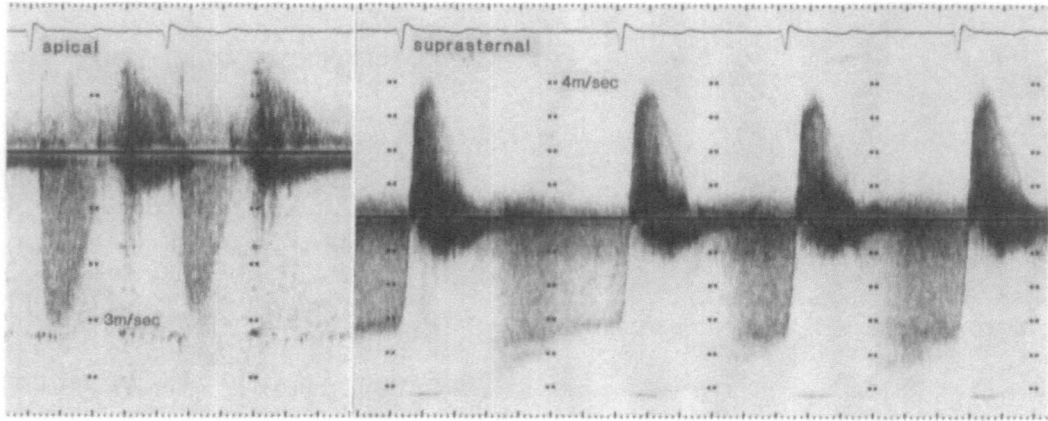

Figure 3.45. CW Doppler recordings of a patient with aortic stenosis and regurgitation. The left image is obtained from the apical approach and the right one from the suprasternal approach. In this patient, the suprasternal approach demonstrates a higher peak velocity due to aortic stenosis than does the apical approach.

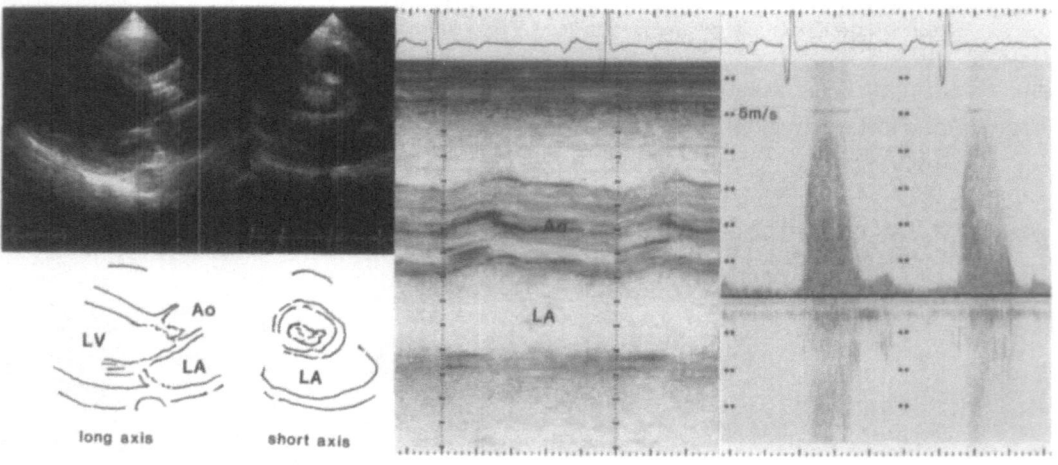

Figure 3.46. Parasternal long and short axis, M-mode and CW Doppler echocardiogram of a patient with severe aortic stenosis. The two-dimensional and M-mode echocardiograms cannot demonstrate the stenotic aortic valve area. CW Doppler from the suprasternal approach can show the increased peak velocity (about 5 m/s) and provide the evaluation of the pressure gradient (about 100 mm Hg).

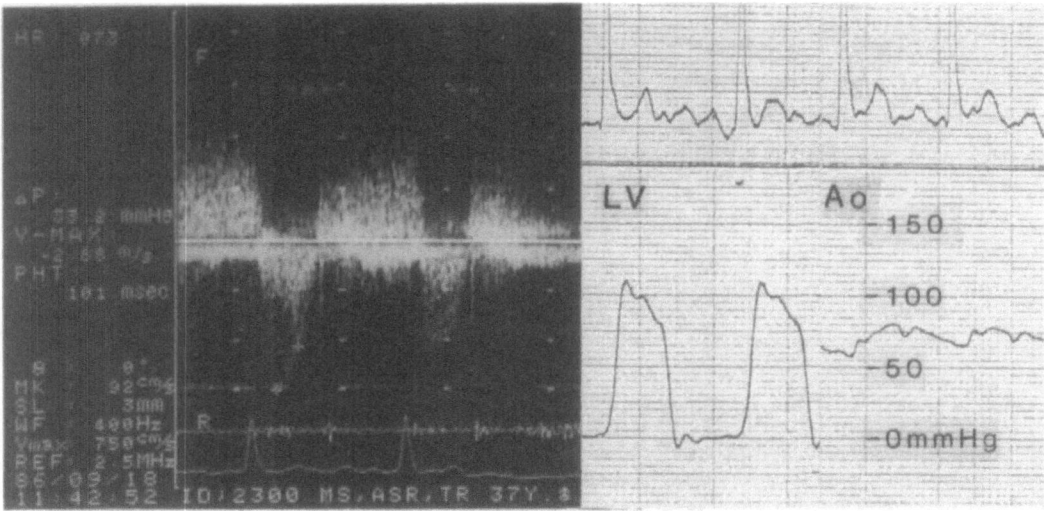

Figure 3.47. CW Doppler echocardiogram and left ventricular and aortic pressure tracings of a patient with aortic stenosis. One sees a peak velocity of approximately 3 m/sec. Using a simplified Bernoulli equation ($p = 4V^2 = 36$ mm Hg), it is possible to obtain a very similar pressure gradient as obtained by cardiac catheterization.

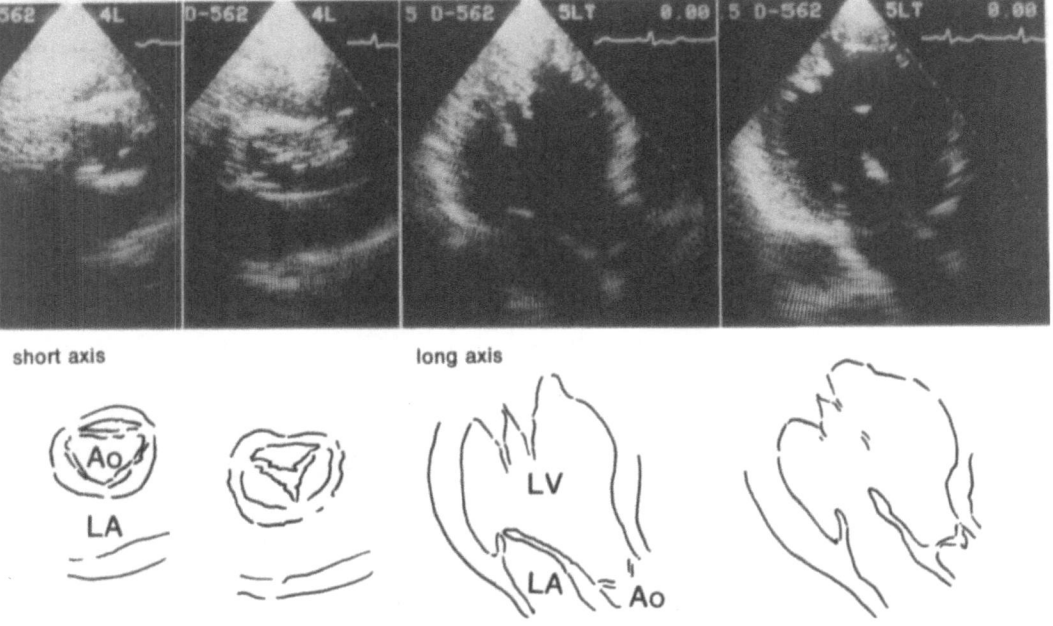

Figure 3.48. parasternal short axis and apical long axis view of a patient with severe aortic regurgitation. A mild increase in echo intensity of aortic cusp (arrow) and circular LV dilatation are observed.

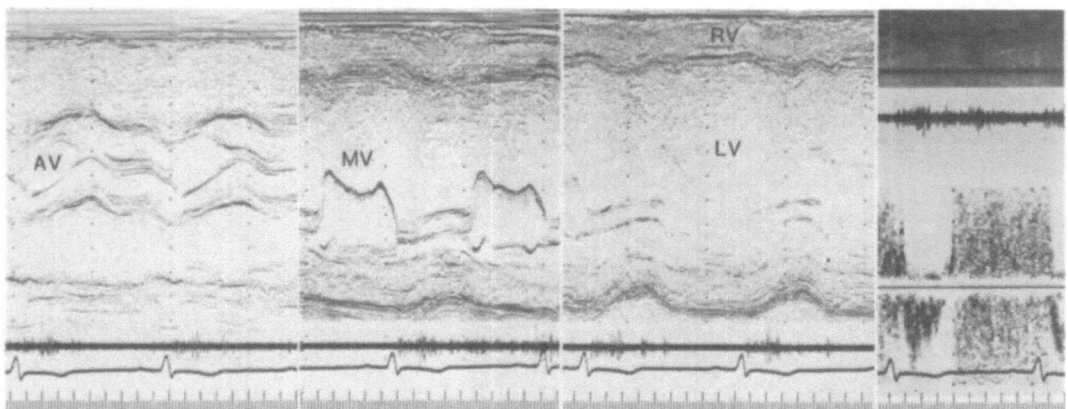

Figure 3.49. M-mode and pulsed Doppler echocardiogram of a patient with severe aortic regurgitation. The left panel shows a prominent diastolic aortic valve echo. The middle panel shows a severe LV dilatation without abnormal mitral valve motion, since the regurgitant jet is not directed toward the mitral valve (see Figure 3.56). The right panel shows a diastolic turbulent flow in the LV outflow tract.

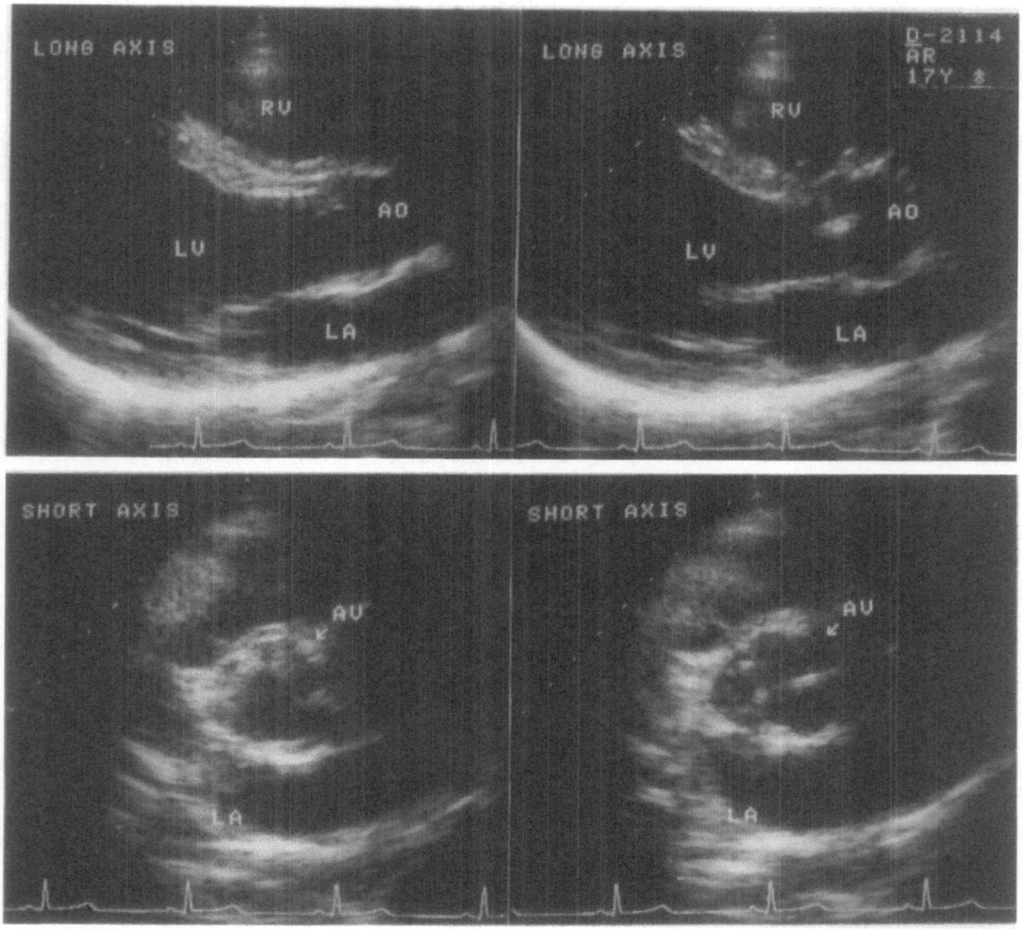

Figure 3.50. Parasternal long and short axis view demonstrating LV dilatation, with almost normal closure of the aortic valve in a patient with moderate aortic regurgitation. Aortic valve echoes show slightly increased echo intensity.

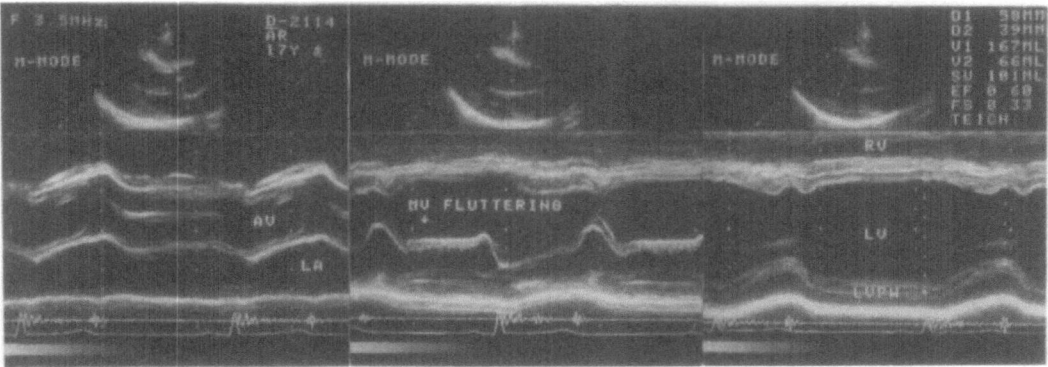

Figure 3.51. M-mode echocardiogram of a patient with moderate aortic regurgitation. Diastolic mitral valve fluttering and LV dilatation are shown.

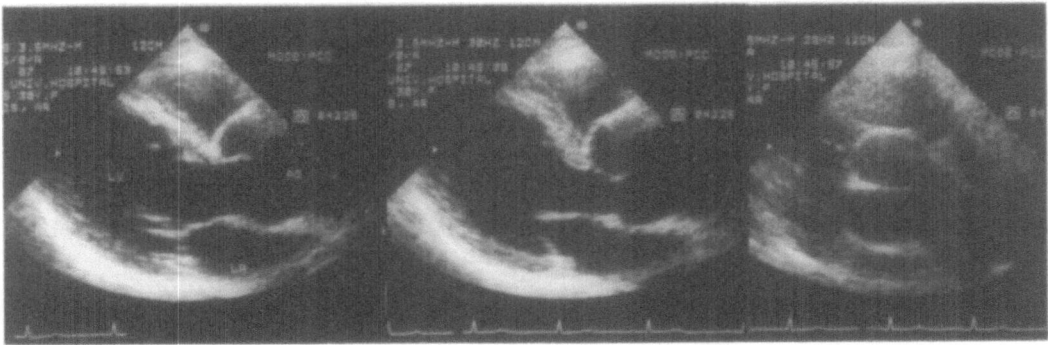

Figure 3.52. Parasternal long and short axis view of a patient with aortitis syndrome. A progressive dilatation of the ascending aorta is demonstrated.

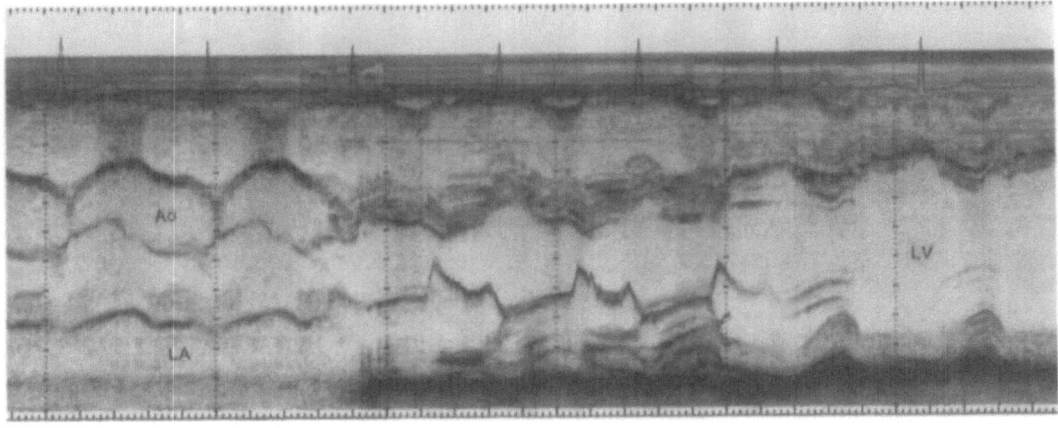

Figure 3.53. M-mode illustrating a progressive dilatation of the ascending aorta and mitral valve fluttering due to aortic regurgitation.

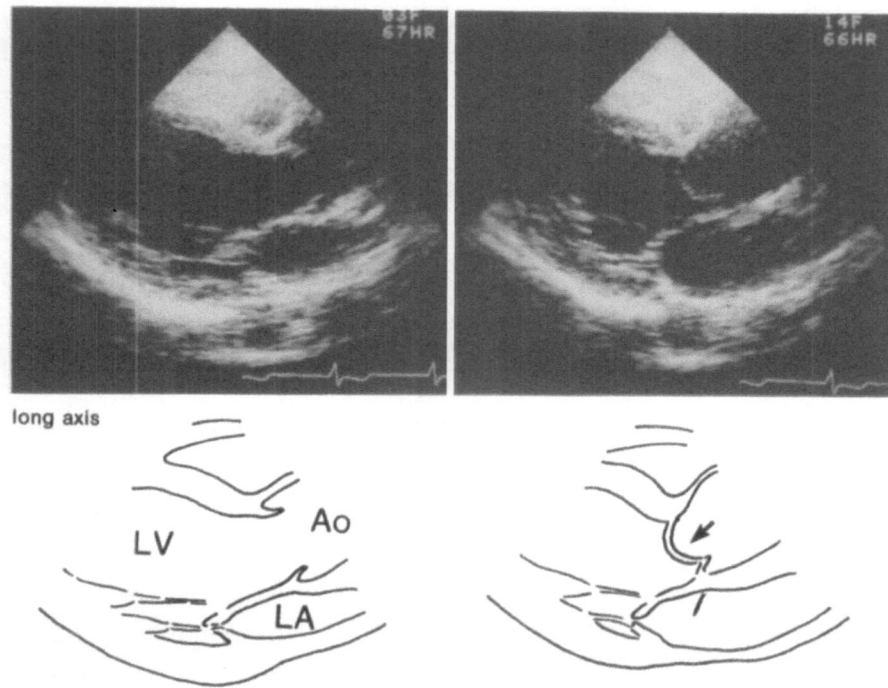

Figure 3.54.   Parasternal long axis view of a patient with aortic valve prolapse of the right coronary cusp (arrow).

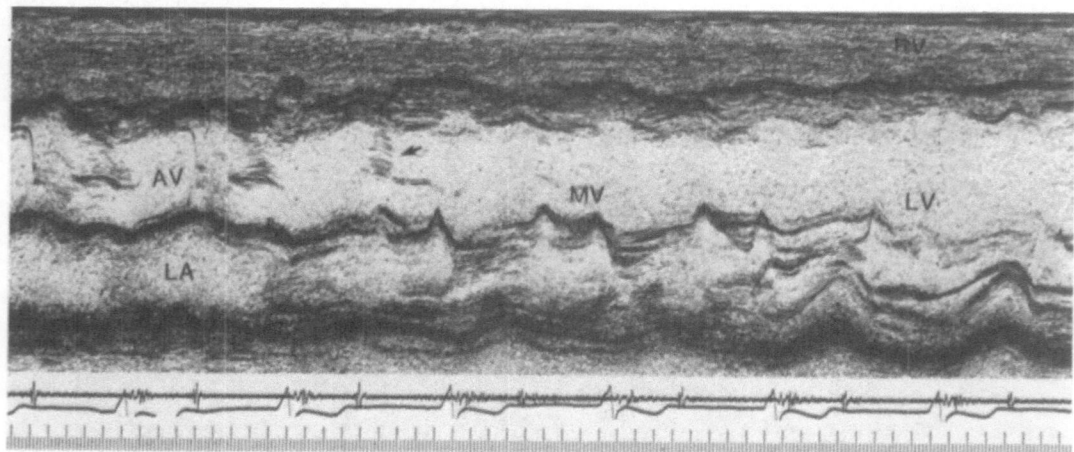

Figure 3.55.   M-mode scan of a patient with aortic valve prolapse and mild aortic regurgitation. Abnormal diastolic echoes of the aortic valve in LV outflow tract (arrow) can be seen.

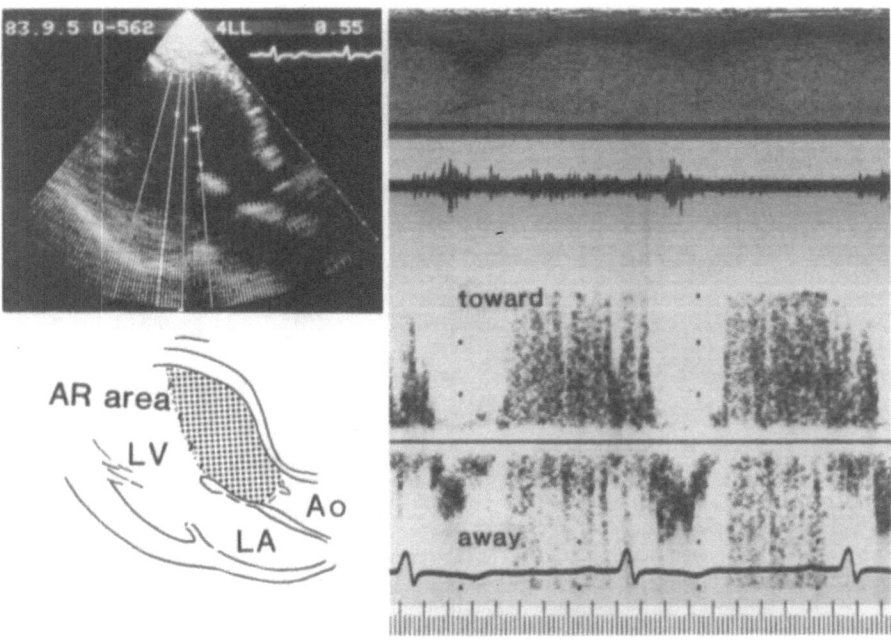

Figure 3.56. Flow mapping evaluation of aortic regurgitation using pulsed Doppler echocardiography. The left panel illustrates the location of the regurgitant flow area. The right one demonstrates the turbulent diastolic flow from the aortic regurgitation.

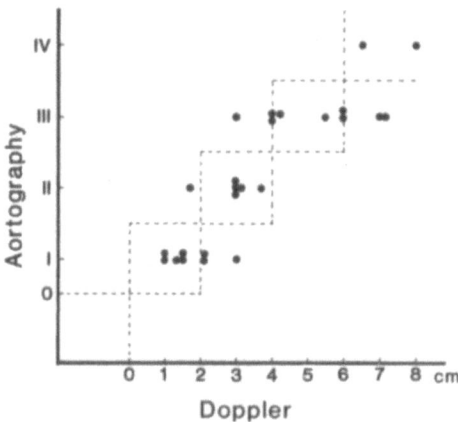

Figure 3.57. Correlation of pulsed Doppler flow mapping and aortography in quantitating the degree of aortic regurgitation (by angiographic Sellers grade).

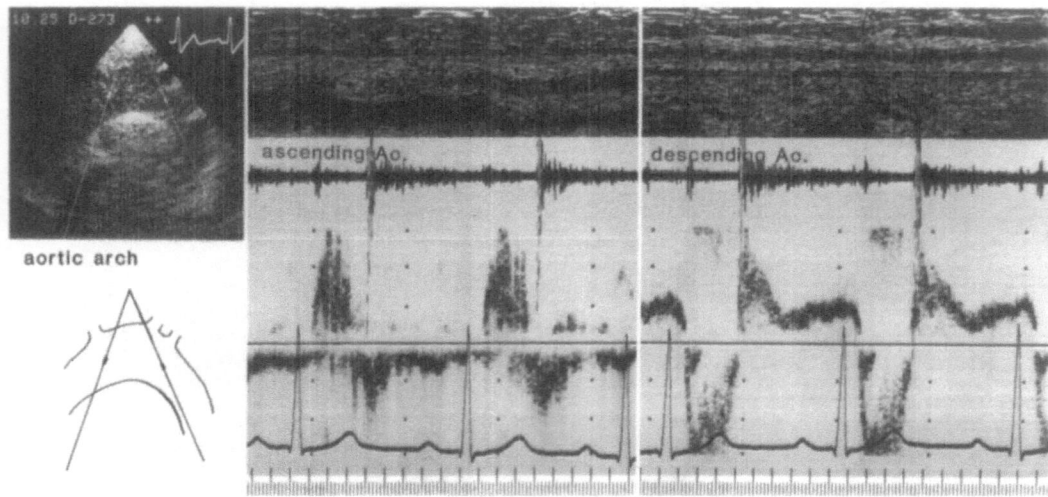

Figure 3.58. Pulsed Doppler echocardiogram of aortic regurgitant flow recorded from the suprasternal notch transducer position. When the sample volume is located in the ascending or descending aorta, a lower retrograde flow velocity is observed than that obtained in the left ventricle.

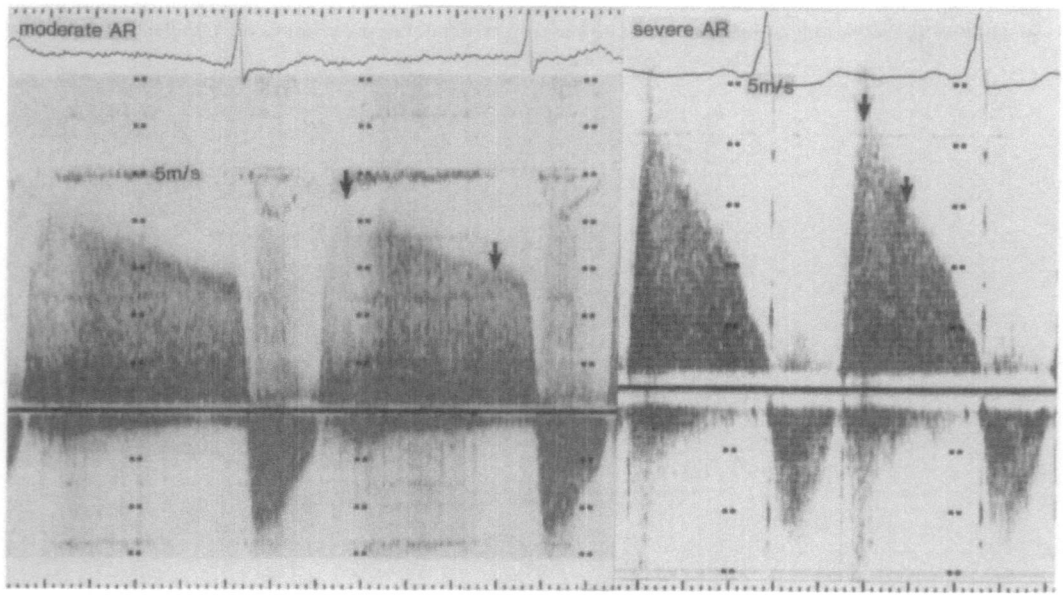

Figure 3.59. CW Doppler echocardiograms of aortic regurgitant flow in moderate and severe cases recorded from the apical approach. The time-course of aortic regurgitant flow is prolonged (pressure half-time is 700 msec) on the left, indicating a normal LV end-diastolic pressure. The pressure half-time measured is 200 msec on the right. This decreased pressure-half time indicates an increased LV end-diastolic pressure.

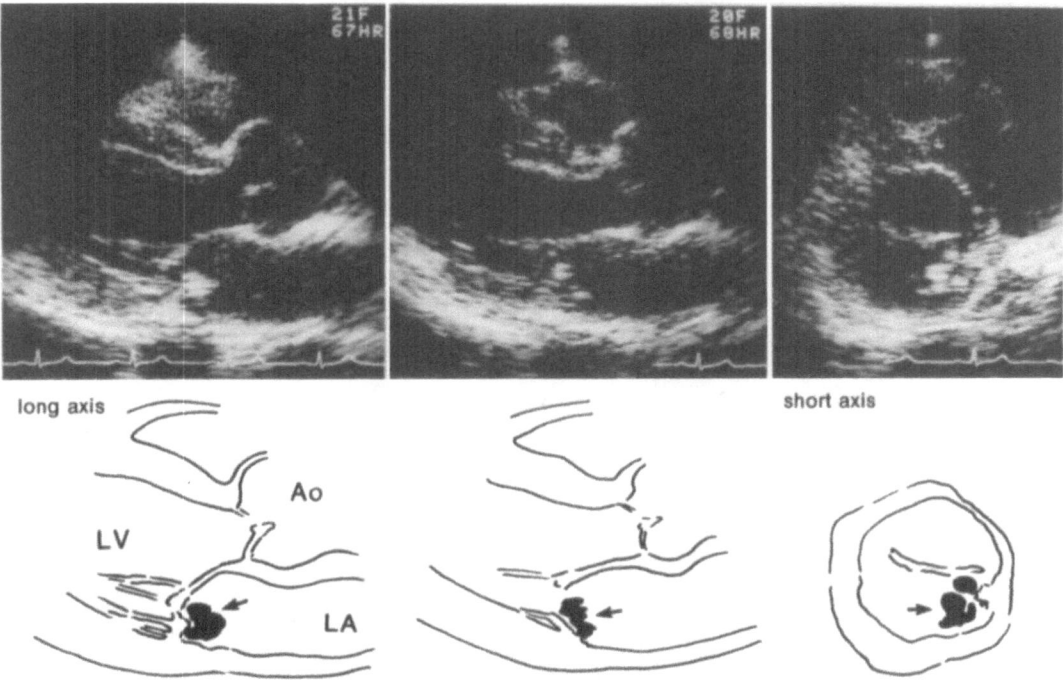

Figure 3.60. Parasternal long and short axis view illustrating a vegetation (arrow) located on the posterior mitral leaflet.

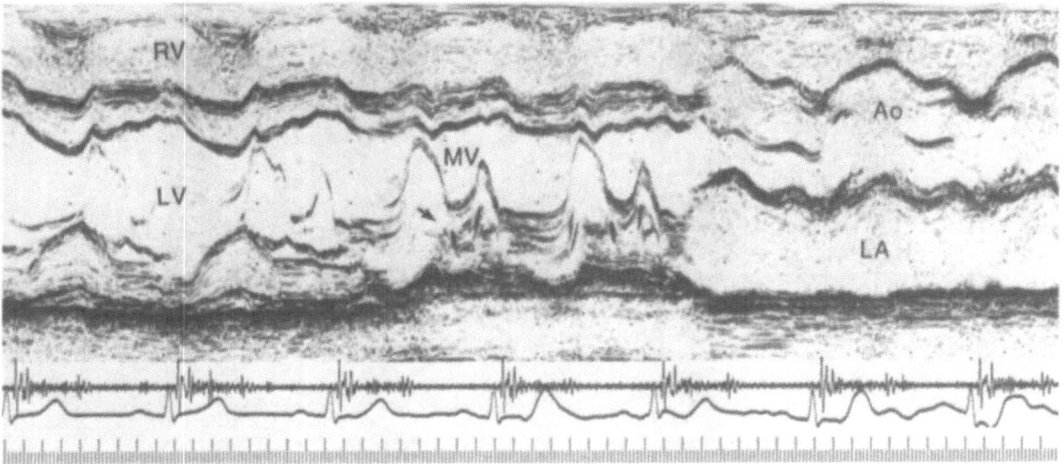

Figure 3.61. M-mode scan of a patient with infective endocarditis. Abnormal echoes on the posterior mitral leaflet (vegetation) are shown by arrows.

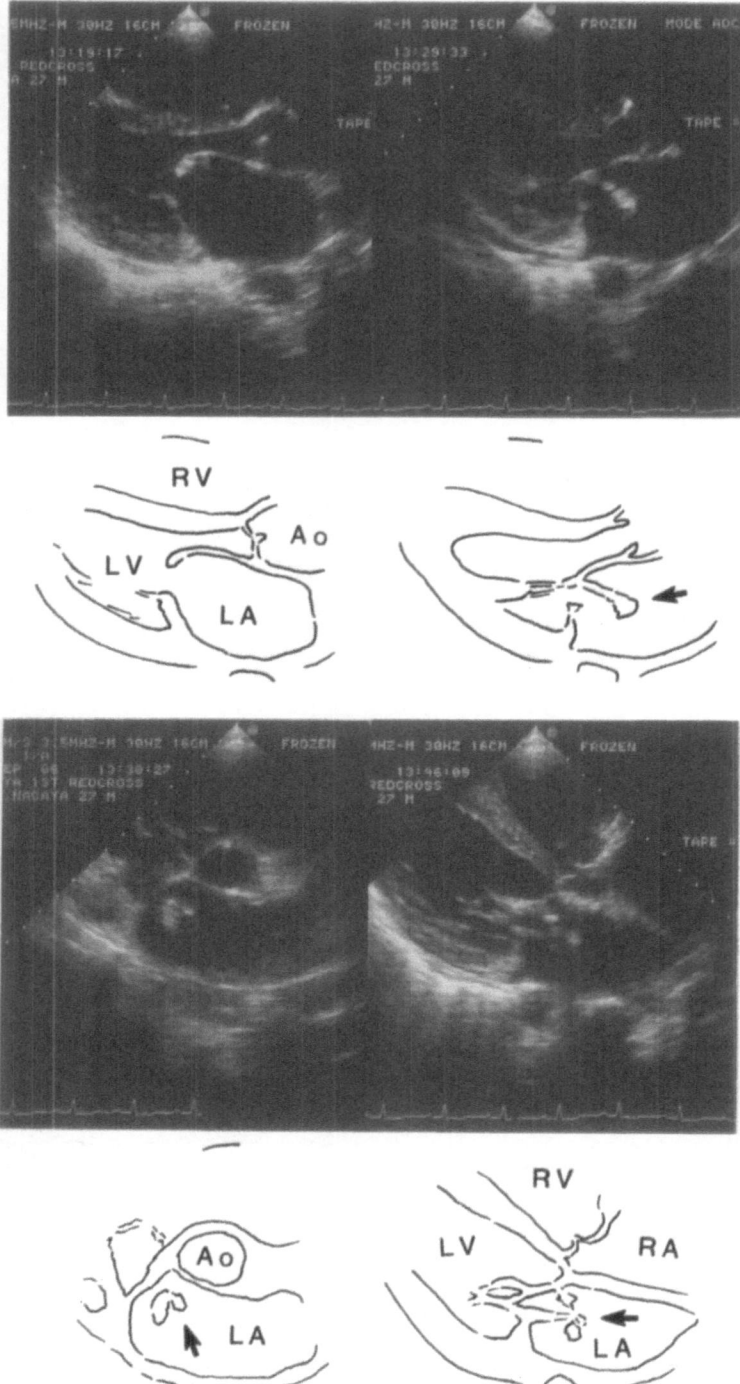

Figure 3.62.   Parasternal long and short axis and four-chamber view of a patient with mitral stenosis and infective endocarditis. In the long axis view, we can see the stenotic changes of mitral valve with vegetation (arrow) attached to anterior leaflet on the atrial side. The short axis and four-chamber views clearly show the vegetation (arrow).

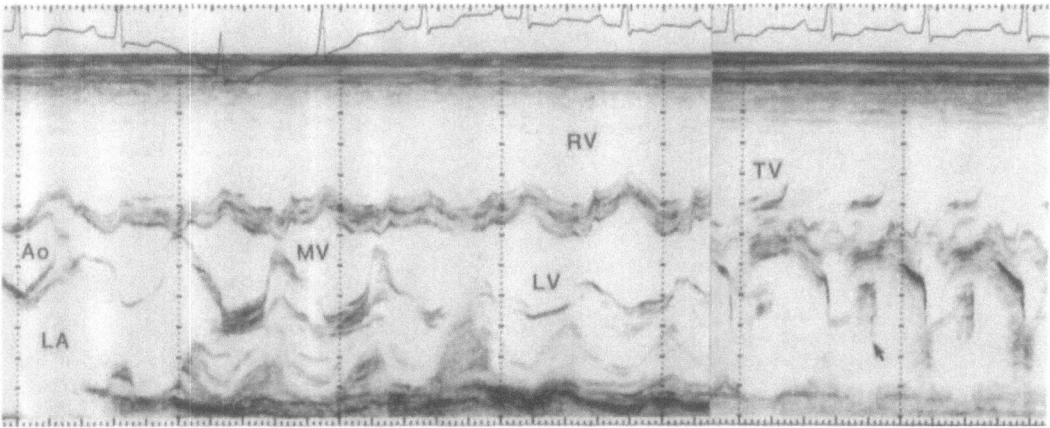

Figure 3.63. M-mode scan illustrating abnormal echoes during systole on the mitral valve due to vegetation. The panel on the right shows the M-mode tracing recorded from a parasternal four-chamber view (see Figure 3.62) which more clearly demonstrates the abnormal echoes due to vegetation (arrow).

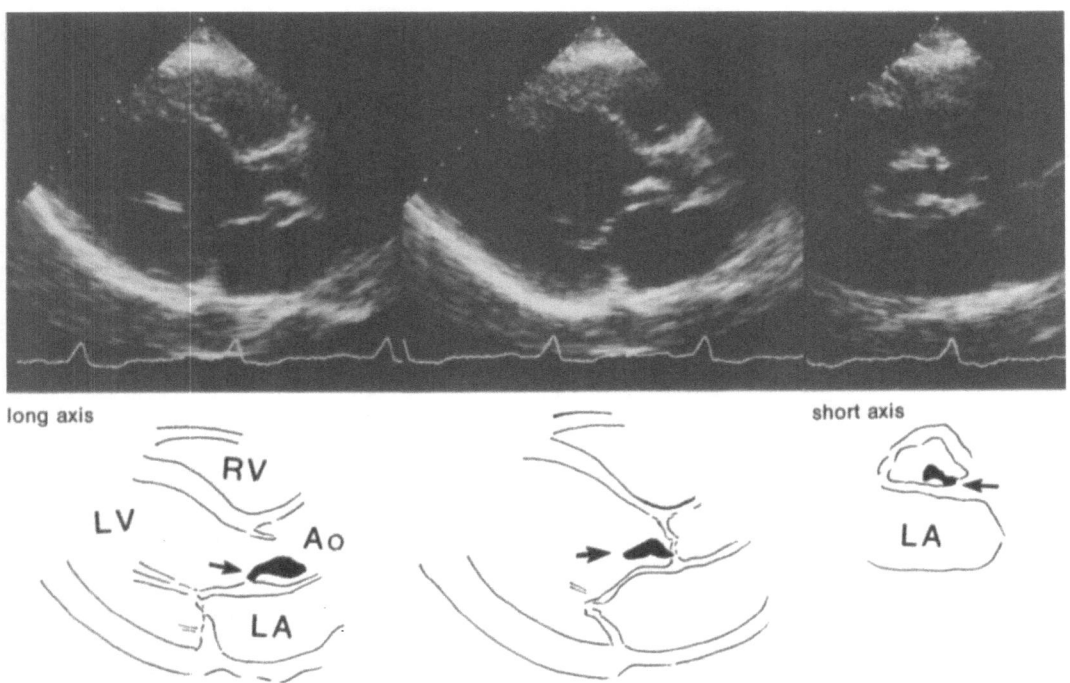

Figure 3.64. Parasternal long and short axis view demonstrating a mobile vegetation (arrow) on the aortic valve.

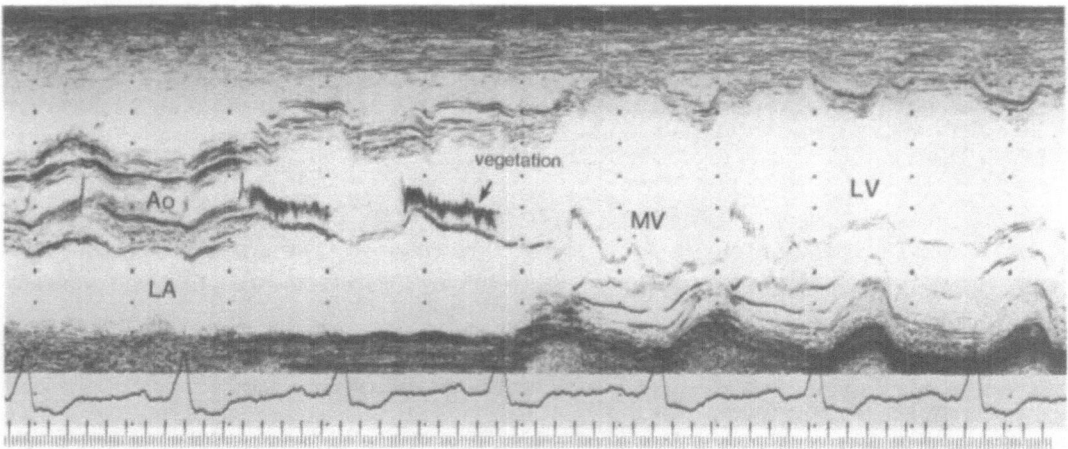

Figure 3.65.   M-mode scan showing 'shaggy' echoes (arrow) during diastole in the left ventricular outflow tract. Mitral valve fluttering and severe LV dilatation secondary to aortic regurgitation can also be seen.

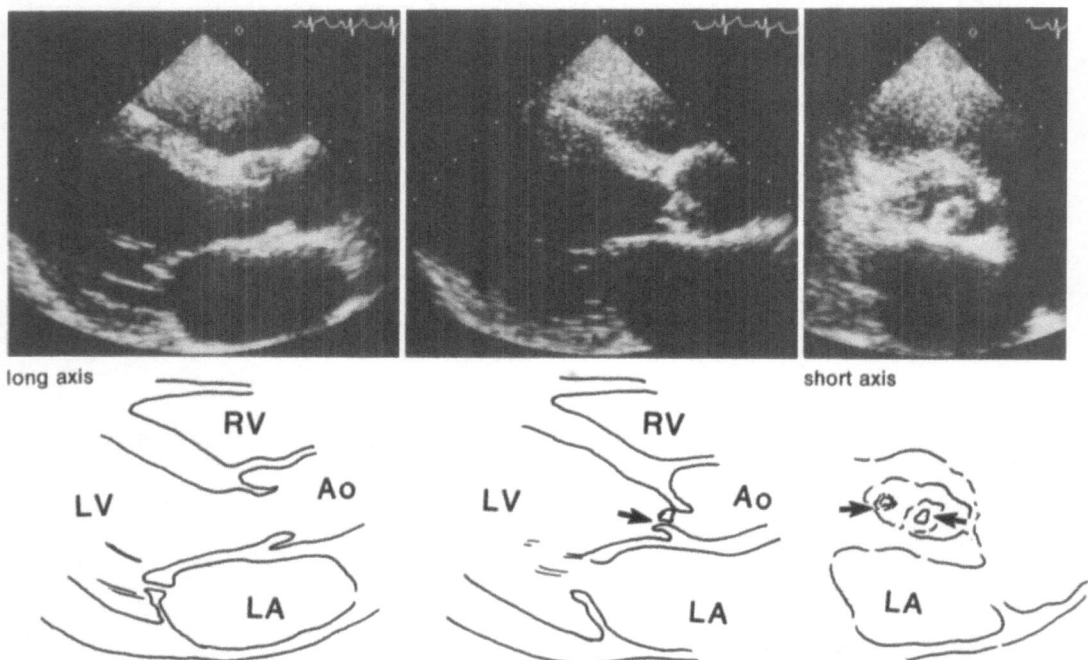

Figure 3.66.   Parasternal long and short axis view of a patient with infective endocarditis and aortic valve perforation (arrow). In this patient, a regurgitant flow signal was also demonstrated by color flow mapping (see Figure 11.20).

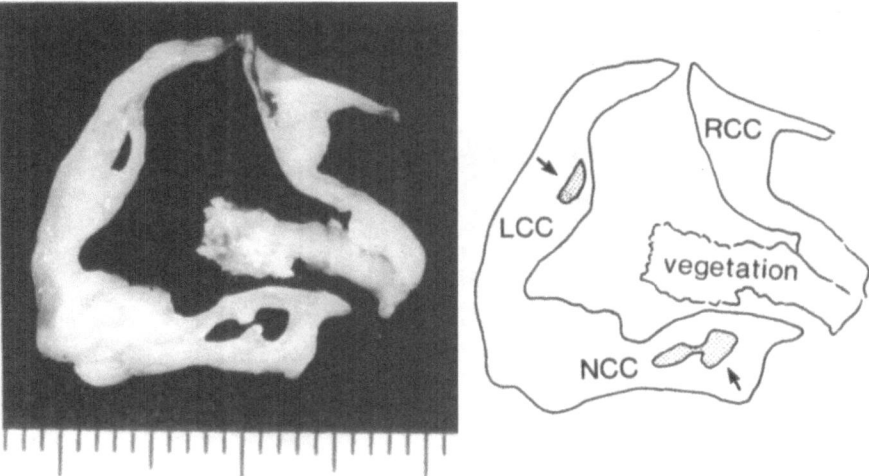

Figure 3.67.   Aortic valve specimen of the same patient as Figure 3.66. The aortic valve perforations are indicated by arrows.

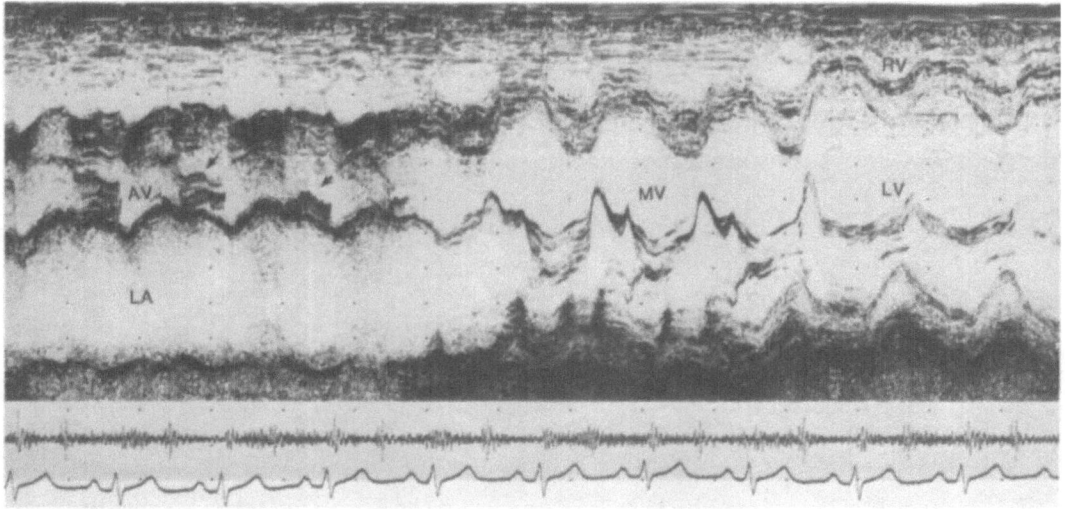

Figure 3.68.   M-mode scan of a patient with infective endocarditis and aortic valve perforation showing abnormal aortic valve echoes during diastole (arrow).

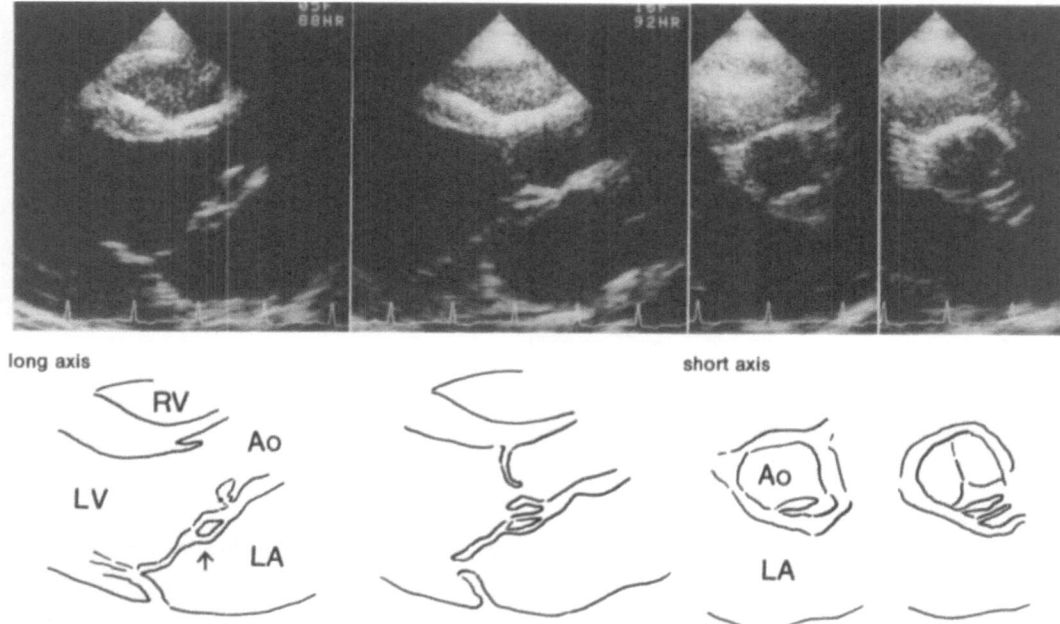

Figure 3.69.   Parasternal long and short axis view of a patient with infective endocarditis and abscess formation in the aortic annulus (arrow) (see Figure 11.21).

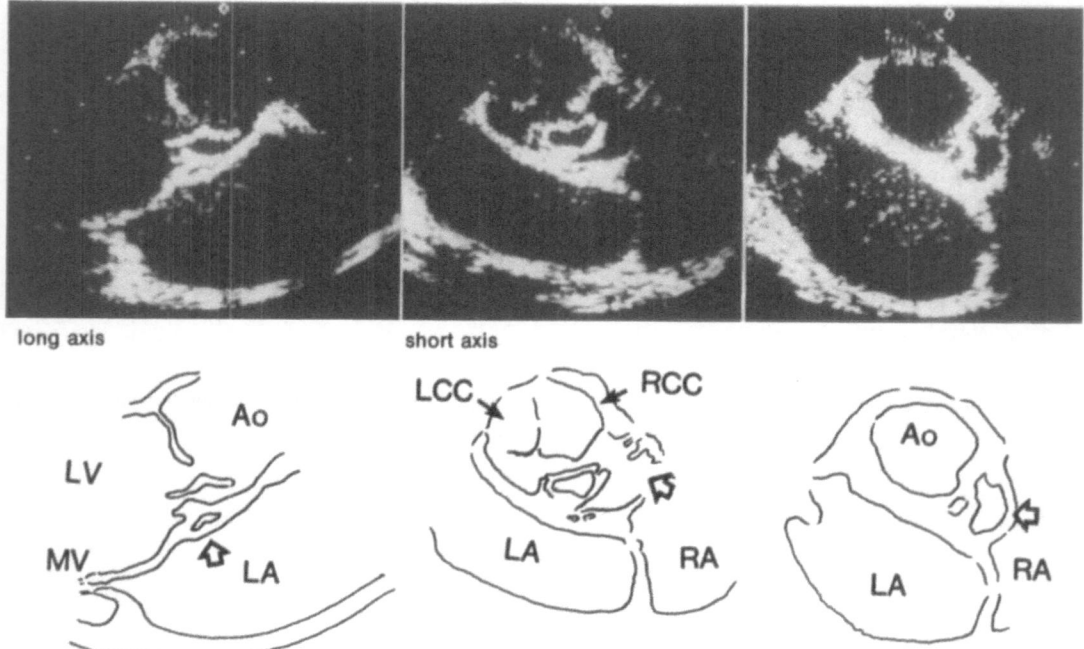

Figure 3.70.   Trans-operative long and short axis view from the same patient as in Figure 3.69 illustrating the abscess formation more clearly in the aortic annulus (arrow) (see Figure 11.22).

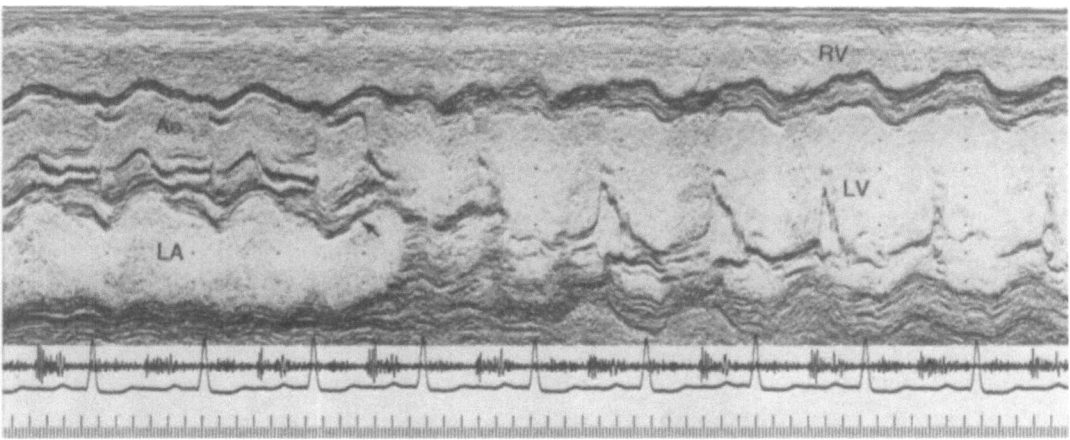

Figure 3.71. M-mode scan of the same patient as in Figure 3.69 demonstrating the double echoes (arrow) on the posterior aortic wall due to abscess formation.

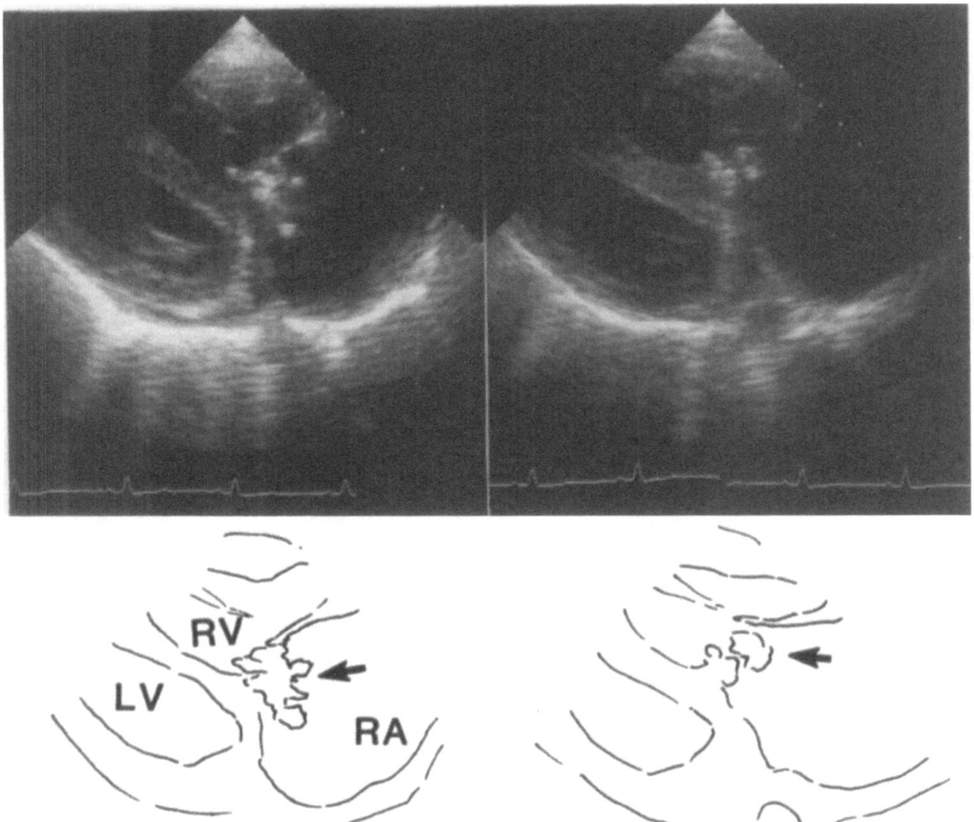

Figure 3.72. Parasternal right ventricular inflow view showing a large vegetation (arrow) attached to the atrial side of the tricuspid septal leaflet in a patient with infective endocarditis and a VSD.

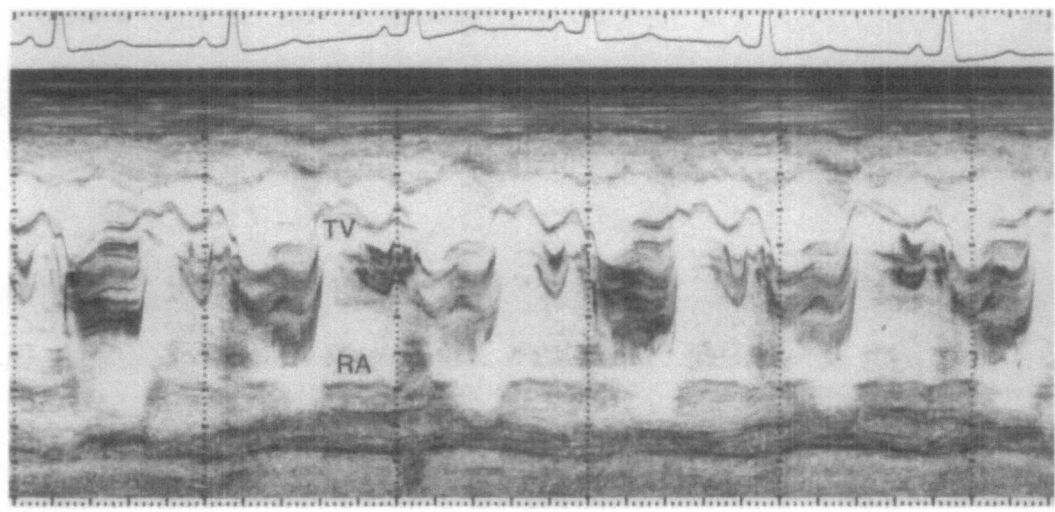

Figure 3.73. M-mode echocardiogram of tricuspid valve demonstrating 'shaggy' echoes in a patient with infective endocarditis and a VSD.

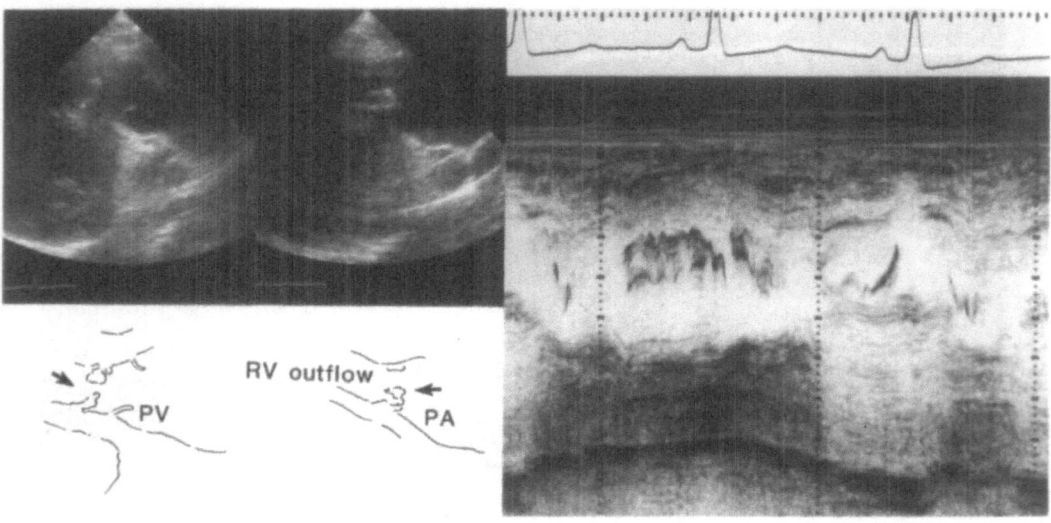

Figure 3.74. Parasternal right ventricular outflow view and M-mode echocardiogram of a patient with a VSD and a vegetation in the pulmonary subvalvular region of the right ventricular outflow tract (arrow). M-mode clearly demonstrates the 'shaggy' echoes due to vegetation.

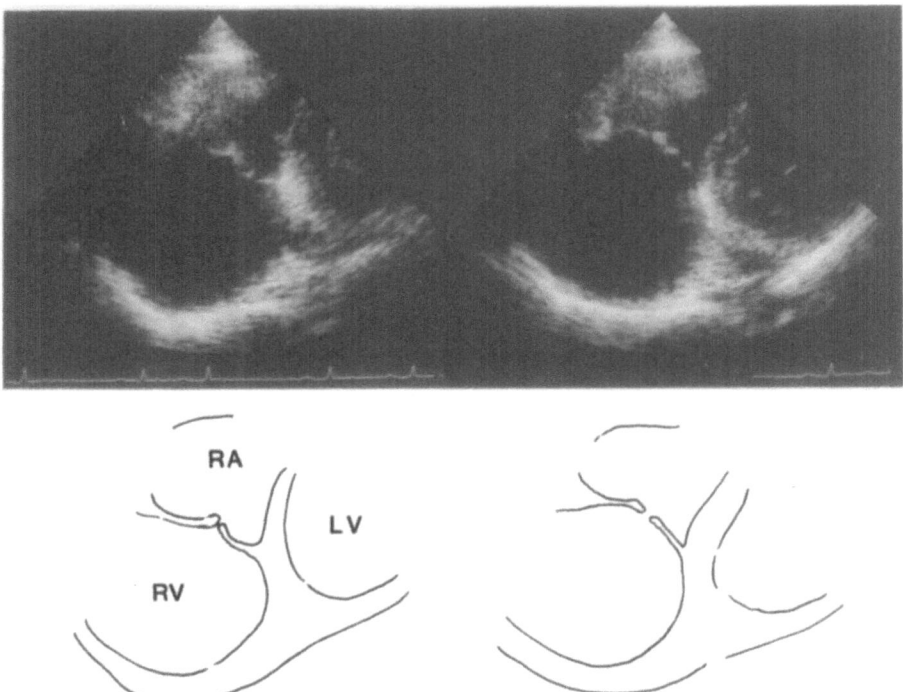

Figure 3.75. Parasternal right ventricular inflow view of a patient with rheumatic tricuspid stenosis. Tricuspid valve doming with increased echo intensity and right atrial (RA) dilatation are evident.

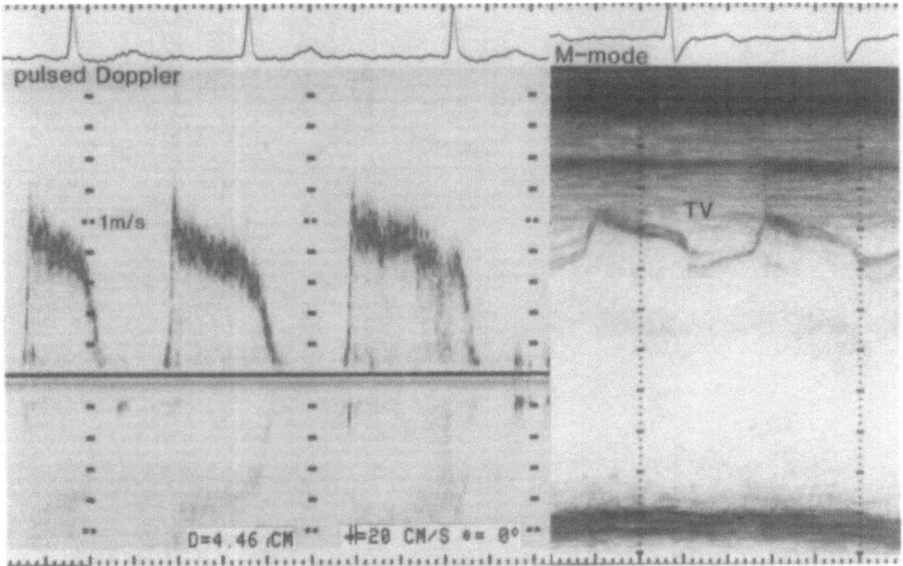

Figure 3.76. Pulsed Doppler and M-mode echocardiogram of a patient with mitral and tricuspid stenosis. The pulsed Doppler echocardiogram demonstrates an increased peak velocity and a prolonged pressure half-time. M-mode shows a limited excursion and decreased E–F slope of the tricuspid valve with increased echo intensity.

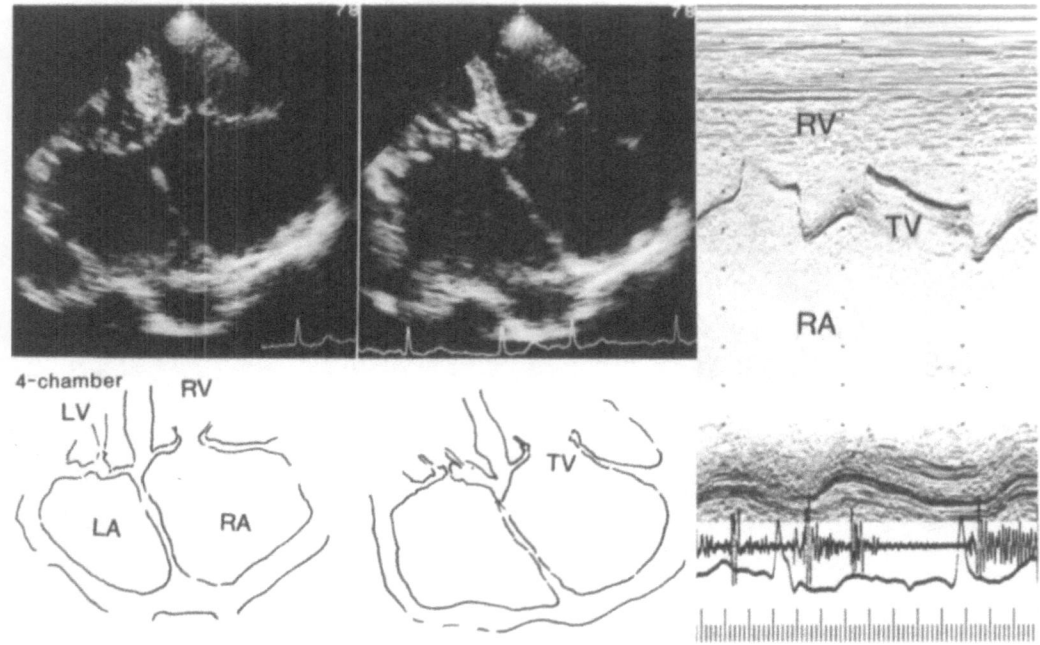

Figure 3.77. Apical four-chamber view and M-mode echocardiogram of a patient with mitral stenosis and tricuspid regurgitation. Two-dimensional echocardiogram illustrates the incomplete closure of tricuspid valve with normal opening. In M-mode the tricuspid valve motion is very similar to those with tricuspid stenosis (see Figure 3.76).

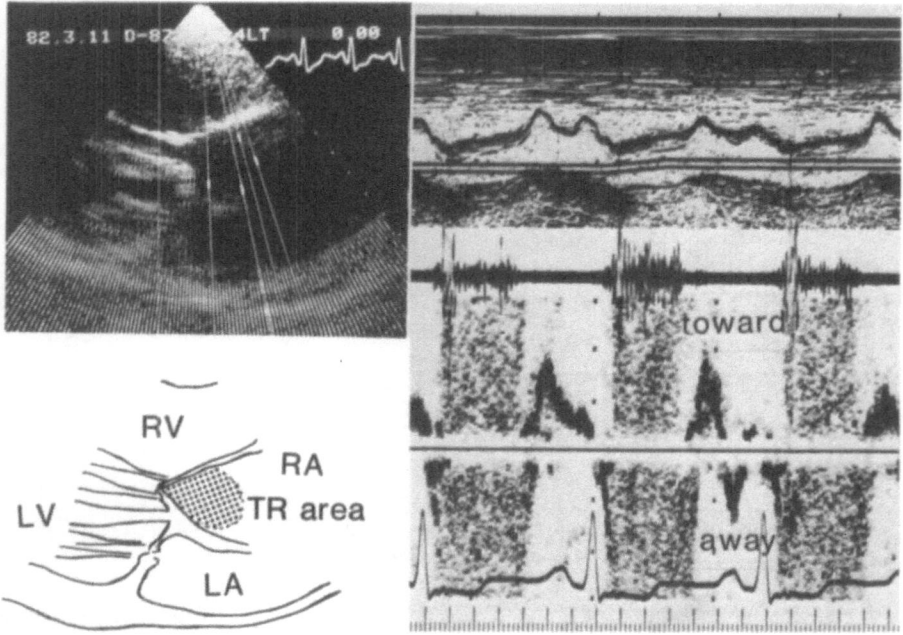

Figure 3.78. Pulsed Doppler echocardiogram of a patient with tricuspid regurgitation. The left panel shows the flow mapping of tricuspid regurgitant flow (TR area). The right panel shows the systolic turbulent flow in the right atrium.

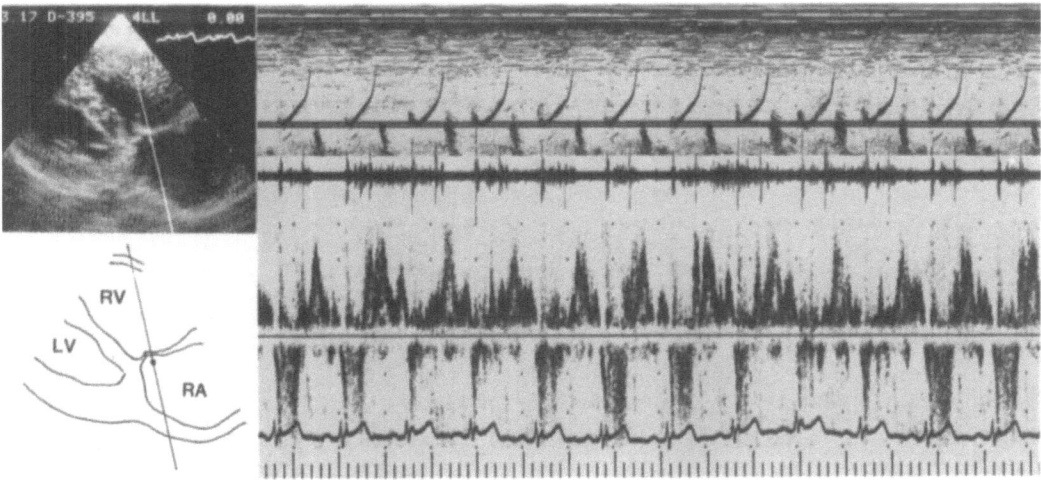

Figure 3.79. Pulsed Doppler echocardiogram illustrating the Doppler changes of tricuspid regurgitant signal with respiratory cycle.

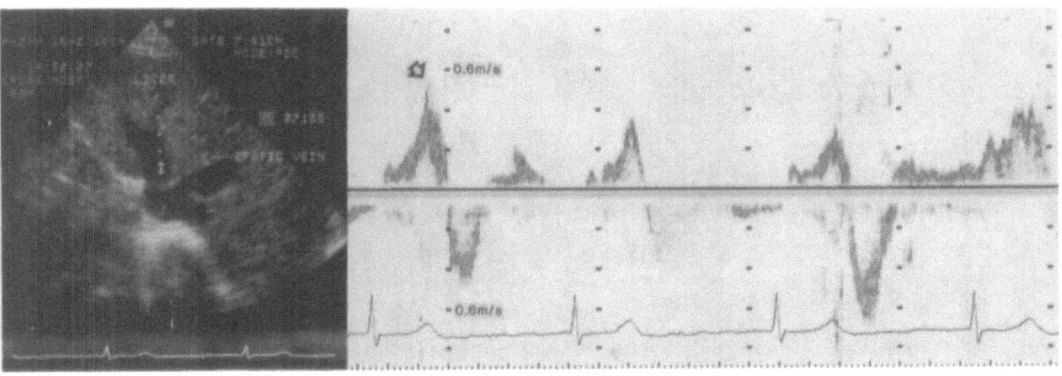

Figure 3.80. Pulsed Doppler echocardiogram of hepatic vein flow in severe tricuspid regurgitation. Systolic flow reversal is observed (arrow) and diastolic flow is accentuated.

9. Tricuspid valve stenosis

Tricuspid stenosis (TS) is a rare acquired valvular heart disease that usually is accompanied with other rheumatic valvular alterations, especially mitral stenosis. A two-dimensional echocardiogram can demonstrate stenosis of the tricuspid valve as a doming formation with increased echo intensity (Figure 3.75). Associated with this, right atrial dilatation with normal or relatively small right ventricle can occur, which reflects the stenotic condition. In M-mode, a decreased amplitude and E–F slope of the tricuspid valve with increased echo intensity are common, but the same findings are also observed in pure tricuspid regurgitation. Doppler echocardiography can provide information about stenotic conditions, such as an increased peak velocity and prolonged pressure half-time (Figure 3.76). In this entity, tricuspid regurgitation is frequently observed as well.

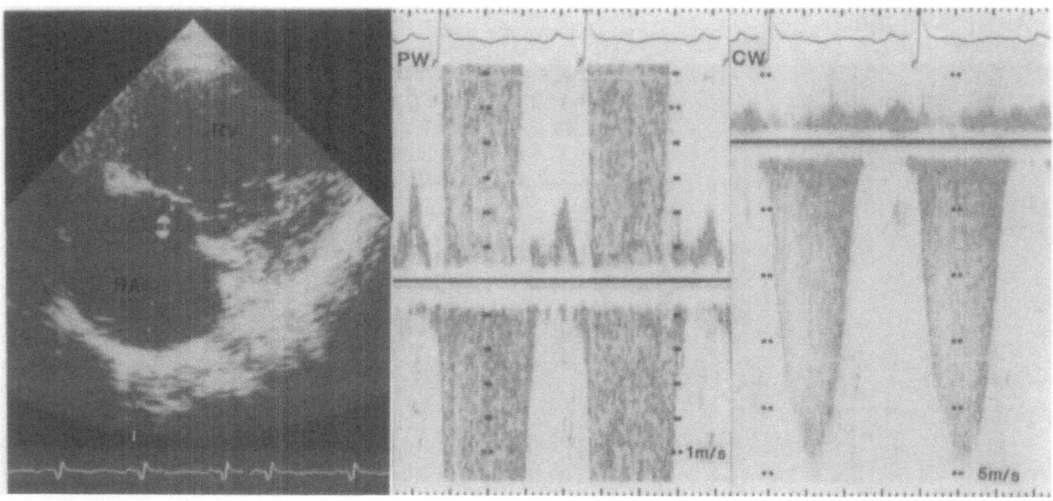

Figure 3.81. Pulsed and CW Doppler echocardiogram of a patient with tricuspid regurgitation. Pulsed wave Doppler (PW) shows the systolic turbulence of tricuspid regurgitation while continuous wave Doppler (CW) demonstrates the peak velocity (about 5 m/sec).

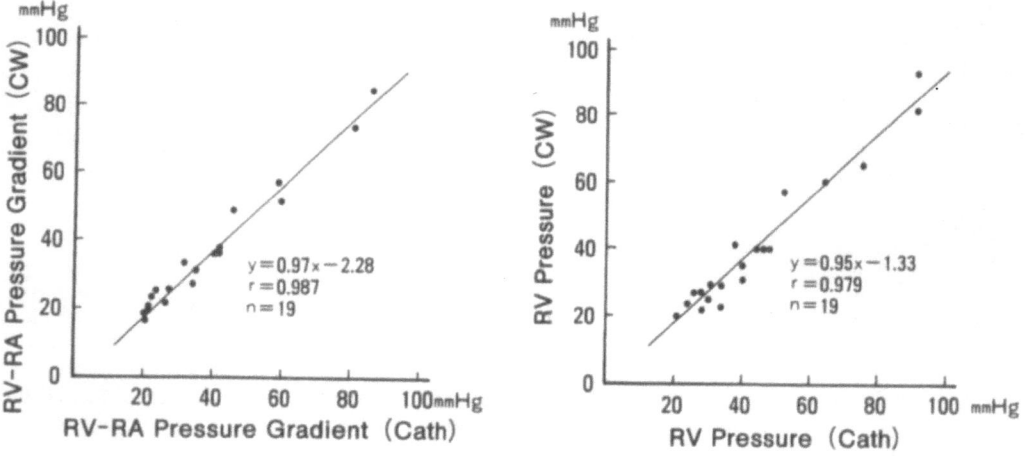

Figure 3.82. Correlation between CW Doppler and cardiac catheterization in patients with tricuspid regurgitation. In the left panel, a very good correlation ($r = 0.987$) of right ventricular/atrial pressure gradient obtained by catheterization and the Doppler technique is demonstrated. The right panel also shows a very good correlation ($r = 0.979$) of right ventricular pressure. We assume a right atrial pressure of 5 mm Hg in patients with normal respiratory changes in the size of inferior vena cava and 10 mm Hg in patients without respiratory changes in the inferior vena cava.

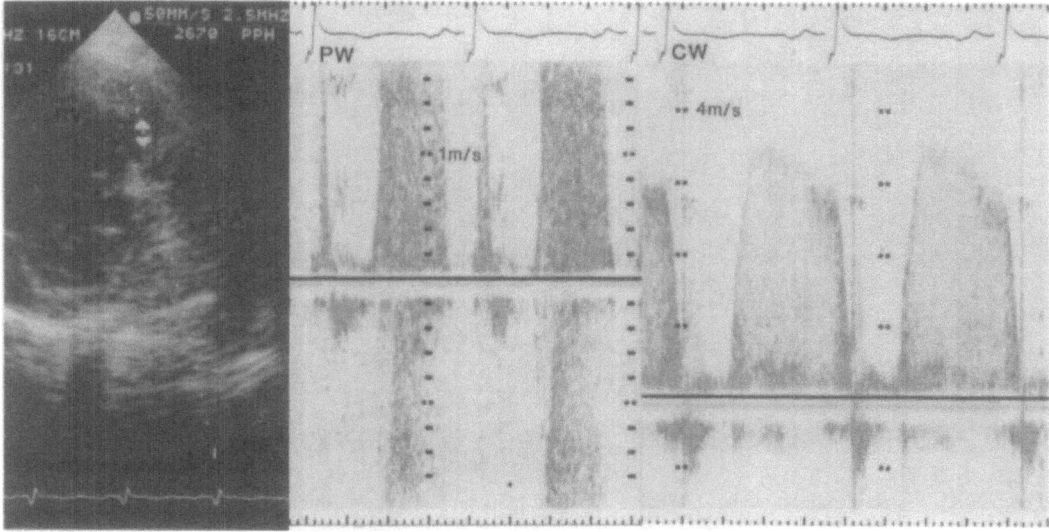

Figure 3.83. Pulsed and CW Doppler echocardiogram of a patient with pulmonary hypertension and pulmonary regurgitation. One can see the increased regurgitant flow velocity in early diastole (about 3.6 m/sec) and end-diastole (about 3 m/sec) indicating that the diastolic pulmonary artery pressure is elevated.

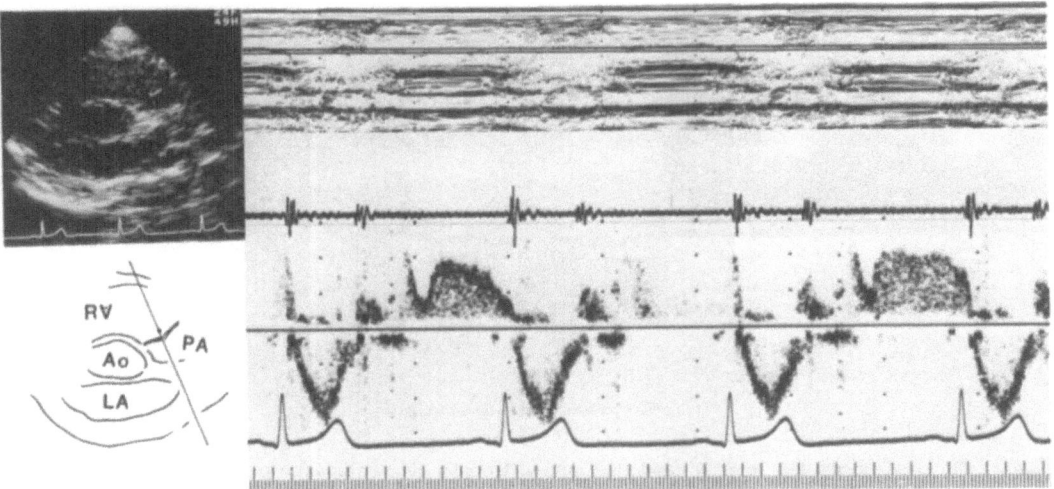

Figure 3.84. Pulsed Doppler echocardiogram of a patient with idiopathic pulmonary regurgitation. The sample volume is located in the right ventricular outflow tract, a normal ejection flow and a turbulent diastolic flow with low peak velocity mainly in late diastole can be observed.

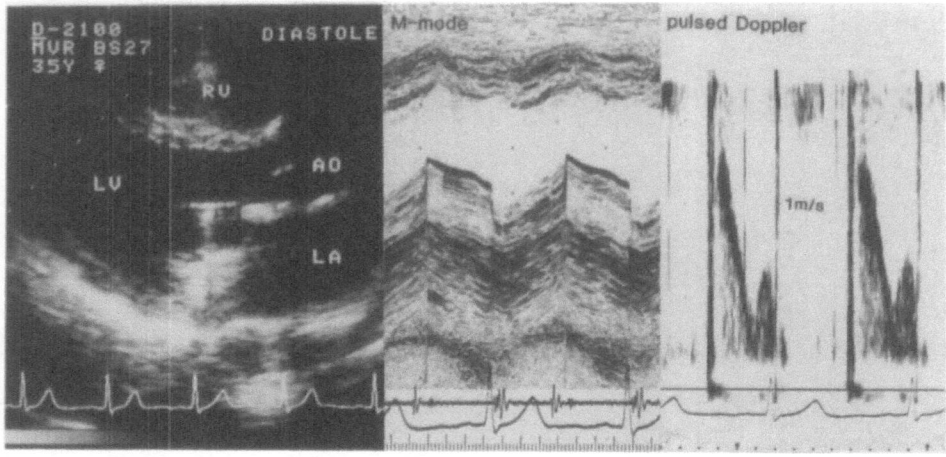

Figure 3.85. Parasternal long axis, M-mode and pulsed Doppler echocardiograms of a patient with a Bjork-Shiley valve in the mitral position with normal function. The two-dimensional echocardiogram shows the opening of the prosthetic valve and the M-mode illustrates the prominent acoustic shadow behind the prosthetic valve during diastole. The pulsed Doppler echocardiogram demonstrates a slightly increased peak velocity of the transprosthetic valve flow with a normal pressure half-time. This suggests that a mild pressure gradient across the prosthetic valve exists, which is often noted in normally functioning valve prosthesis.

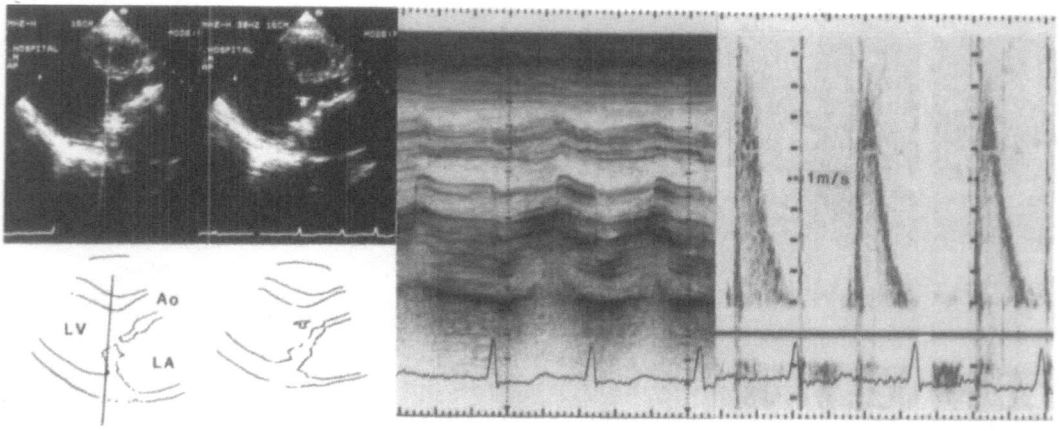

Figure 3.86. Parasternal long axis, M-mode and pulsed Doppler echocardiogram of a patient with a St. Jude Medical valve in mitral position with normal function. The two-dimensional echocardiogram shows the prominent acoustic shadow during systole and the opening of prosthetic valve. The M-mode illustrates the prominent acoustic shadow behind the prosthetic valve during diastole. The pulsed Doppler echocardiogram illustrates a slightly increased peak velocity of transprosthetic valve flow with a normal pressure half-time, which suggests a mild pressure gradient in the prosthetic valve.

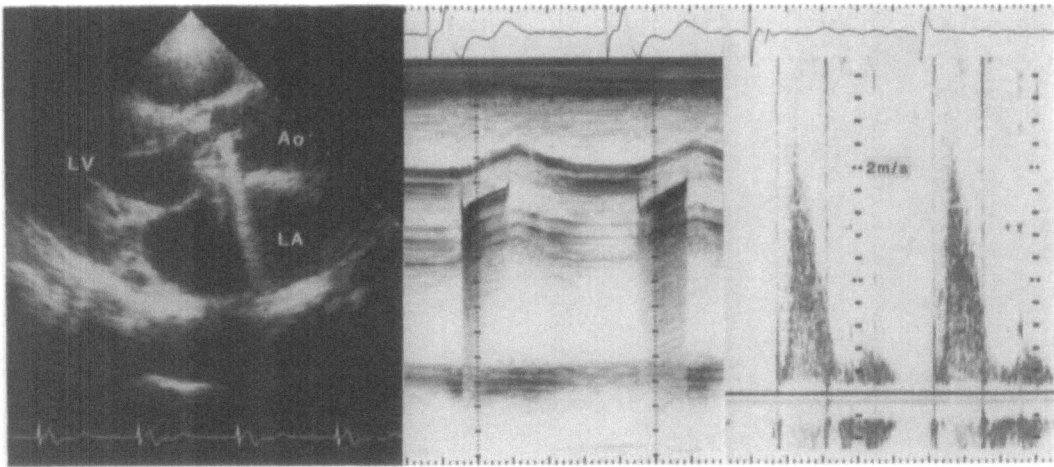

Figure 3.87. Parasternal long axis, M-mode and CW Doppler echocardiogram from a patient with a Bjork-Shiley valve in the aortic position with a normal function. Two-dimensional and M-mode echocardiograms show the opening of prosthetic valve as the prominent acoustic shadow behind the prosthetic valve during systole. The CW Doppler echocardiogram recorded from the suprasternal approach illustrates an increased peak velocity of transprosthetic valve flow, which suggests a mild pressure gradient in the prosthetic valve.

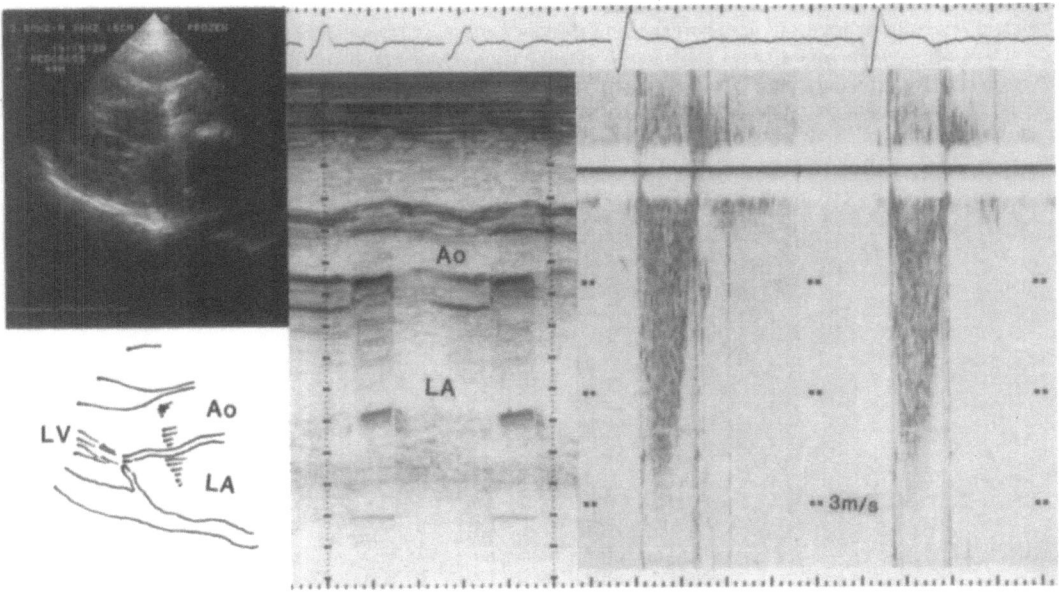

Figure 3.88. Parasternal long axis, M-mode and CW Doppler echocardiogram of a patient with a St. Jude Medical valve in the aortic position with a normal function. The two-dimensional echocardiogram shows the opening of two prosthetic leaflet but the M-mode can not reveal this. The CW Doppler echocardiogram recorded from the apical approach illustrates increased peak velocity of the transprosthetic valve flow, which suggests a mild pressure gradient in the prosthetic valve.

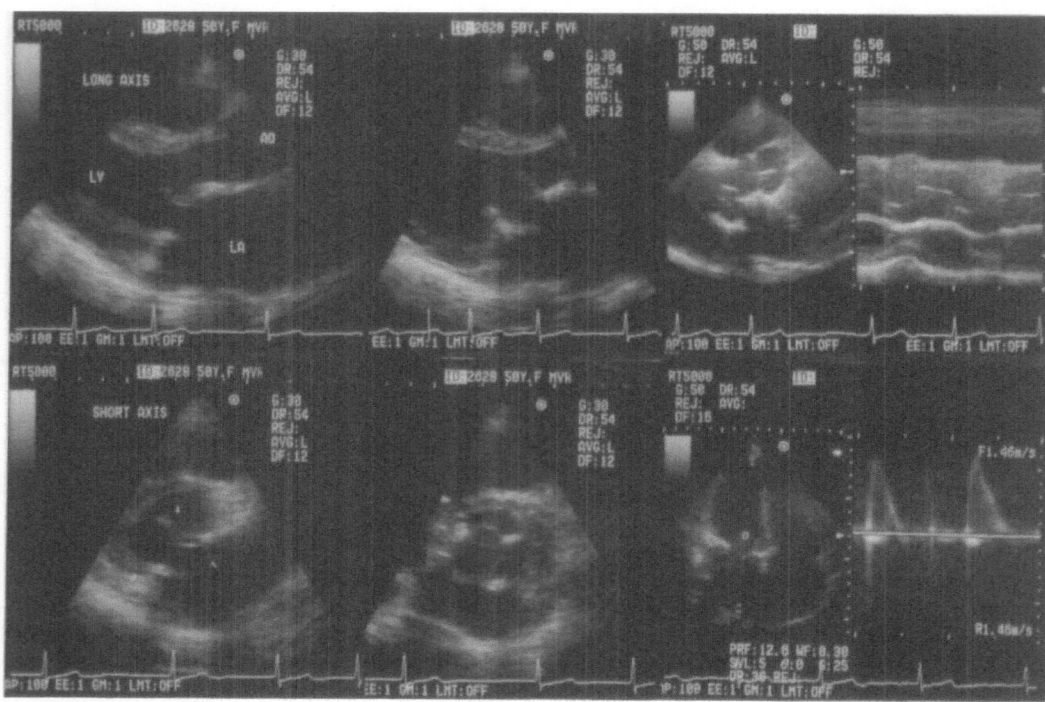

Figure 3.89. Parasternal long and short axis view, M-mode and pulsed Doppler echocardiogram from a patient with a bio-prosthetic (Ionesque-Shiley) valve in the mitral position. One can identify the movement of three leaflets (arrow) in the two-dimensional short axis view. The M-mode echocardiogram shows the movement of leaflets. Pulsed Doppler demonstrates a slightly increased peak velocity of the transprosthetic valve flow with a normal pressure half-time.

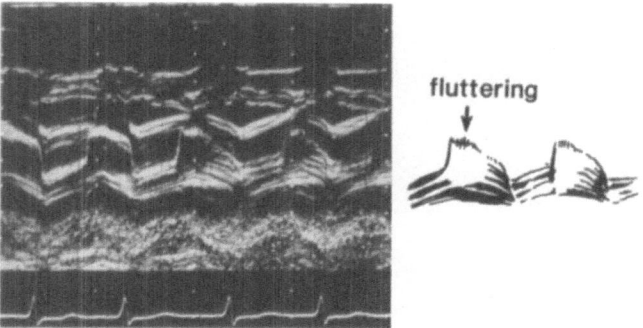

Figure 3.90. M-mode echocardiogram illustrating diastolic fluttering of a bioprosthetic valve (Hancock) in the mitral position due to valve 'tear'.

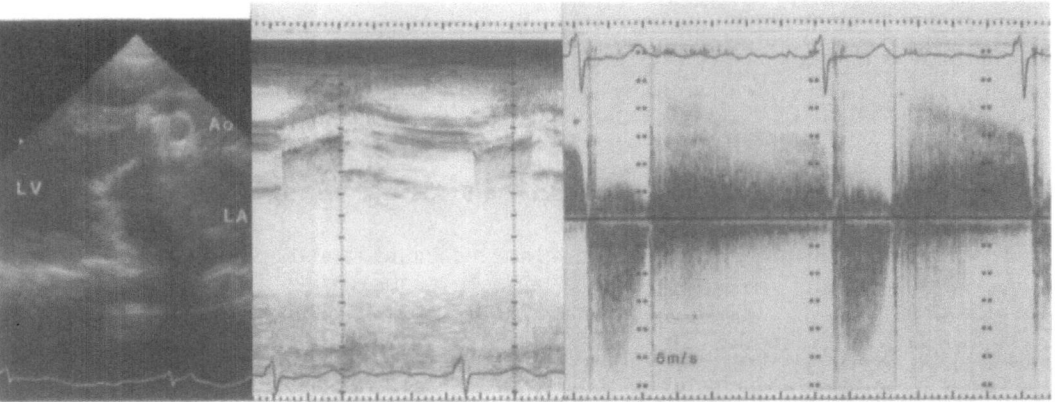

Figure 3.91. Parasternal long axis, M-mode and CW Doppler echocardiogram from a patient with a malfunctioning Starr-Edwards ball prosthetic valve in the aortic position. The two-dimensional echocardiogram shows the leading edge of the cage, but does not illustrate malfunctioning. CW Doppler demonstrates the stenotic and regurgitant flow due to malfunctioning.

10. Tricuspid valve regurgitation

Tricuspid regurgitation (TR) is usually a functional alteration that mainly occurs concomitantly with mitral valvular disease but, in rare cases, organic changes can be demonstrated. Using two-dimensional echocardiography, an incomplete closure of tricuspid leaflets with right atrial and ventricular dilatation are observed (Figure 3.77). In M-mode, the tricuspid valve motion in the case of tricuspid regurgitation is usually very similar to that in tricuspid stenosis, because the enlarged right ventricle restricts the valve's motion. Until recently, contrast echocardiography has been used to evaluate the presence and severity of tricuspid regurgitation (see Figure 2.8). Pulsed Doppler echocardiography and color flow mapping more readily demonstrate the presence and direction of tricuspid regurgitant flow and can also evaluate its severity (Figure 3.78). The Doppler signal of tricuspid regurgitation can be influenced by respiratory cycles with augmentation during the inspiratory phase (Figure 3.79). Flow patterns in the hepatic veins and the vena cava also are affected by the presence of moderate to severe tricuspid regurgitation. Systolic flow reversal and the diastolic antegrade accentuated flow can be observed (Figure 3.80). Using CW Doppler echocardiography, we can obtain the peak velocity of the tricuspid regurgitant flow (Figure 3.81) and assess the systolic pressure gradient between right ventricle and right atrium by a simplified Bernoulli equation. By adding the estimated right atrial pressure to the calculated gradient, the right ventricular systolic pressure can be estimated noninvasively (Figure 3.82).

11. Pulmonary valve regurgitation

Pulmonary regurgitation (PR) is usually secondary to pulmonary hypertension, infective endocarditis or post-surgical valvotomy, but sometimes it can be idiopathic. Pulsed Doppler echocardiography and color flow mapping readily identify the presence of pulmonary regurgitation. In the case of pulmonary hypertension, the peak velocity of the regurgitant jet is very high, which suggest elevated pulmonary diastolic pressure (Figure 3.83). In contrast, patients with normal pulmonary artery pressure, the regurgitant jet usually recorded in mid- to end-diastole with low velocity and respiratory changes (Figure 3.84).

12. Prosthetic valve

There are primarily two types of prosthetic valves: mechanical and bioprosthesis. Mechanical valves consisted of three types; the ball-cage variety (the Starr-Edwards type), the disc-cage valve and the tilting disc valve. The Bjork-Shiley valve is the most common tilting disc valve. The St. Jude Medical valve has two semicircular discs. Until recently, echocardiography has been used to evaluate valve function, although there are many technical problems in detecting prosthetic valve motion. The most frequent limitation is due to prominent acoustic shadowing, especially in mechanical prostheses (Figures 3.85, 86, 87, 88). In bioprosthetic valves one can see the movements of three leaflets by using two-dimensional echocardiography (Figure 3.89). In patients with bioprosthesis, the fluttering of the valve may indicate valve dysfunction (Figure 3.90). Doppler echocardiography can be used to evaluate the normal function of the prosthetic valve. Since the flow is not through the center of the Bjork-Shiley valve, the absolute velocities cannot be estimated. The St. Jude valve and bioprosthetic valve are probably more suitable for evaluating flow patterns since the flow is through the center of the valve. Because the prosthetic valve is mildly stenotic, the Doppler recording usually shows the mildly increased peak velocity with normal pressure half-time in the mitral position (Figures 3.85, 86, 89) and moderately increased peak velocity in the aortic position (Figures 3.87, 88) depending on the pressure gradient. Its dysfunction, such as stenotic conditions and valvular or paravalvular regurgitation, can also be detected by the Doppler technique (Figure 3.91 and also Figures 11.12, 13). These studies are performed as in the diseased native valves.

CHAPTER 4

Congenital heart disease

1. Atrial septal defect

Atrial septal defects (ASD) are one of the most frequent congenital heart diseases in the adult patient. Atrial septal defects are classified according to site of the defect. The three types are: (1) ostium secundum, (2) ostium primum and (3) sinus venosus. In clinical practice the secundum defect is the most common type of atrial septal defect which is located in the site of foramen ovale. Two-dimensional echocardiography can directly demonstrate this defect in the middle portion of the atrial septum (Figure 4.1). However, in normals, a dropout of atrial septal echo is sometimes observed. Therefore, this finding should not be used as a definitive diagnostic criterion. In addition, the right ventricular and pulmonary artery enlargement with abnormal IVS motion due to right ventricular volume overload are present (Figure 4.2). Using M-mode echocardiography, the IVS motion is usually paradoxical or exhibits flattening (Figure 4.3), but in rare cases normal IVS motion can also occur (Figures 4.5). In primum type atrial septal defect, the defect is located in the inferior portion of atrial septum close to the atrioventricular valves (Figure 4.4), and mitral valve cleft can also occur (Figure 4.6). In sinus venosus type, the atrial defect cannot usually be identified by two-dimensional echocardiography and right ventricular volume overload may be the only finding. Mitral valve prolapse is sometimes associated with an atrial septal defect and can produce mitral regurgitation (Figure 4.7). Using pulsed Doppler and/or color flow mapping, it is possible to illustrate the left-to-right shunt across the defect from the parasternal four chamber view (Figure 4.8 and also Figure 11.28). A better angle to the flow can be usually obtained from the subcostal window which demonstrates more clearly the laminar left-to-right shunt flow (Figure 4.9). The increased flow volume in the right atrium results in augmented flow across the tricuspid and pulmonary valve, and higher than normal peak velocities are recorded. We can estimate the degree of the shunt from Qp/Qs assessment by pulsed Doppler derived left and right ventricular stroke volume (Figure 4.10).

2. Endocardial cushion defect

The endocardial cushion includes the membranous portion of IVS, the primum portion of the atrial septum and septal leaflets of mitral and tricuspid valves. In the setting of an endocardial cushion defect (ECD) these structures are frequently affected. With two-dimensional echocardiography, the primum type of atrial septal defect, one can evaluate the membranous IVS defect and also the altered atrioventricular valves (Figures 4.11, 12).

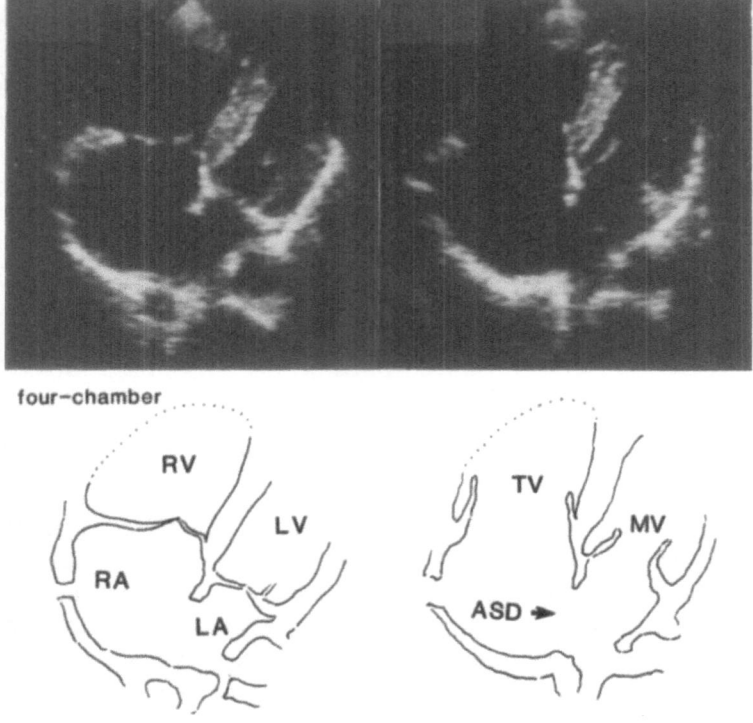

Figure 4.1.   Apical four-chamber view showing a secundum type of atrial septal defect (ASD).

3. Persistent left superior vena cava

Normally, the left superior vena cava is an embryological structure that is connected directly to the coronary sinus. Infrequently this condition may persist without clinical symptoms. The echocardiographic findings include enlargement of the coronary sinus (Figure 4.13), which is opacified by contrast injection from the left cubital vein.

4. Ventricular septal defect

The ventricular septal defect (VSD) is a frequent anomaly which is mainly divided in membranous and muscular type according to the location. Usually, the membranous type may be detected by two-dimensional echocardiography (Figures 4.14, 15). The muscular septal defect however, is relatively difficult to detect. Only a large ventricular septal defect can be demonstrated by M-mode echocardiography (Figure 4.16). Using Doppler techniques, the detection of the left-to-right ventricular shunt may generally be performed. These techniques may be implemented to evaluate the size and location of the ventricular septal defect. The flow across the defect occurs primarily during systole, and is turbulent with a high flow velocity. The peak velocity can be assessed by the CW Doppler technique (Figure 4.17). In the presence of a ventricular septal defect with pulmonary hypertension (Eisenmenger complex), the flow across the defect becomes bidirectional (Figures 4.18, 19). Ventricular

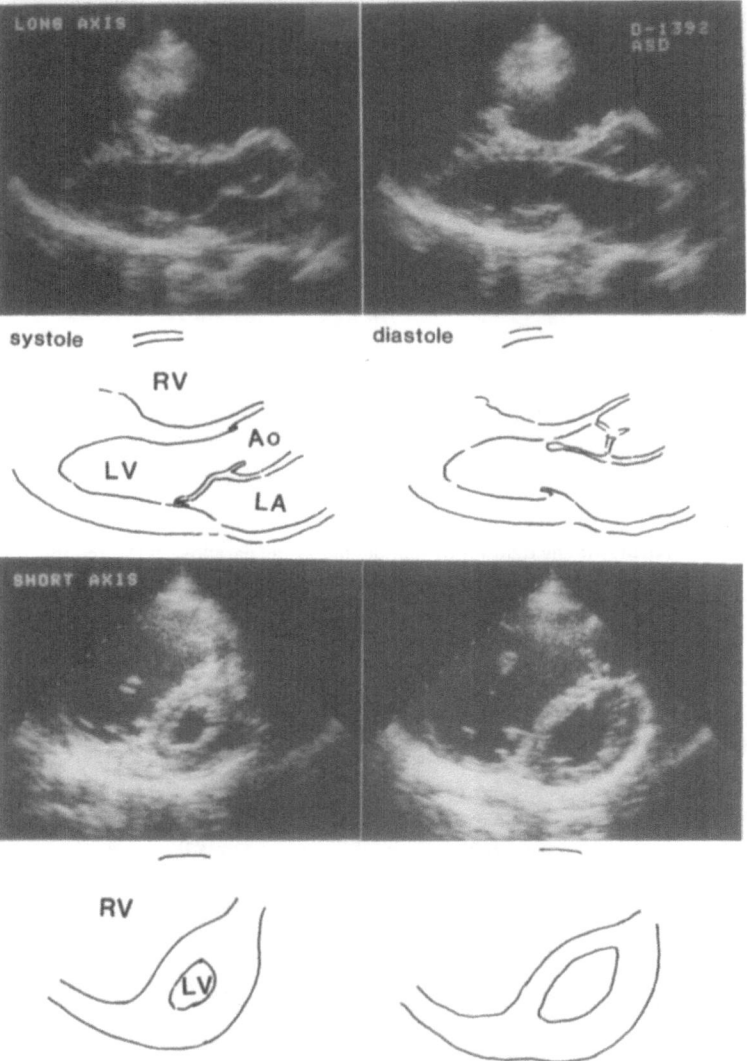

Figure 4.2. Parasternal long and short axis views from a patient with atrial septal defect. Right ventricular enlargement and flattening of IVS in the short axis view in end-diastole are clearly demonstrated.

septal defects are sometimes accompanied with a ventricular septal aneurysm, which may be related with a partial or complete closing process of the ventricular septal defect (Figure 4.20). In rare cases, a large ventricular septal aneurysm occurs and a bulging into the right ventricular outflow tract is demonstrated (Figure 4.21). The membranous type ventricular septal defect is sometimes associated with aortic valve prolapse (right coronary cusp) and aortic regurgitation (Figures 4.22, 23).

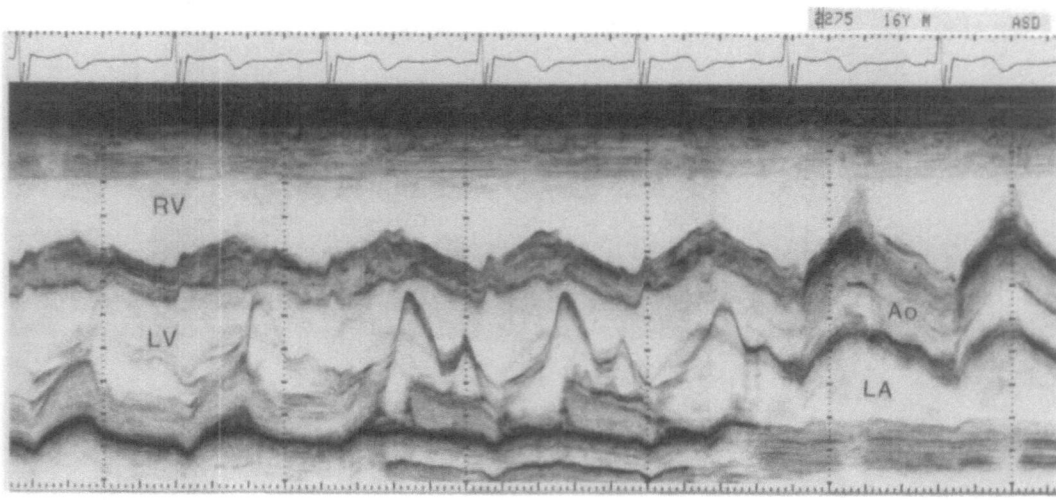

Figure 4.3.   M-mode scan illustrating right ventricular dilatation and paradoxical IVS motion in a patient with atrial septal defect.

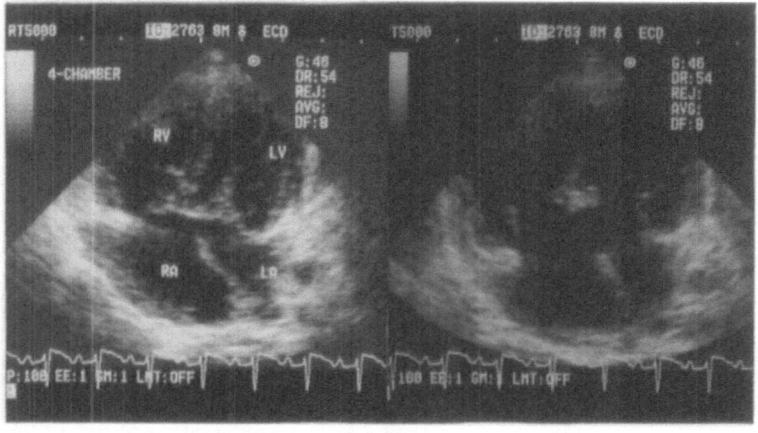

Figure 4.4.   Apical four chamber view illustrating a primum type atrial septal defect.

5. Sinus of Valsalva aneurysm

Sinus of Valsalva aneurysm is a congenital anomaly that is usually associated with a membranous type ventricular septal defect. It is sometimes secondary to thoracic trauma or infective endocarditis. The echocardiographic finding consists of an aneurysmatic protrusion of the coronary sinus into the right ventricle (Figures 4.24, 25). Pulsed Doppler and color flow mapping techniques can demonstrate the left-to-right shunt during the entire cardiac cycle in patients with rupture of a Valsalva aneurysm.

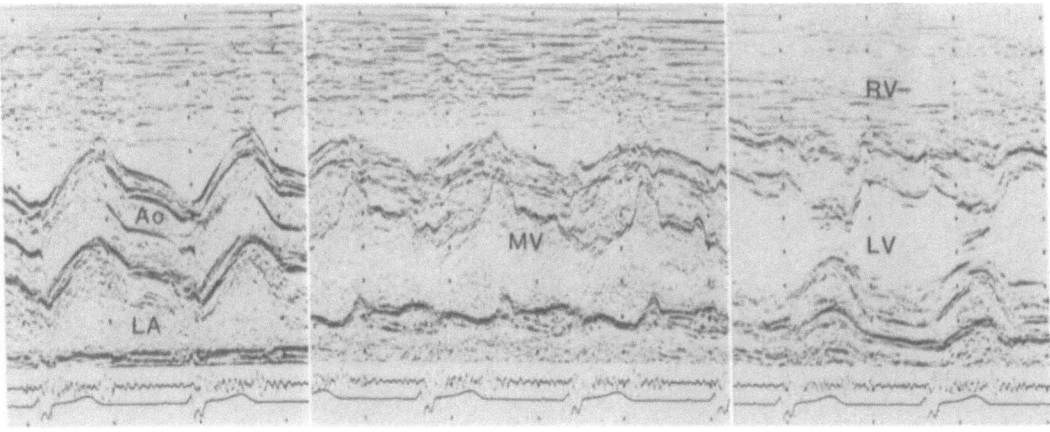

Figure 4.5. M-mode echocardiogram of a patient with primum type atrial septal defect. Right ventricular dilatation without paradoxical motion of IVS is observed.

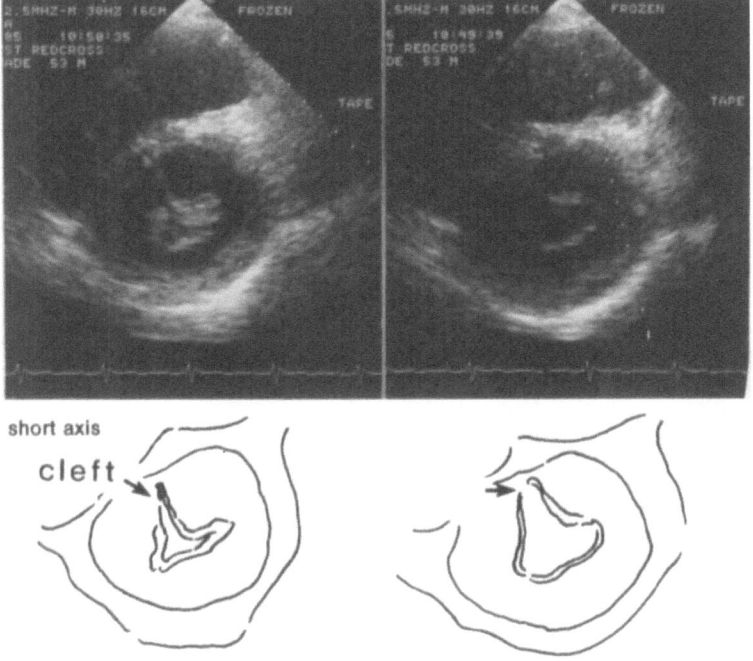

Figure 4.6. Parasternal short axis view illustrating cleft of mitral valve (arrow) in a patient with primum type atrial septal defect.

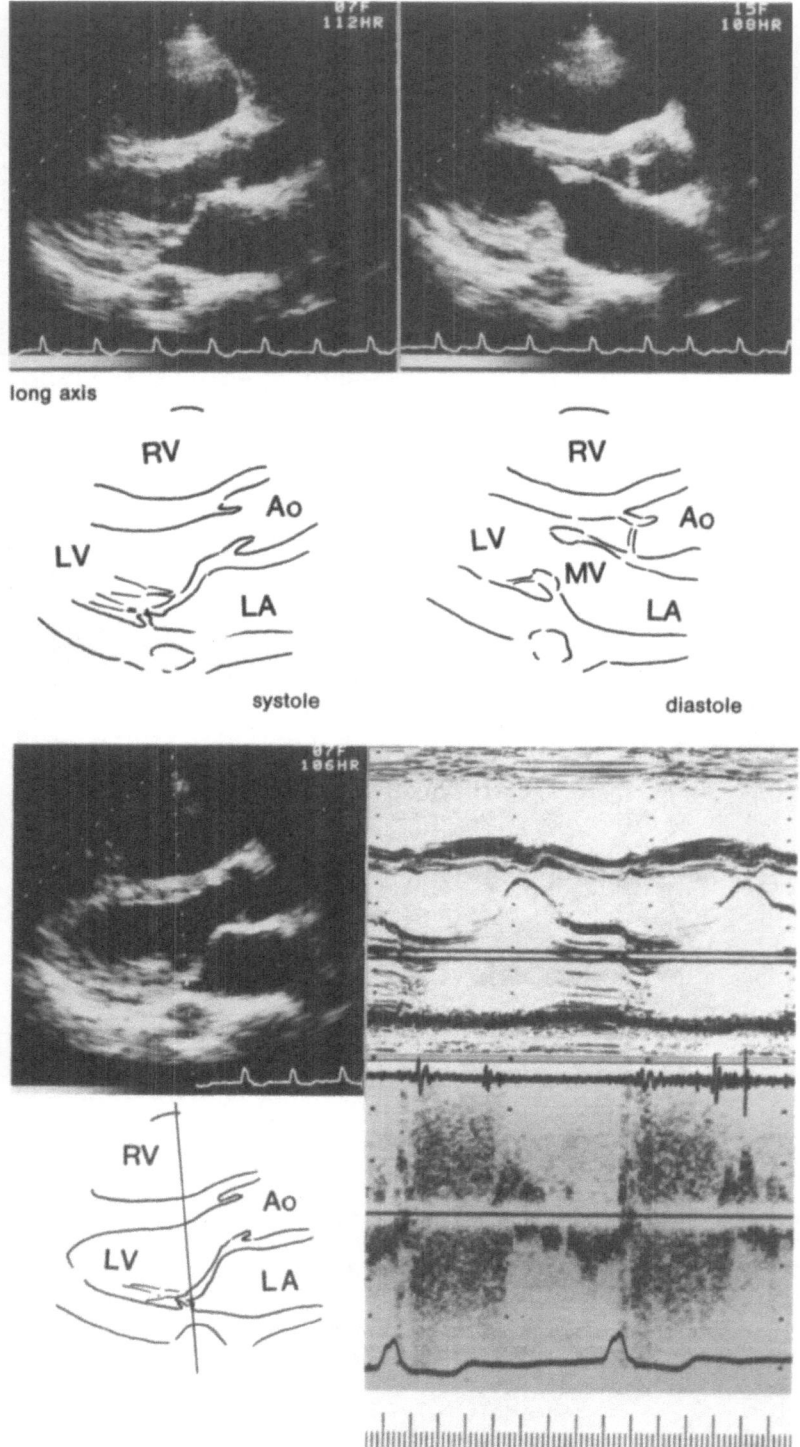

Figure 4.7.   Parasternal long axis view and pulsed Doppler echocardiogram from a patient with atrial septal defect. Anterior mitral valve prolapse and mitral regurgitation are observed.

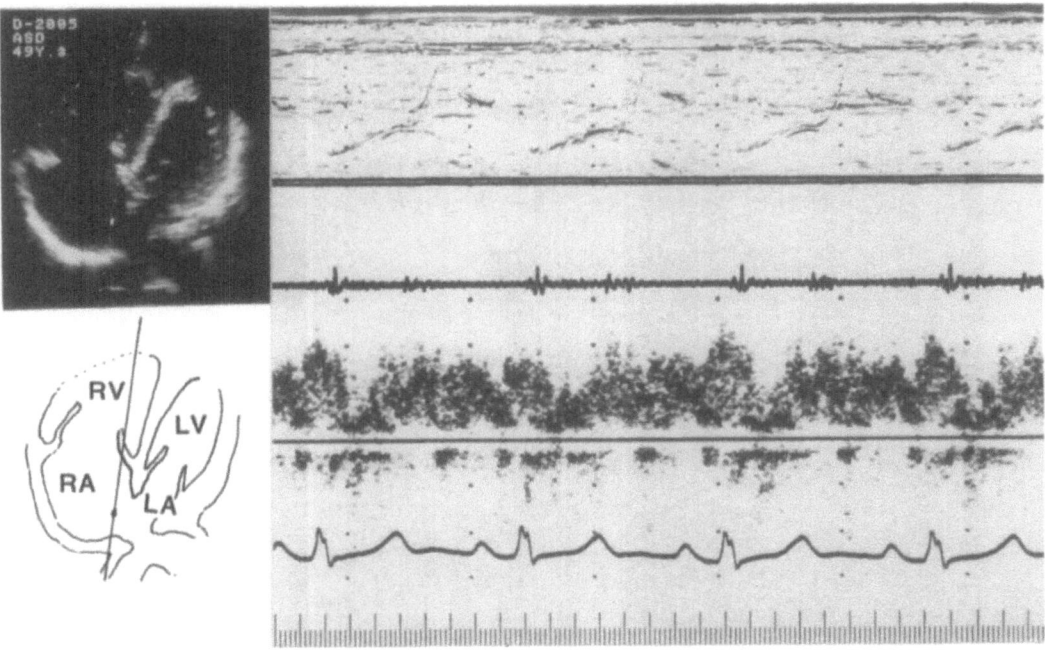

Figure 4.8.   Pulsed Doppler echocardiogram of a patient with atrial septal defect recorded from the parasternal window. The sample volume is located on the right side of the defect and flow across the defect (toward the transducer) is demonstrated during all cardiac cycles.

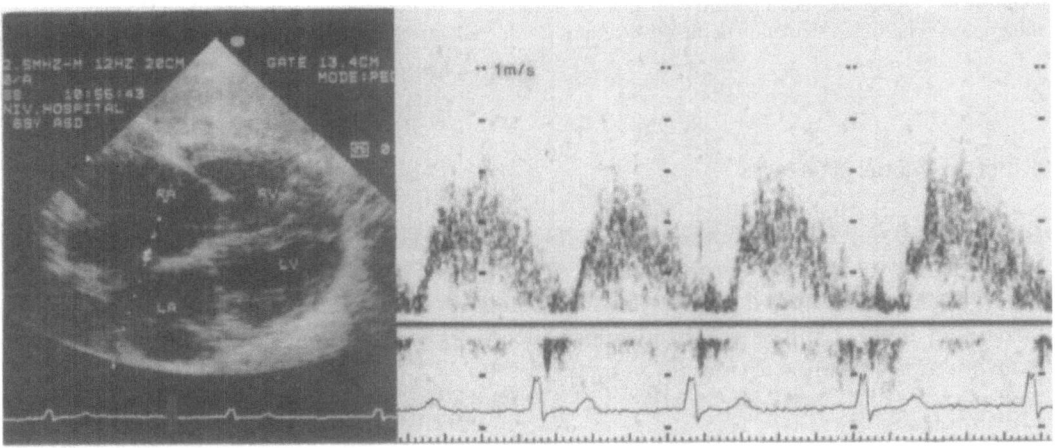

Figure 4.9.   Pulsed Doppler echocardiogram of a patient with atrial septal defect recorded from the subcostal window. The sample volume is located on the right side of the defect and laminar left-to-right shunt flow across the defect is demonstrated.

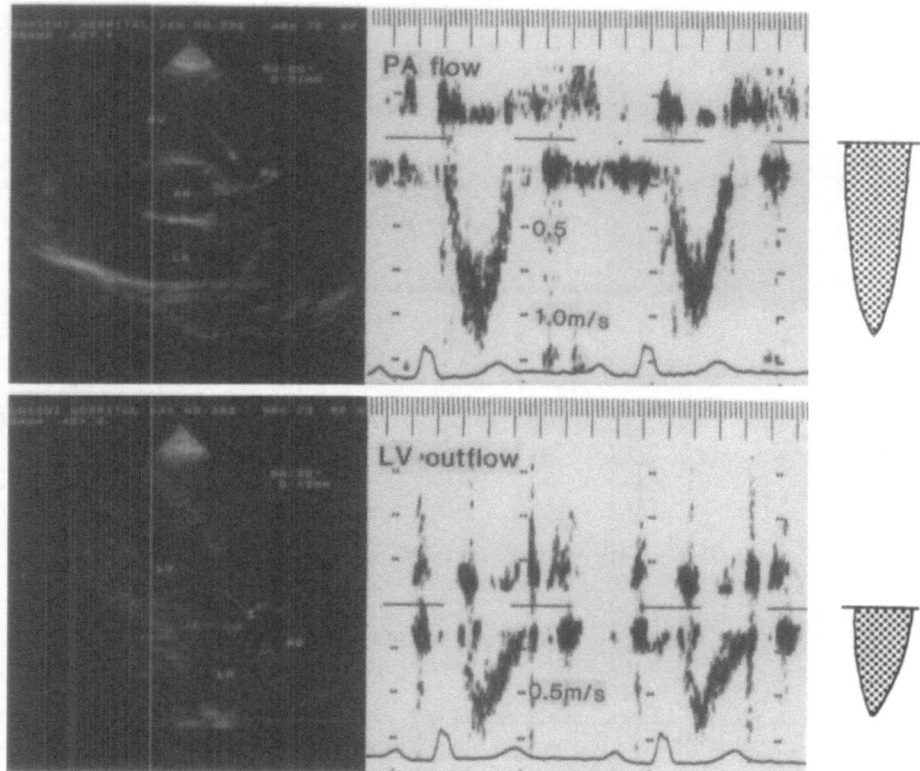

Figure 4.10.   Assessment of a patient with an atrial septal defect by two-dimensional and pulsed Doppler echocardiography permits the calculation of the *Qp/Qs* ratio. (For details see Chapter 8, Measurement of Cardiac Output.)

6. Patent ductus arteriosus

In utero, the descending thoracic artery and the left pulmonary artery are connected by a ductus arteriosus which is normally closed after birth. The two-dimensional echocardiographic detection of the patent ductus arteriosus is relatively easy in infants and children but may be difficult in adults. Conventional and color coded Doppler technique play an important role in its evaluation (Figure 4.26 and also Figure 11.36).

7. Pulmonary stenosis

Pulmonary stenosis is a frequent congenital heart disease that is frequently asymptomatic. The echocardiographic findings include the dome formation of the pulmonary valve during systole in a two-dimensional echocardiogram, and a prominent *a*-dip in M-mode (Figure 4.27). Pulsed Doppler echocardiography provides information about the post-stenotic turbulent flow in the pulmonary artery and CW Doppler echocardiography is implemented to measure the increased peak flow velocity (Figure 4.28). This velocity is inserted into the Bernouili equation to assess the systolic pressure gradient (Figure 4.29).

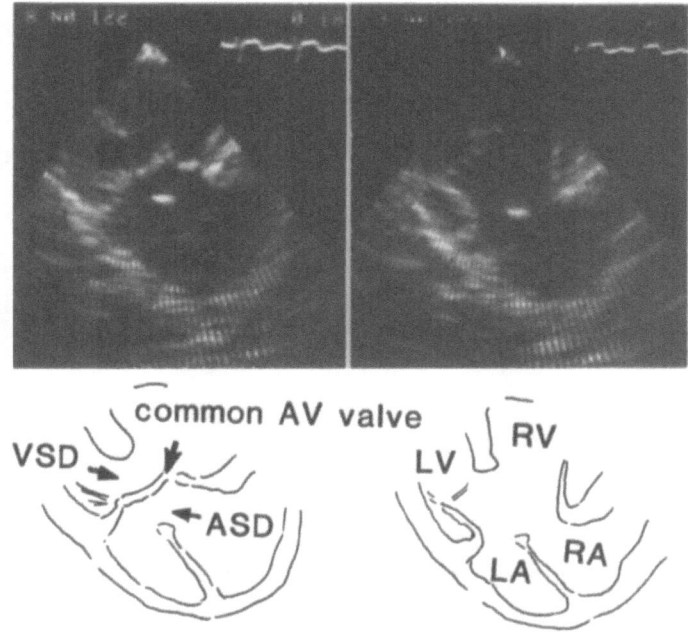

Figure 4.11. Apical four-chamber view demonstrating a complete form of ECD. Ventricular septal defect (VSD), atrial septal defect (ASD) and common atrioventricular (AV) valve are shown during systole and diastole.

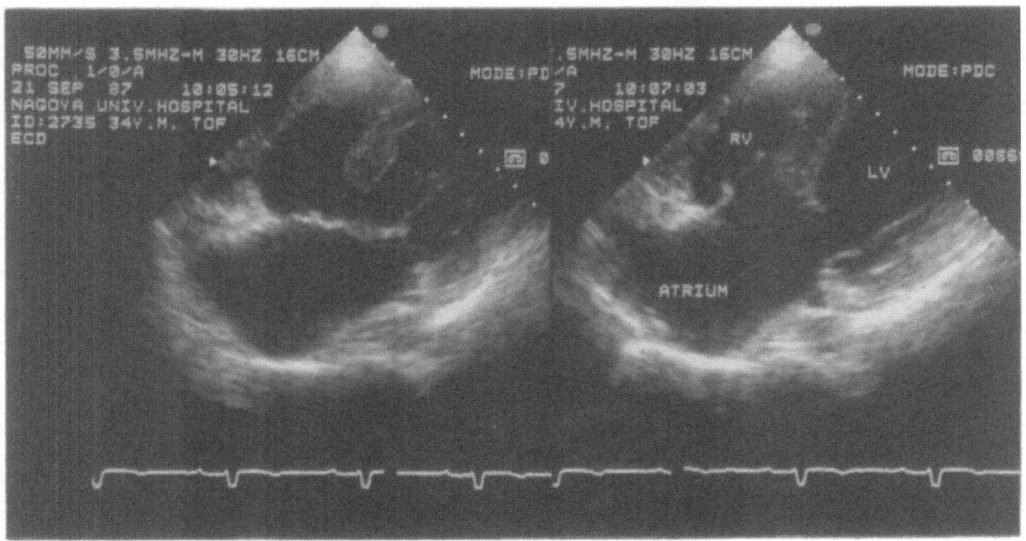

Figure 4.12. Apical four-chamber view demonstrating a complete form of ECD and single atrium. Ventricular septal defect, common atrioventricular valve and single atrium are shown.

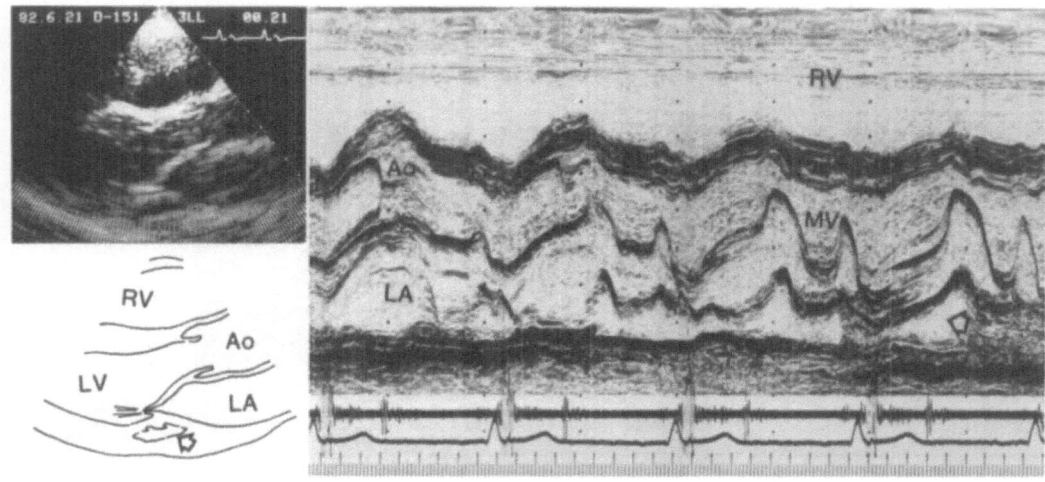

Figure 4.13.   Parasternal long axis view and M-mode scan of a patient with persistent left superior vena cava. An enlarged coronary sinus (arrow) behind the posterior portion of the mitral annulus is shown.

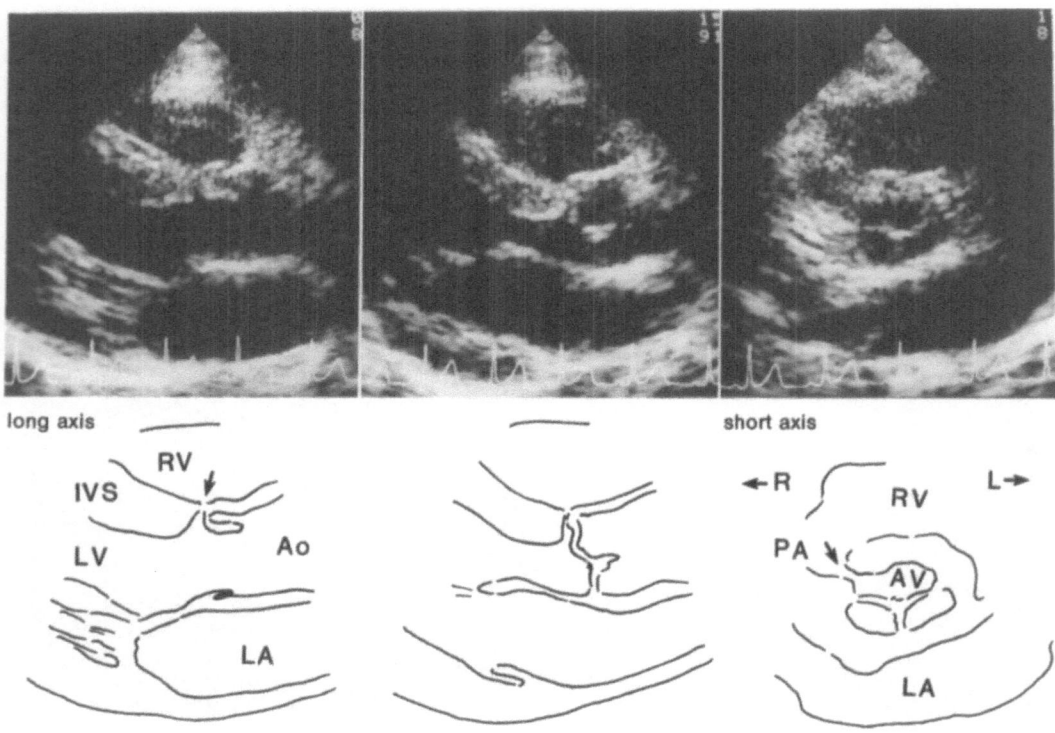

Figure 4.14.   Parasternal long and short axis view showing a membranous type of ventricular septal defect (arrow).

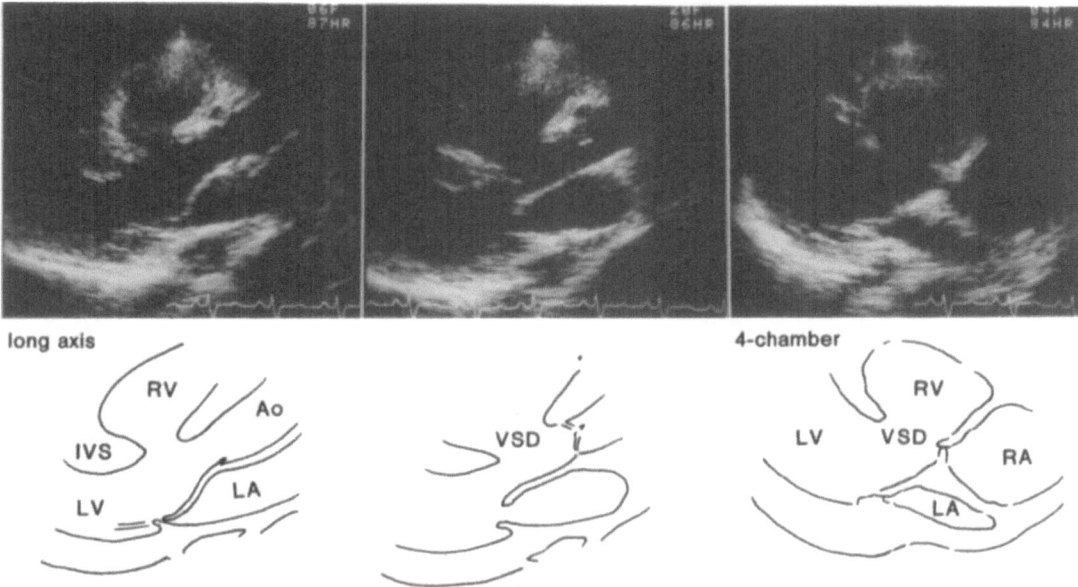

Figure 4.15. Parasternal long axis view and apical four chamber views from a patient with a large ventricular septal defect.

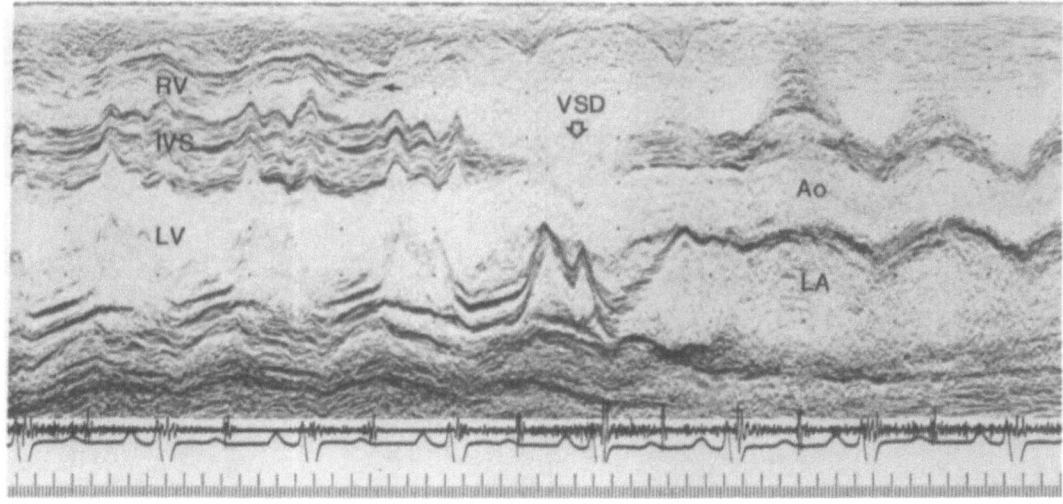

Figure 4.16. M-mode scan illustrating a discontinuity of the IVS in a patient with large ventricular septal defect.

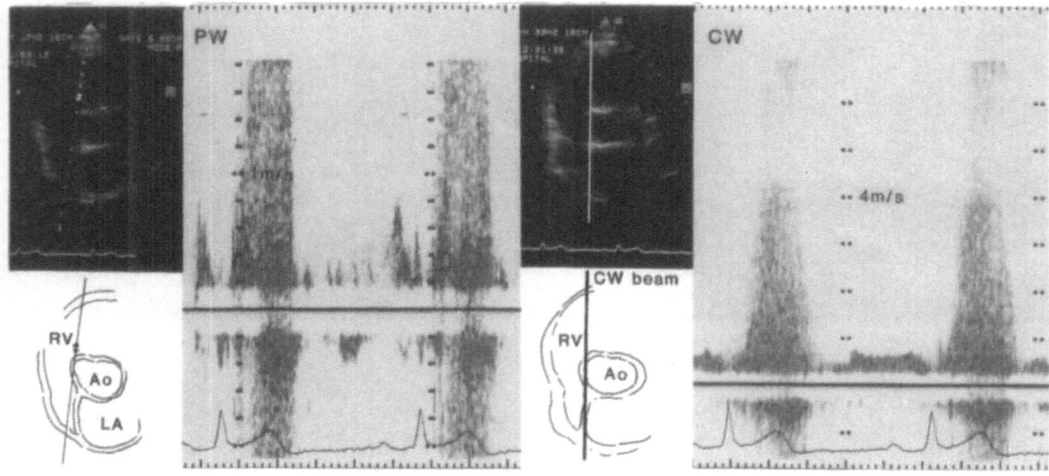

Figure 4.17. Pulsed and CW Doppler echocardiogram of a patient with a small ventricular septal defect. Pulsed Doppler illustrates the systolic turbulent flow in the right ventricle and CW Doppler demonstrates a high velocity flow (peak velocity = 4 m/sec).

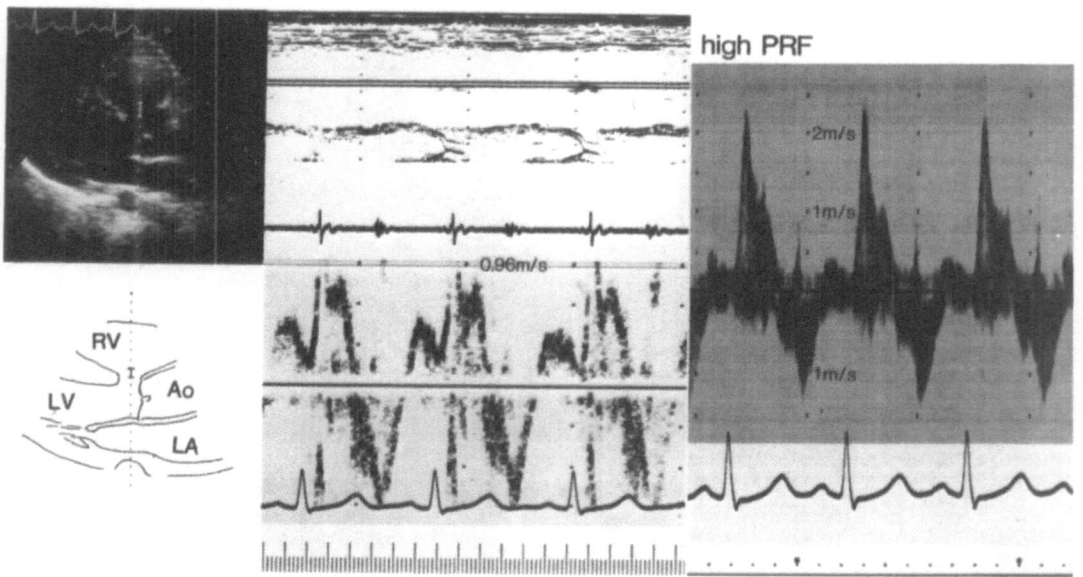

Figure 4.18. Pulsed and high PRF Doppler echocardiogram of a patient with a large ventricular septal defect and an Eisenmenger complex. In this patient, the pulmonary hypertension is moderate and one can see bi-directional flow across the defect.

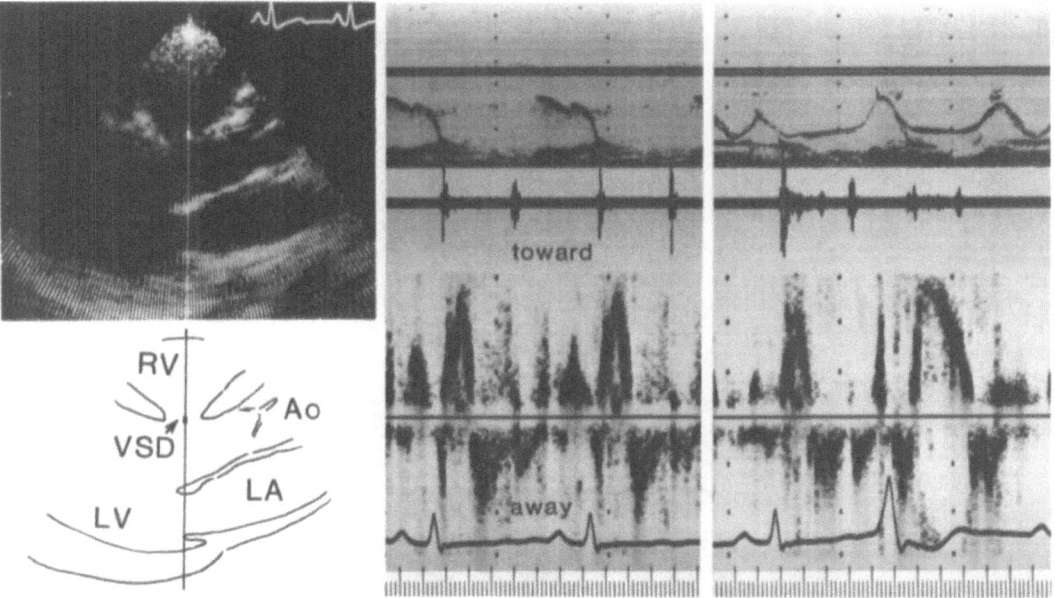

Figure 4.19. Pulsed Doppler echocardiogram of a patient with a large ventricular septal defect and severe pulmonary hypertension. The sample volume is placed in the septal defect, and a bi-directional flow with a peak velocity lower than that shown in Figure 4.16 is clearly demonstrated.

8. Ebstein's anomaly

Ebstein's anomaly is a congenital heart disease in which the insertion of the tricuspid septal leaflet is more apical than the normal position. The basal portion of the right ventricle becomes atrialized (Figure 4.30). The M-mode echocardiogram shows a characteristic delaying in the closure of the tricuspid valve and enlargement of the right side of the heart (Figure 4.31) Using Doppler techniques, it is possible to demonstrate the tricuspid regurgitation which is secondary to the incomplete closure of the tricuspid valve.

9. Tetralogy of Fallot

Tetralogy of Fallot consists of a defect in the membranous portion of the IVS with an overrriding aorta, right ventricular hypertrophy and pulmonic stenosis. Using two-dimensional echocardiography (Figures 4.32, 34), these abnormalities can usually be detected. However, the evaluation of pulmonary stenosis in these patients is sometimes difficult. M-mode can also demonstrate these findings (Figure 4.33, 35). Using pulsed Doppler and color flow mapping techniques from the parasternal long axis view, bidirectional flow is detected through the ventricular septal defect (Figure 4.36 and also Figure 11.34).

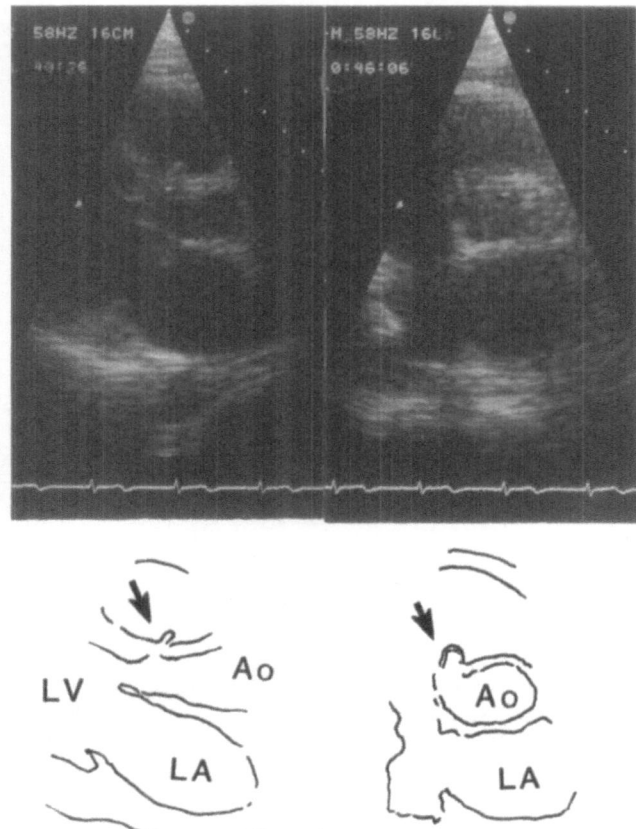

Figure 4.20.   Parasternal long and short axis view illustrating a small ventricular septal aneurysm (arrow).

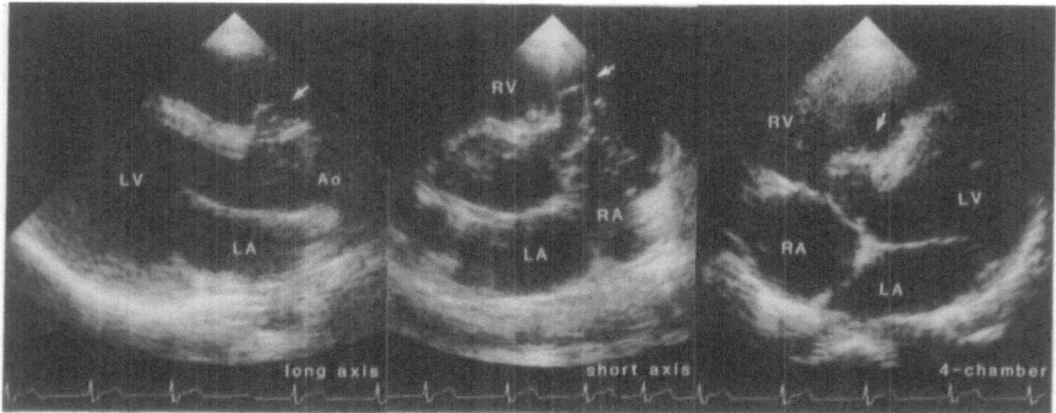

Figure 4.21.   Parasternal long and short axis and four-chamber view of a patient with large ventricular septal aneurysm. An aneurysmal bulging into the right ventricular outflow tract is shown by the arrow.

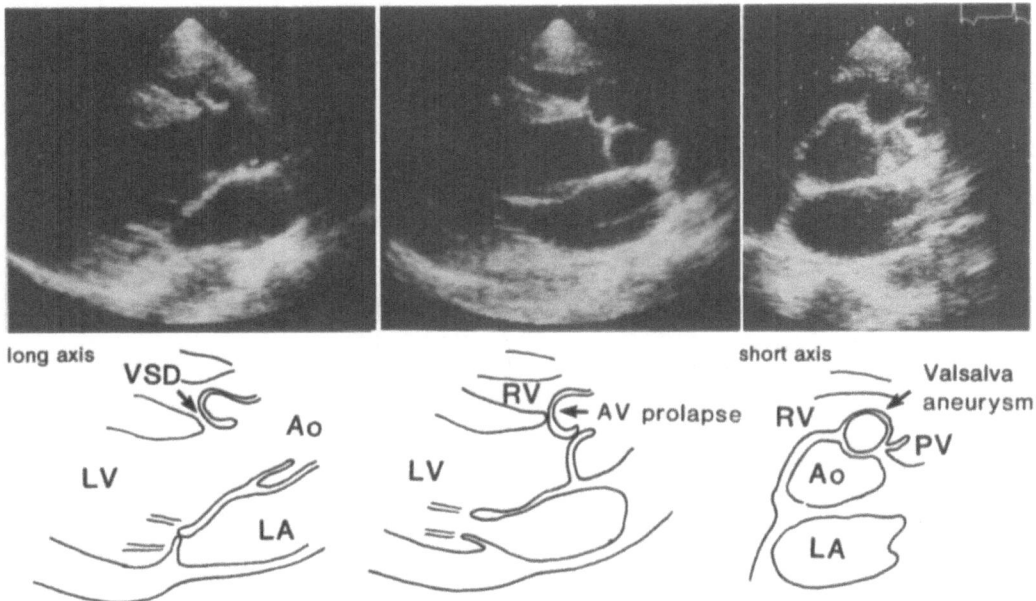

Figure 4.22.   Parasternal long axis view showing a membranous ventricular septal defect and aortic valve prolapse of the right coronary cusp.

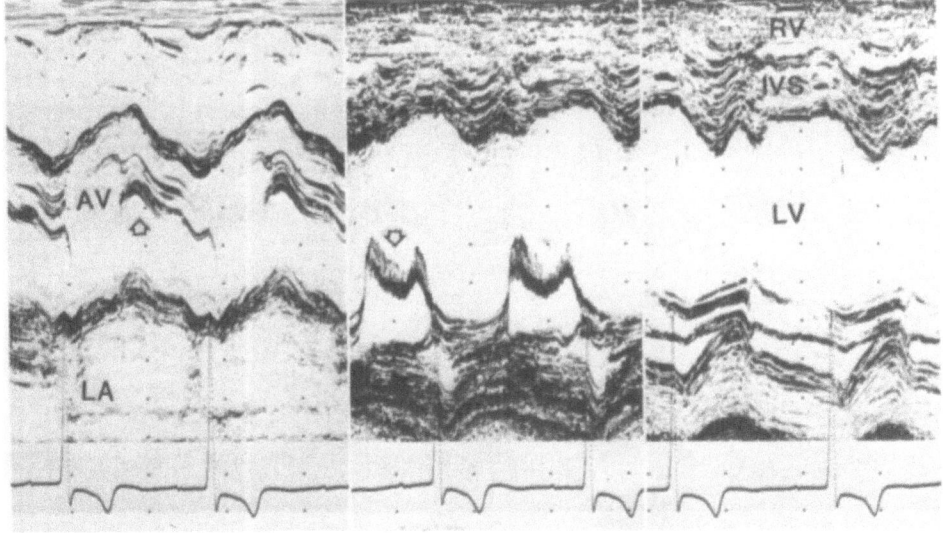

Figure 4.23.   M-mode echocardiogram from a patient with a membranous ventricular septal defect and aortic regurgitation due to aortic valve prolapse. The panel on the left demonstrates an anterior displacement of the aortic valve closure due to prolapse (arrow). The middle panel illustrates an anterior mitral valve fluttering and the right panel shows left ventricular enlargement due to volume overload.

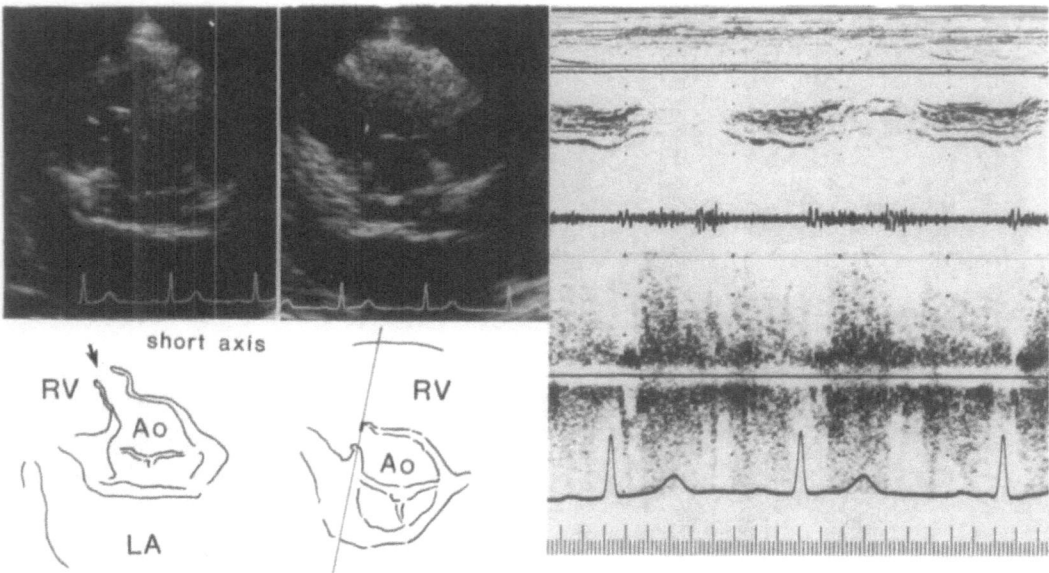

Figure 4.24. Parasternal short axis view and pulsed Doppler echocardiography demonstrating a ruptured right Valsalva sinus aneurysm (arrow) and systolic and diastolic turbulent flow across the rupture.

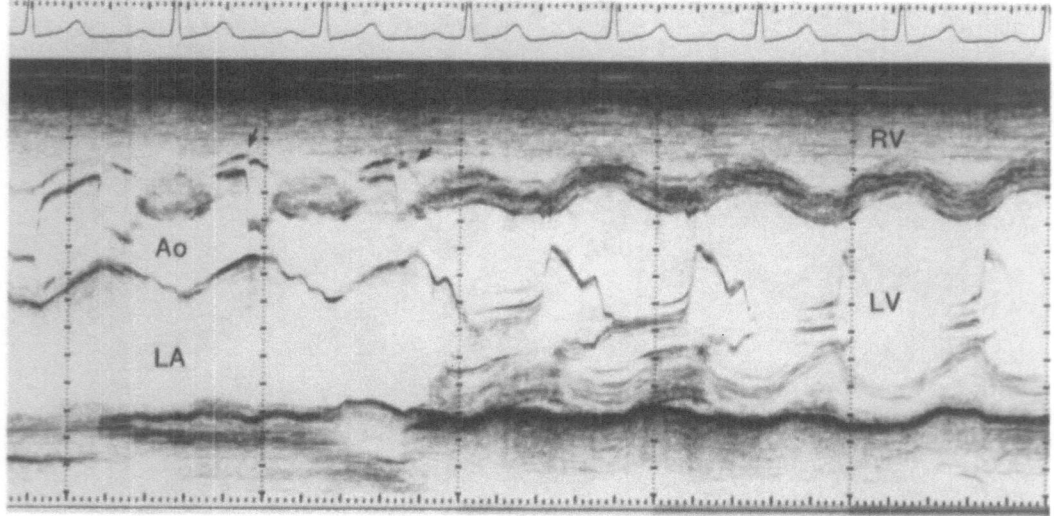

Figure 4.25. An M-mode scan of a patient with an aneurysm of the right sinus of Valsalva. The anterior displacement of sinus is shown by the arrow.

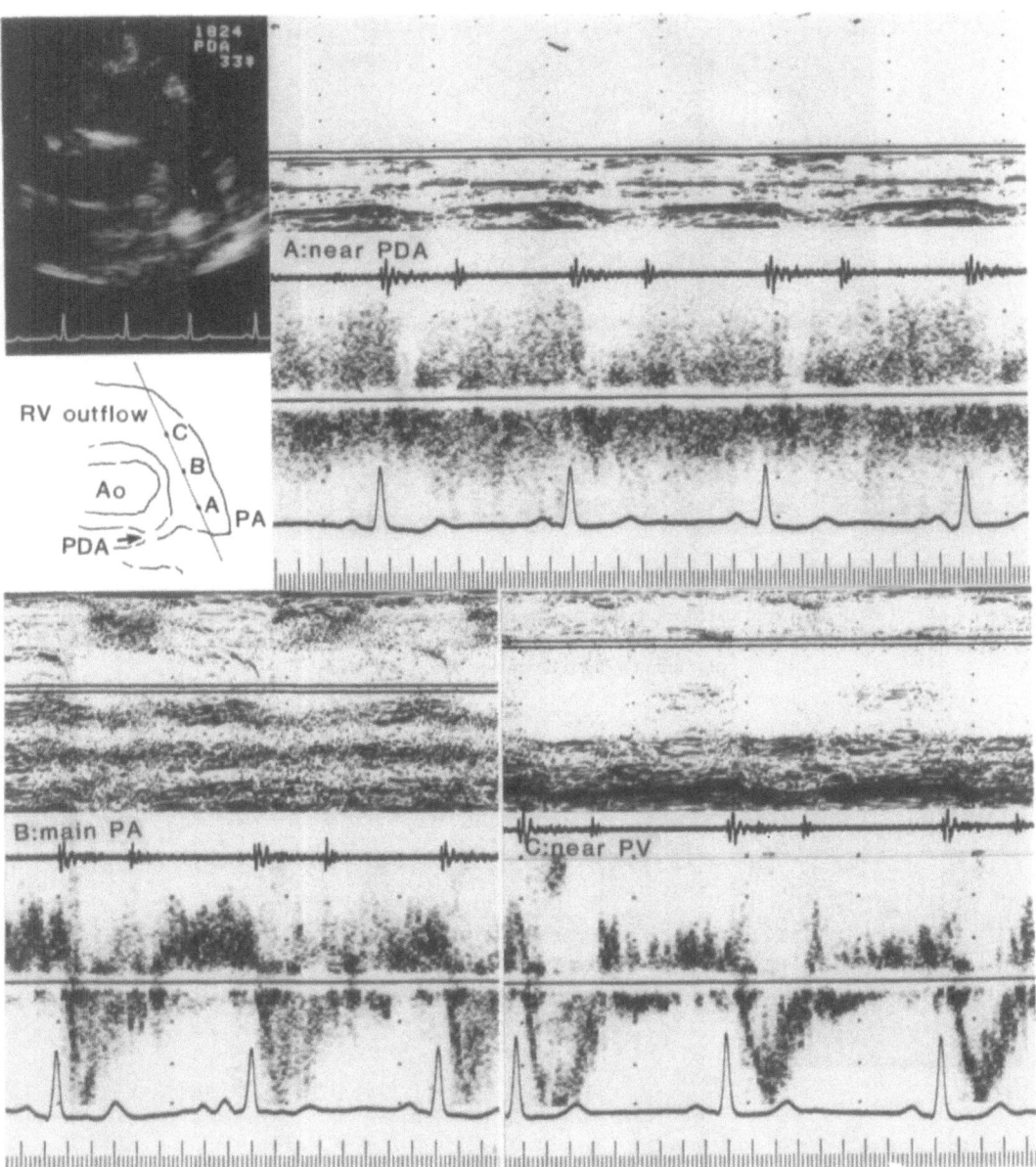

Figure 4.26. Parasternal short axis view and pulsed Doppler echocardiogram on three different sample points in a 34 year-old patient with patent ductus arteriosus. The patent ductus arteriosus is shown by the arrow. The sample point located near the patent ductus arteriosus (A) illustrates the typical systolic and diastolic turbulent flow. In the main pulmonary artery (PA) and near the pulmonic valve (PV), only a diastolic turbulent flow is demonstrated.

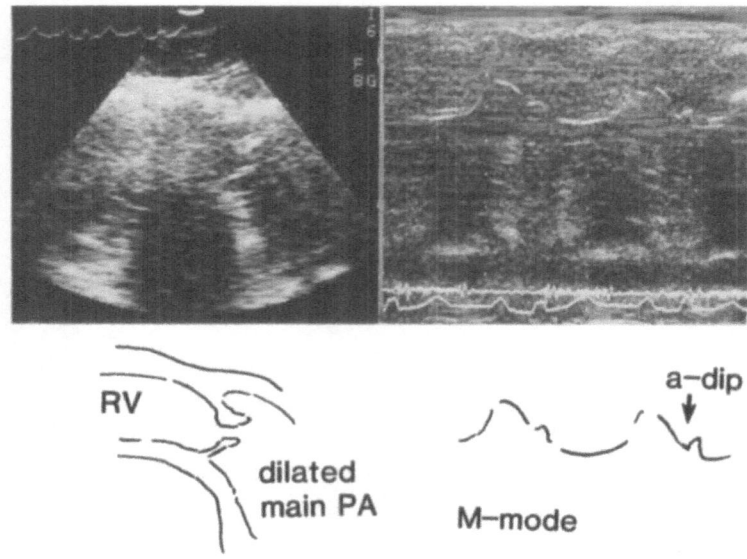

Figure 4.27. Two-dimensional and M-mode echocardiogram of a patient with pulmonary stenosis. Dome formation of the pulmonic valve with poststenotic dilatation of the pulmonary artery are illustrated. In the M-mode, a prominent *a*-dip is demonstrated by the arrow.

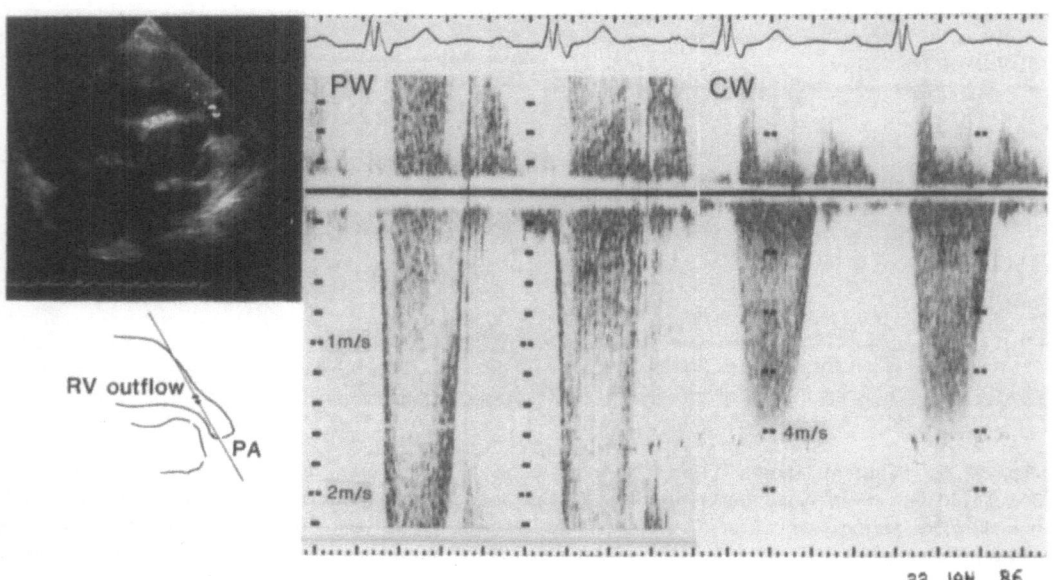

Figure 4.28. Pulsed and CW Doppler echocardiogram of a patient with pulmonary stenosis. Pulsed (PW) Doppler shows a systolic flow turbulence in the pulmonary artery and CW Doppler demonstrates the peakk velocity (4 m/sec).

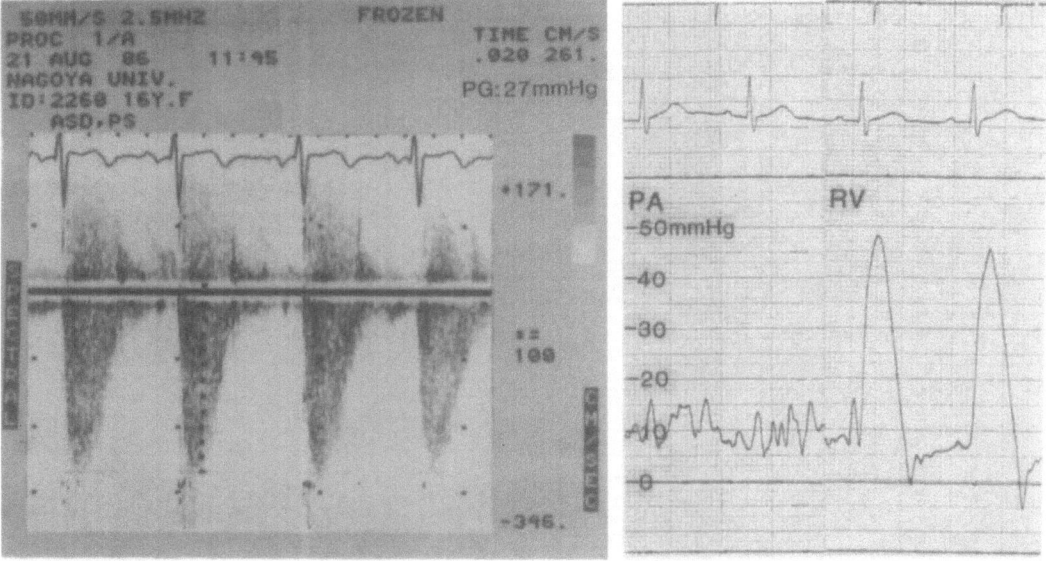

Figure 4.29. CW Doppler, right ventricular and pulmonary arterial pressure tracings from a patient with pulmonary stenosis. The pressure gradient (PG) obtained by CW Doppler-derived peak velocity (2.6 m/sec) is 27 mm Hg, which is very close to that obtained by cardiac catheterization (32 mm Hg).

10. Double outlet of the right ventricle

Double outlet of the right ventricle (DORV) is present when both great arteries arise from the right ventricle with systemic circulation through a membranous ventricular septal defect. Two-dimensional echocardiographic diagnosis is based on the detection of both great arteries arising anterior to the IVS (Figure 4.37).

11. Single ventricle

Single ventricle is a condition in which a single pumping ventricle receives blood from both the left and right atrium without atrioventricular valve atresia. Two-dimensional echocardiographic characteristics consist of a large and trabeculated single ventricle with normal right and left atrioventricular valves (Figure 4.38). These findings may also be detected by M-mode echocardiography (Figure 4.39). When this finding is associated with some degree of pulmonic stenosis, dual M-mode can be used to demonstrate the delayed closure of pulmonic valve (Figure 4.40).

12. Corrected transposition of great arteries

When the aorta and pulmonary artery do not arise from the proper ventricles in assocation with atrio-ventricular discordance, it is called corrected transposition of the great artery, which allows for normal blood circulation. Normally the pulmonary artery is more anterior than the aorta. In the presence of transposition of the great arteries, the pulmonary artery is

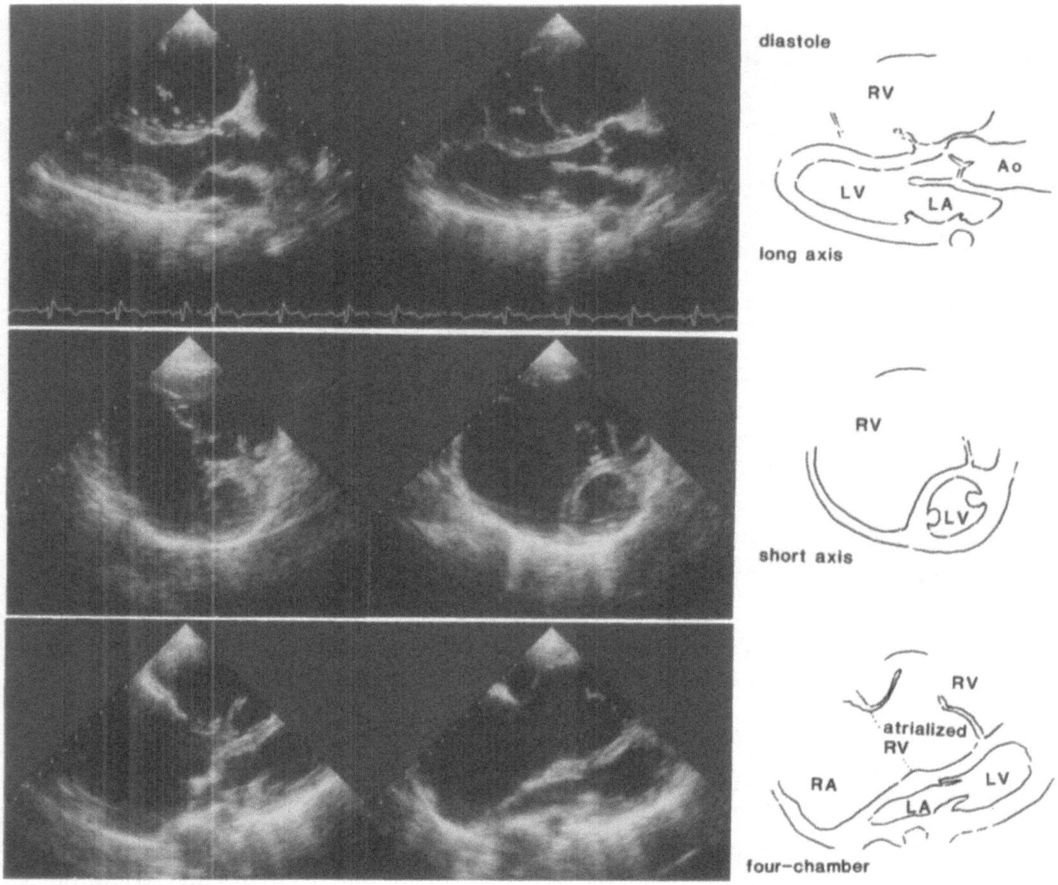

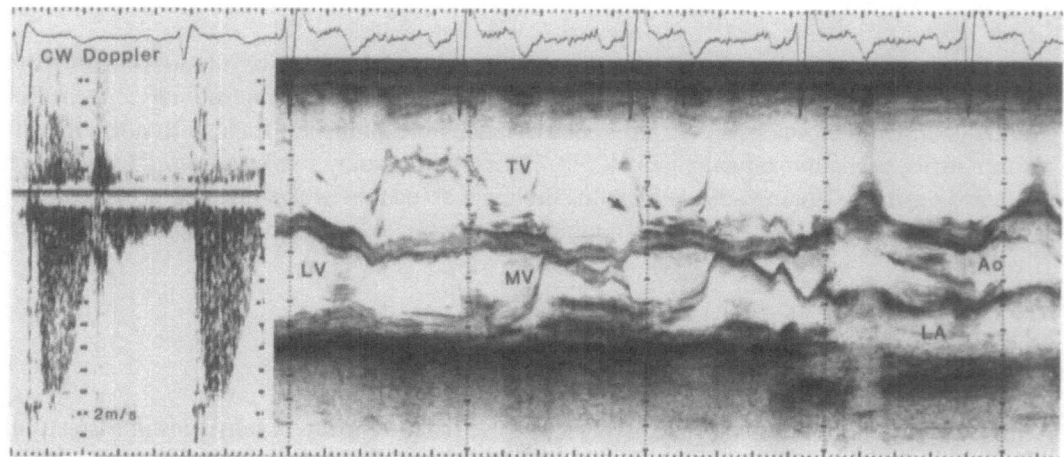

Figure 4.30. Parasternal long and short axis and apical four-chamber views from a patient with Ebstein's anomaly. A right ventricular enlargement with abnormal displacement of the tricuspid valve's septal leaflet and longated anterior leaflet are illustrated. The right ventricular atrialized portion is also demonstrated.

Figure 4.31. M-mode scan and CW Doppler echocardiogram of a patient with Ebstein's anomaly. Delayed closure of tricuspid valve to mitral valve (arrow), right ventricular dilatation and paradoxical motion of IVS are clearly seen. CW Doppler echocardiography illustrates a tricuspid regurgitant flow.

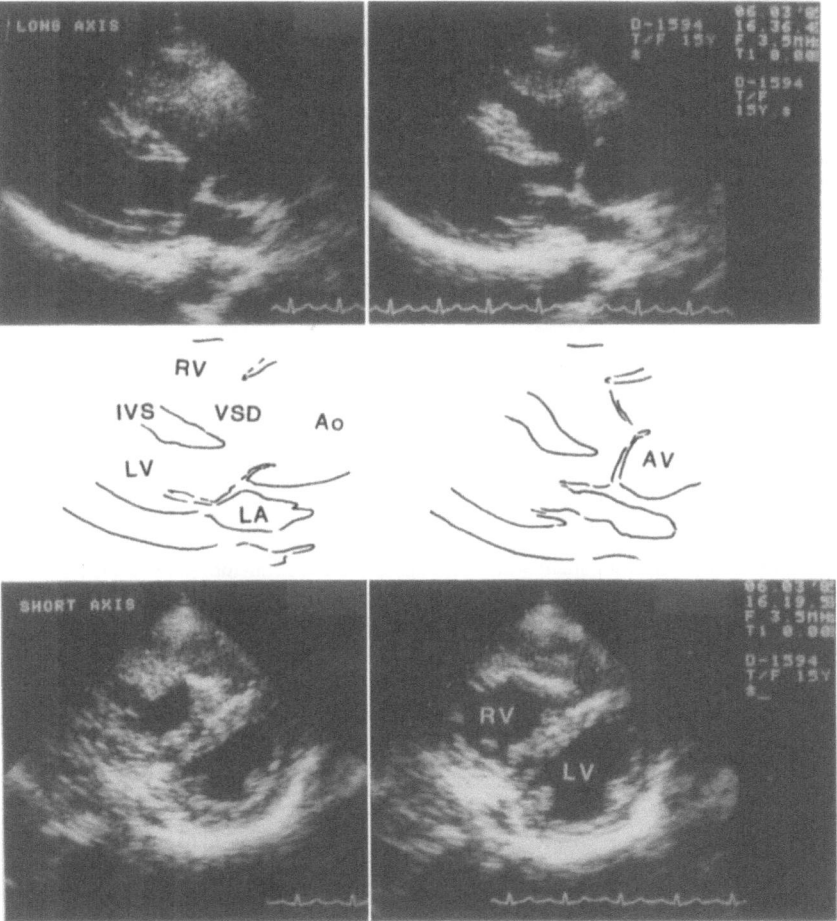

Figure 4.32. Parasternal long and short axis view showing a large ventricular septal defect with overriding of aorta and right ventricular hypertrophy in a patient with Tetralogy of Fallot. The flattening motion of IVS is present throughout the whole cardiac cycle due to right ventricular pressure overload.

located more posterior than the aorta and this finding can be demonstrated using contrast echocardiography (Figure 4.41). The determination of right ventricular morphology depends on the presence of a muscular portion (crista supraventricularis) between the semilunar and atrioventricular valve (Figure 4.42), the finding of which suggest the anatomic right ventricle. Sometimes a three leaflet valve is demonstrated in the left cardiac chamber (Figure 4.43, 44), this finding indicates atrioventricular discordance and incompetence frequently occurs (Figure 4.45).

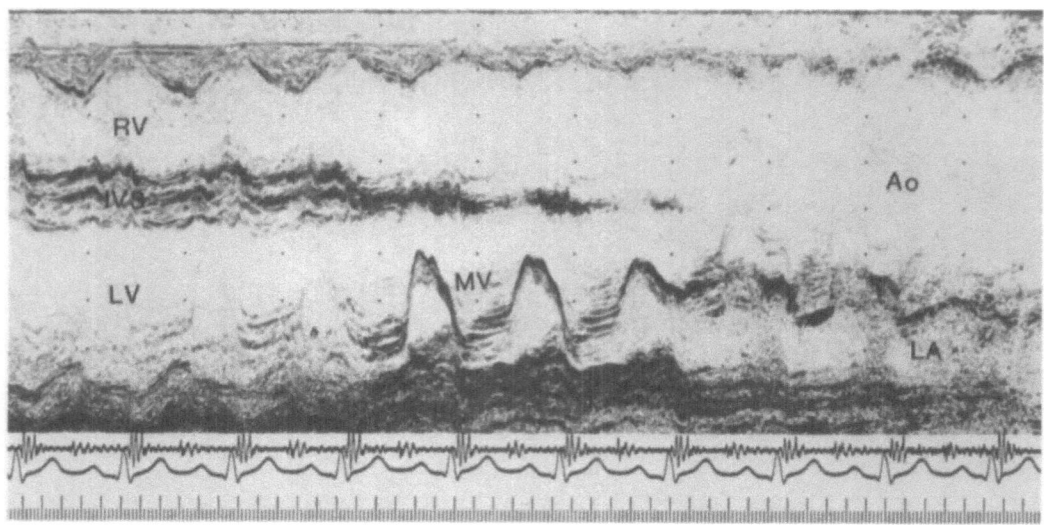

Figure 4.33. M-mode scan of a patient with Tetralogy of Fallot. A membranous ventricular septal defect with overriding of the aorta are clearly seen. Right ventricular hypertrophy (anterior wall) and flattening of the IVS motion are also demonstrated.

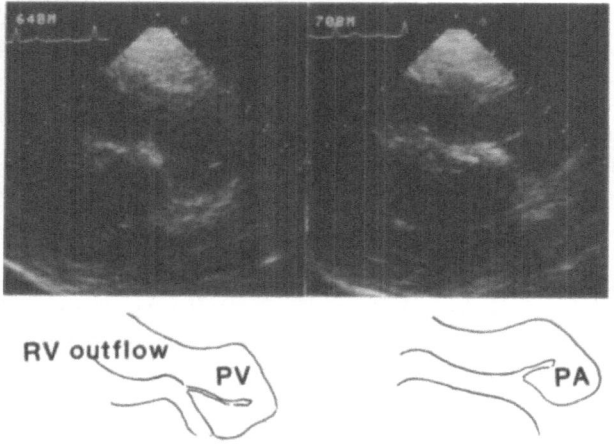

Figure 4.34. Parasternal right ventricular outflow view illustrating the dome formation of the pulmonary valve (pulmonary stenosis) in a patient with Tetralogy of Fallot.

13. Tricuspid atresia

Tricuspid atresia refers to the absence of an atrioventricular valve in the right cavities which is always associated with other congenital abnormalities such as atrial septal defect, ventricular septal defect, patent ductus arteriosus or single atrium. The two-dimensional finding consists of the presence of a dense echo line in the tricuspid position (Figure 4.46). The M-mode can also demonstrate the abnormality (Figure 4.47).

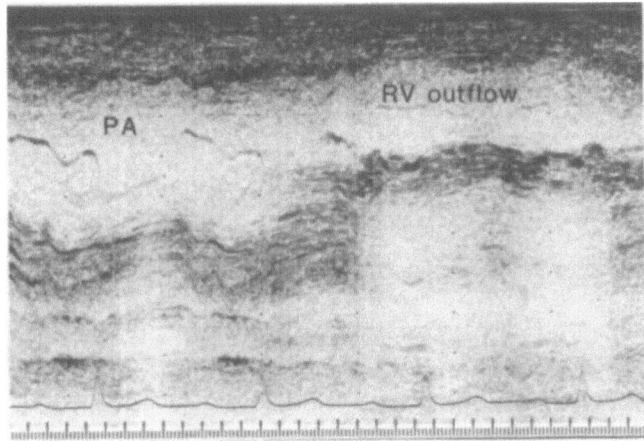

Figure 4.35. M-mode scan of the right ventricular outflow tract and pulmonary artery of a patient with Tetralogy of Fallot. A hypertrophied right ventricular infundibulum (RV outflow) and prominent *a*-dip can be seen.

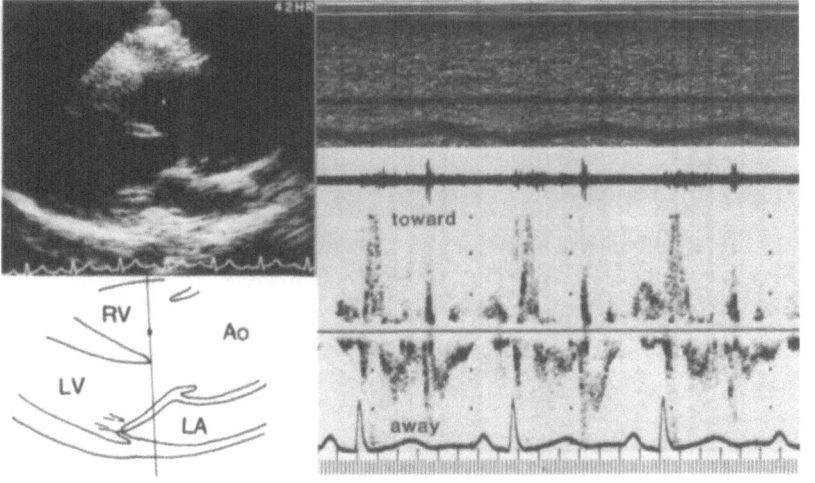

Figure 4.36. Pulsed Doppler echocardiogram of a patient with Tetralogy of Fallot. The sample volume is located in the ventricular septal defect, a bi-directional flow is detected throughout the whole cardiac cycle.

14. Cor triatriatum

Cor triatriatum refers to the presence of a membrane in the left atrium, from the aortic posterior wall to the posterolateral left atrial wall (Figures 4.48, 49). The left atrium is thereby divided into two chambers, and a stenotic condition can occur.

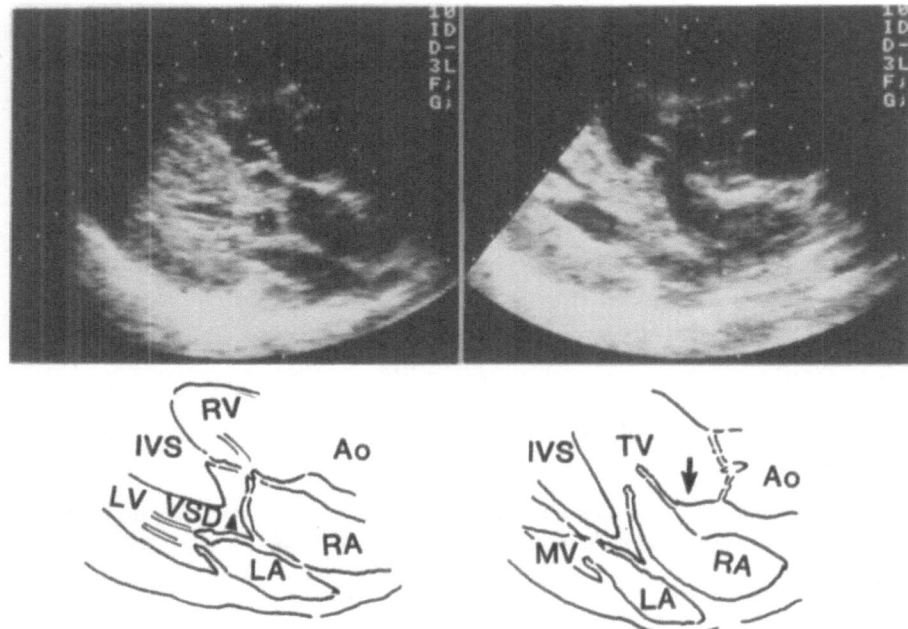

Figure 4.37.   Parasternal long axis view of a patient with a double outlet right ventricle. A discontinuity between IVS and aorta is present. The crista supraventricularis is shown by the arrow. A small left cardiac chamber and membranous ventricular septal defect are also illustrated.

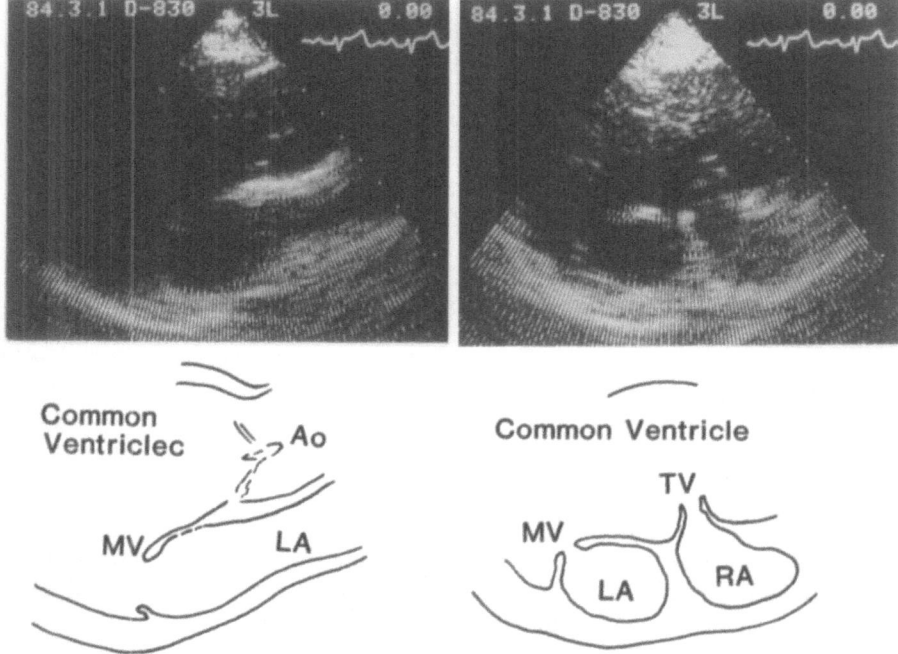

Figure 4.38.   Parasternal and apical long axis view showing a large single ventricle with normal mitral (MV) and tricuspid valve (TV), in a patient with a single ventricle.

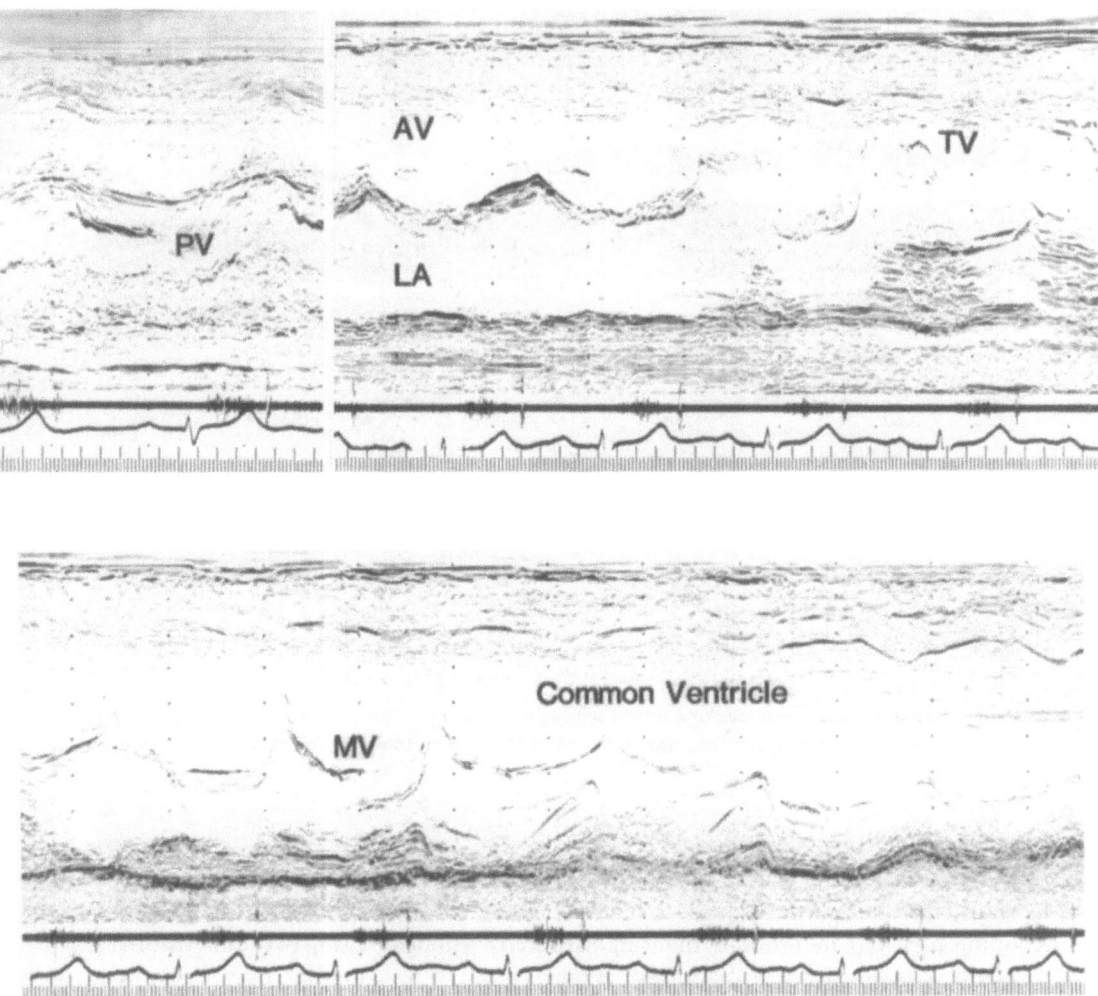

Figure 4.39. M-mode scan of a 16 year-old female with a single ventricle. The aorta is more anterior than the pulmonary artery which suggest transposition of great arteries. A common ventricular chamber with tricuspid (TV) and mitral valve (MV) is clearly illustrated.

15. Bicuspid aortic valve

Normally, the semilunar aortic valve has three cusps. However, the presence of only two cusps may sometimes occur (bicuspid aortic valve), and may be associated with aortic stenosis and/or regurgitation. Using two-dimensional echocardiography, one can directly visualize the presence of only two leaflets with an eccentric closure (Figure 4.50).

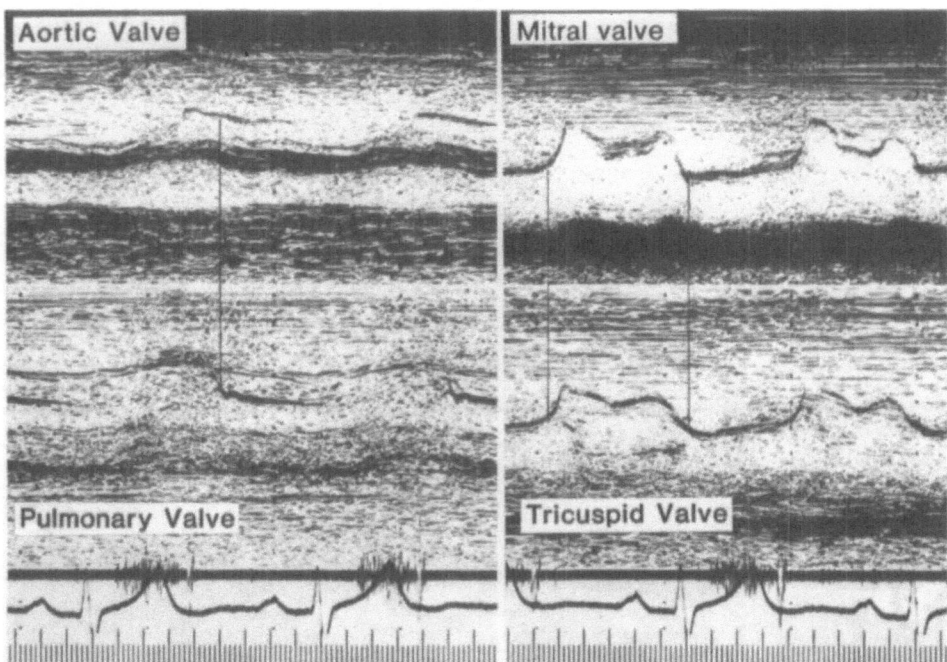

Figure 4.40. Dual M-mode echocardiogram of a patient with a single ventricle. The left panel shows the delayed closure of the pulmonary valve. The right panel shows the similar motion of mitral and tricuspid valves.

16. Supravalvular aortic stenosis

The supravalvular aortic stenosis is characterized by a narrowing of one portion of the ascending aorta of a membrane, that can be directly visualized using two-dimensional (Figure 4.51) and M-mode echocardiography (Figure 4.52). CW Doppler may be implemented quantitatively to evaluate the systolic pressure gradient across this obstruction (Figure 4.53).

17. Coronary artery fistula

Coronary artery fistula is a rare congenital abnormality, which consists of an abnormal communication between the coronary arteries and venous systems with left to right shunting. By two-dimensional echocardiography, dilatation of the coronary artery near the aortic root may indicate the presence of this anomaly (Figure 4.54). Pulsed Doppler echocardiography provides information pertaining to the turbulent flow in the connected portion (Figure 4.55). Sometimes a dilated coronary artery can be demonstrated from many acoustic windows (Figures 4.56, 57).

$\longrightarrow$

Figure 4.41. M-mode scan and M-mode contrast echocardiogram of a patient with corrected transposition of great artery. The posterior pulmonary artery is clearly identified by contrast opacification.

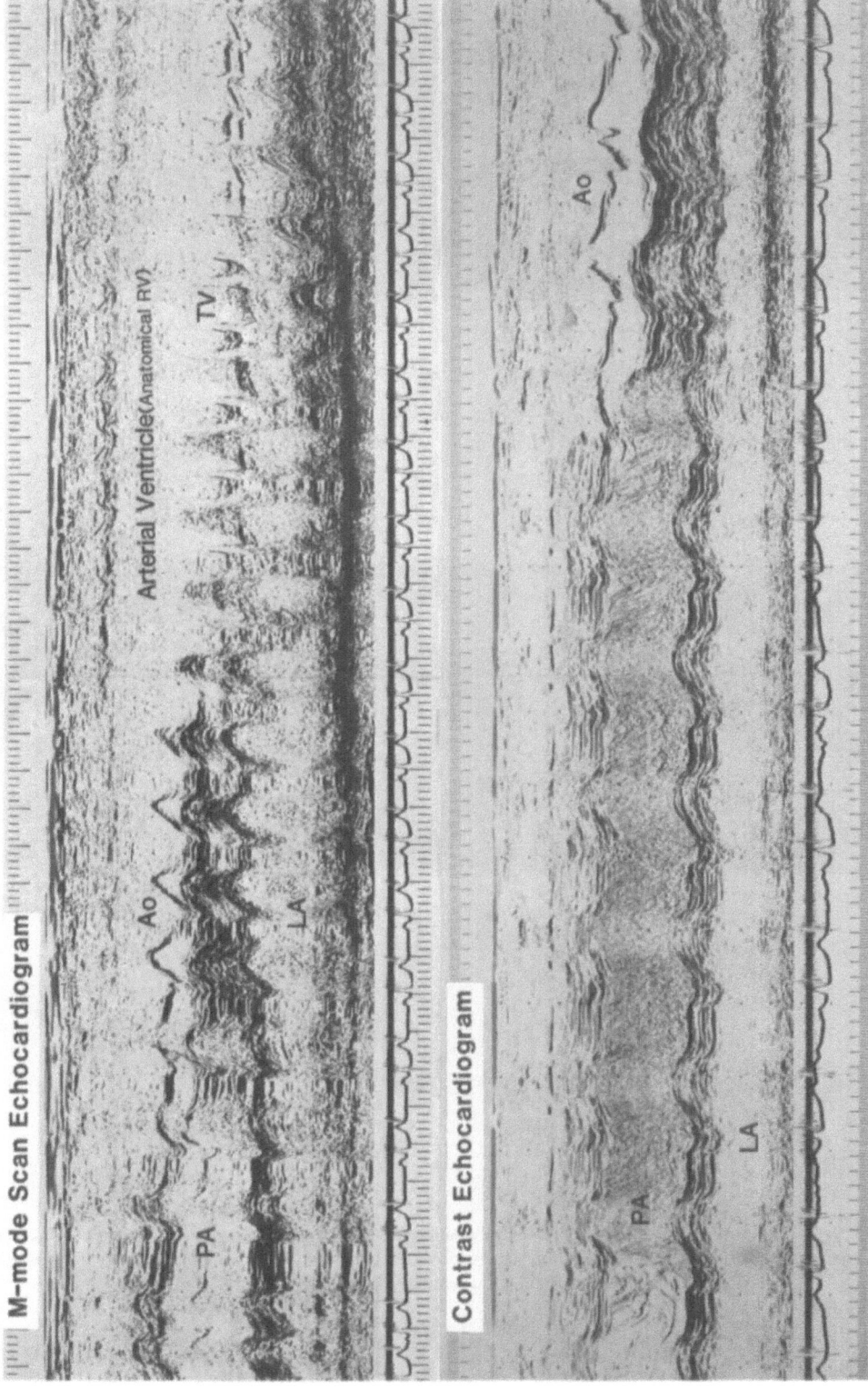

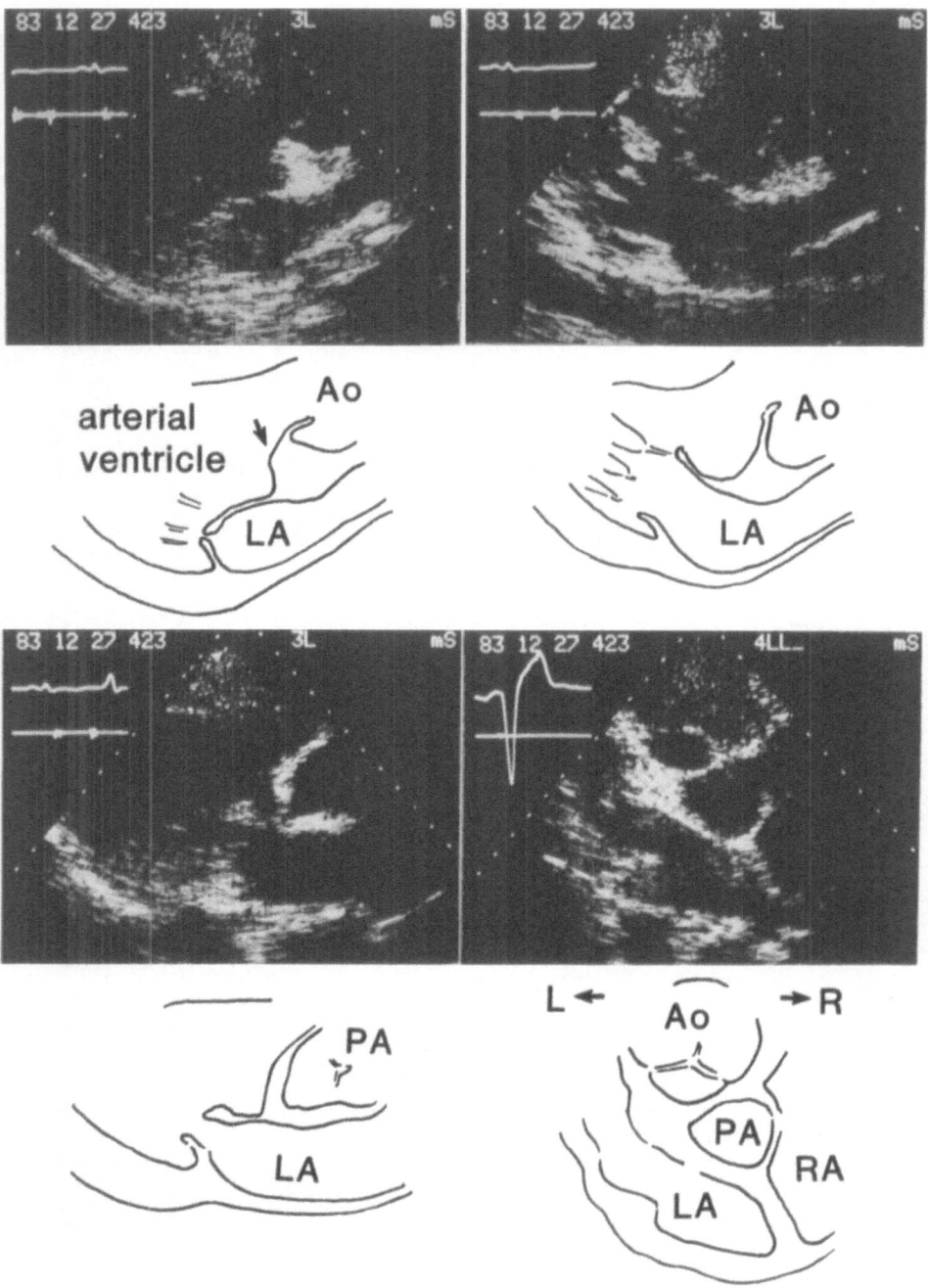

Figure 4.42. Parasternal long and short axis view of a patient with corrected transposition of the great arteries. The crista supraventricularis between the semilunar and atrioventricular valve is shown by the arrow. The pulmonary artery (PA) has a postero-medial position.

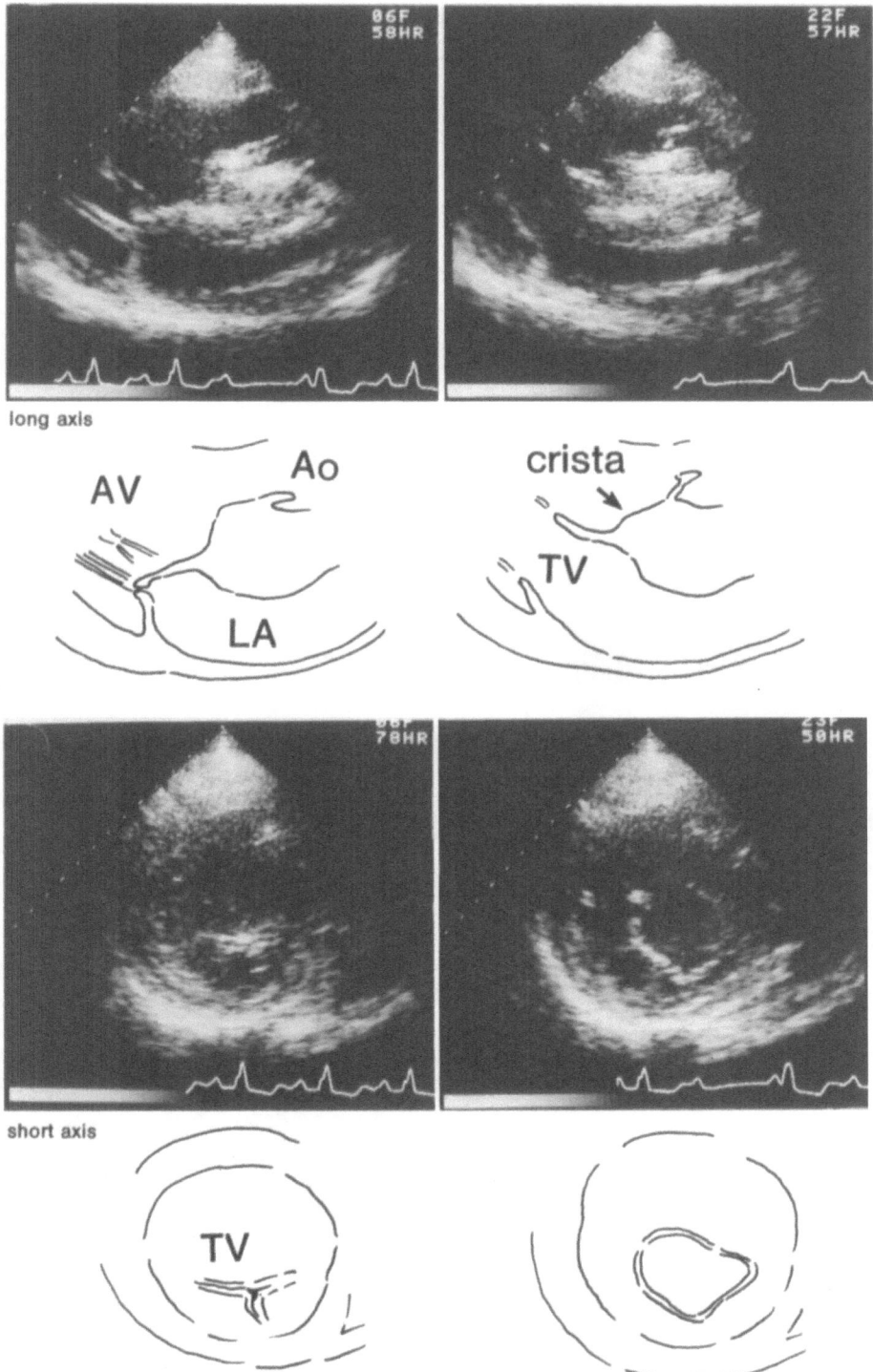

Figure 4.43. Parasternal long and short axis view illustrating the anatomic right ventricle with the muscular portion (crista supraventricularis) behind the aortic valve. The short axis view showing three leaflets (tricuspid) valve in the arterial ventricle in a patient with corrected transposition of great artery.

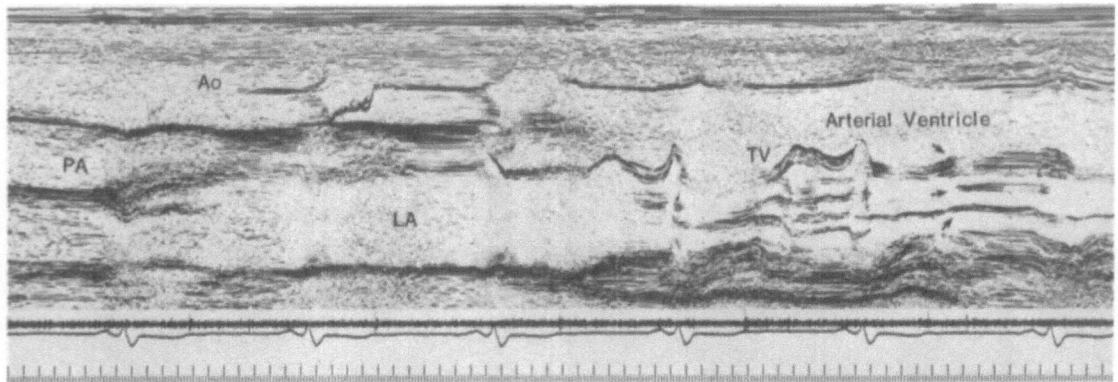

Figure 4.44. M-mode scan of a patient with corrected transposition of the great arteries. The aorta is located more anterior than the pulmonary artery and the tricuspid valve is identified by three different echoes (arrow) in the arterial ventricle.

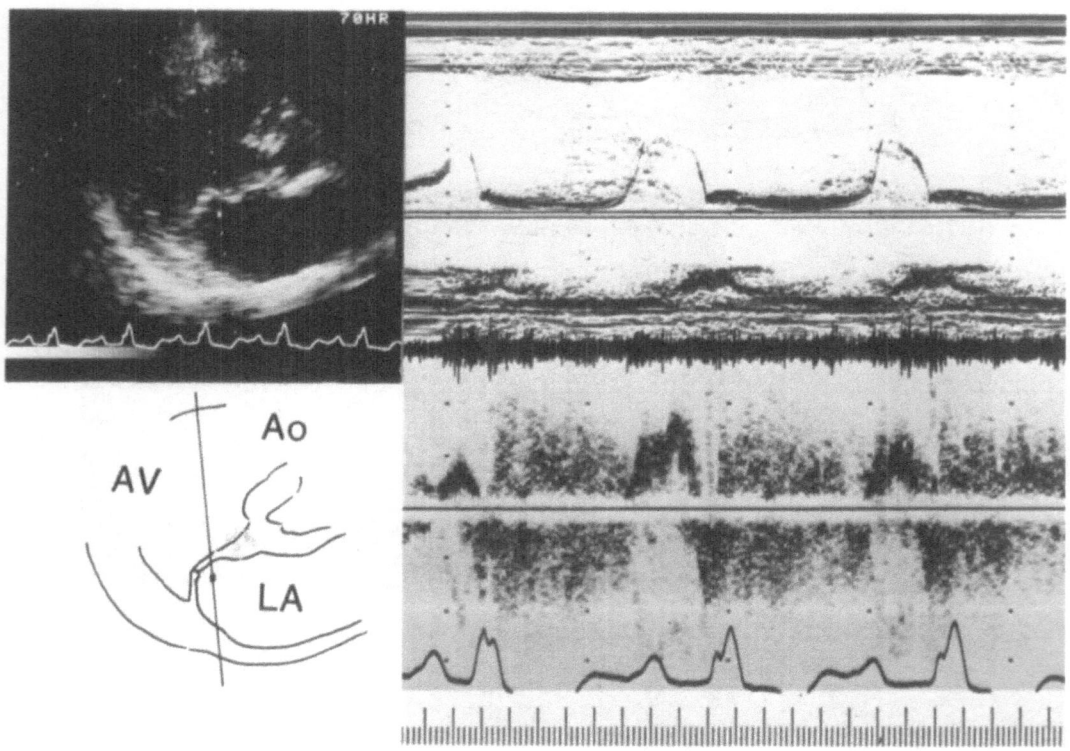

Figure 4.45. Pulsed Doppler echocardiogram illustrating a systolic turbulent flow in the left atrium through the tricuspid valve in a patient with corrected transposition of the great arteries.

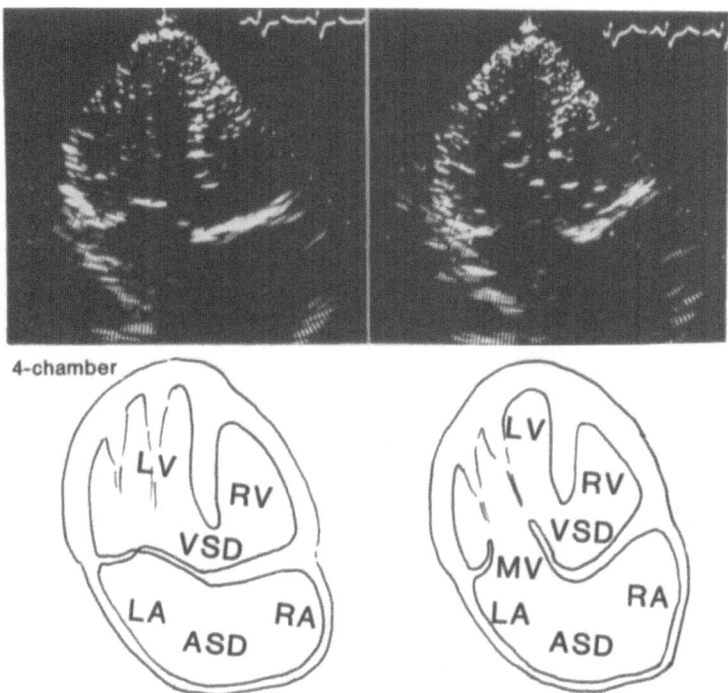

Figure 4.46. Apical four-chamber view of a patient with tricuspid atresia and large atrial septal defect and ventricular septal defect. A dense echo line is found in the tricuspid position (arrow).

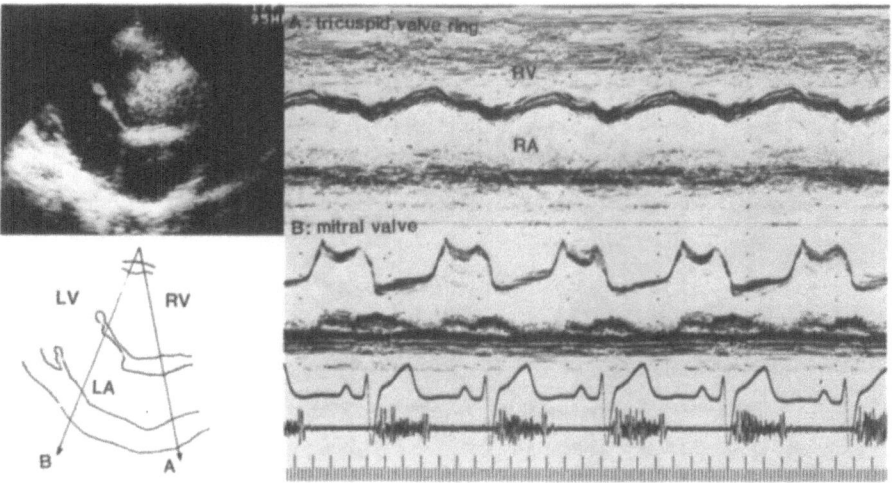

Figure 4.47. Dual M-mode echocardiogram of a patient with tricuspid atresia. In the tricuspid position, a dense linear echo is clearly demonstrated.

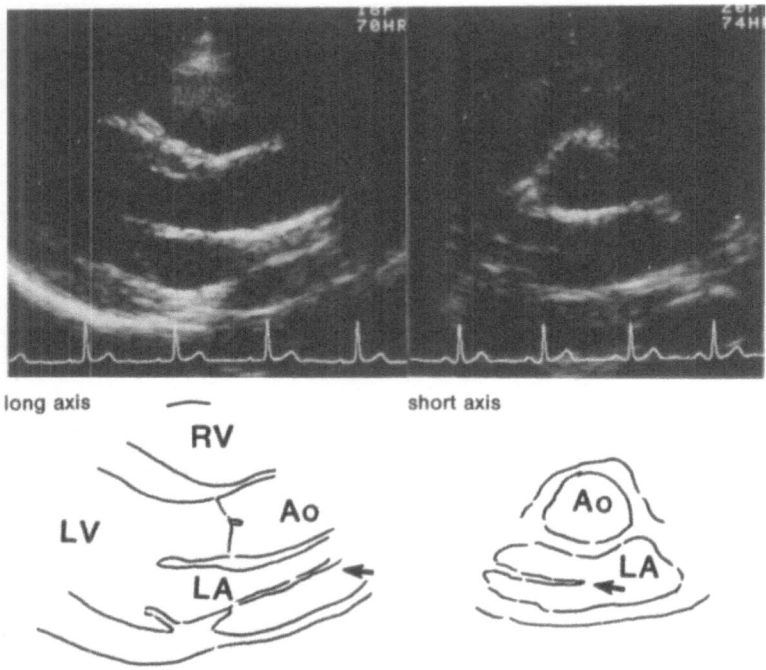

Figure 4.48. Parasternal long and short axis view of a patient with a cor triatriatum. An echo dense line from the posterior aortic wall to posterolateral atrial wall is shown by the arrow.

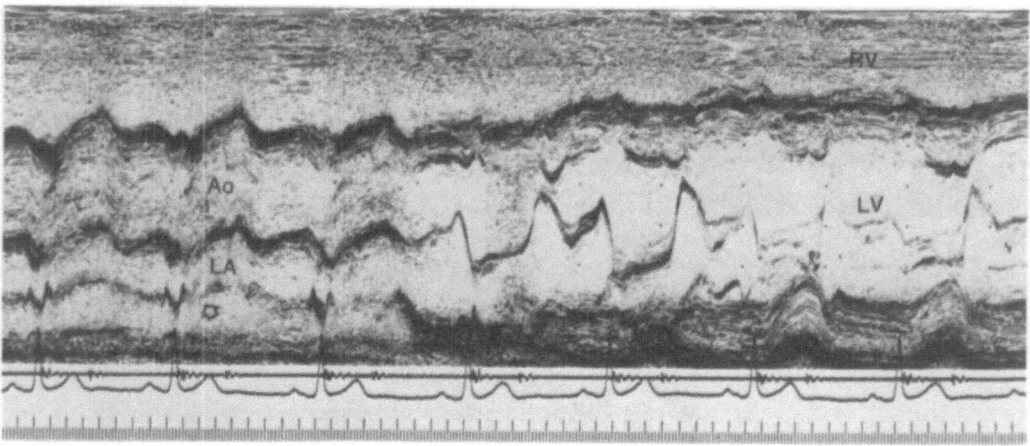

Figure 4.49. M-mode scan illustrating a linear echo in the left atrium (arrow) in a patient with cor triatriatum.

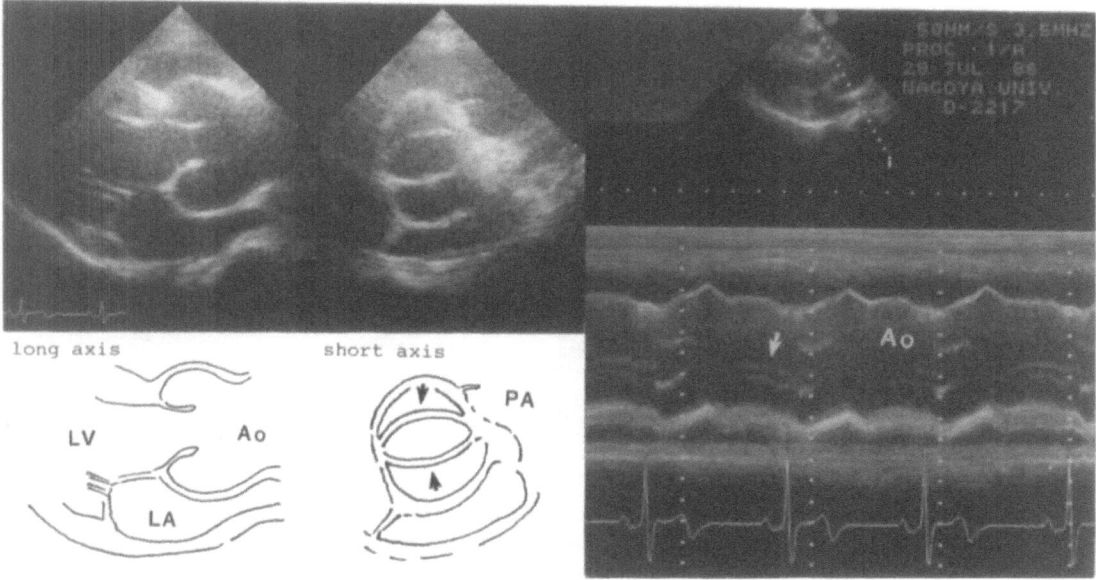

Figure 4.50.   Parasternal long and short axis view and M-mode echocardiogram of a patient with bicuspid aortic valve. In the short axis view one notes only two aortic cusps. In the M-mode, an eccentric and incomplete closure is shown by the arrow.

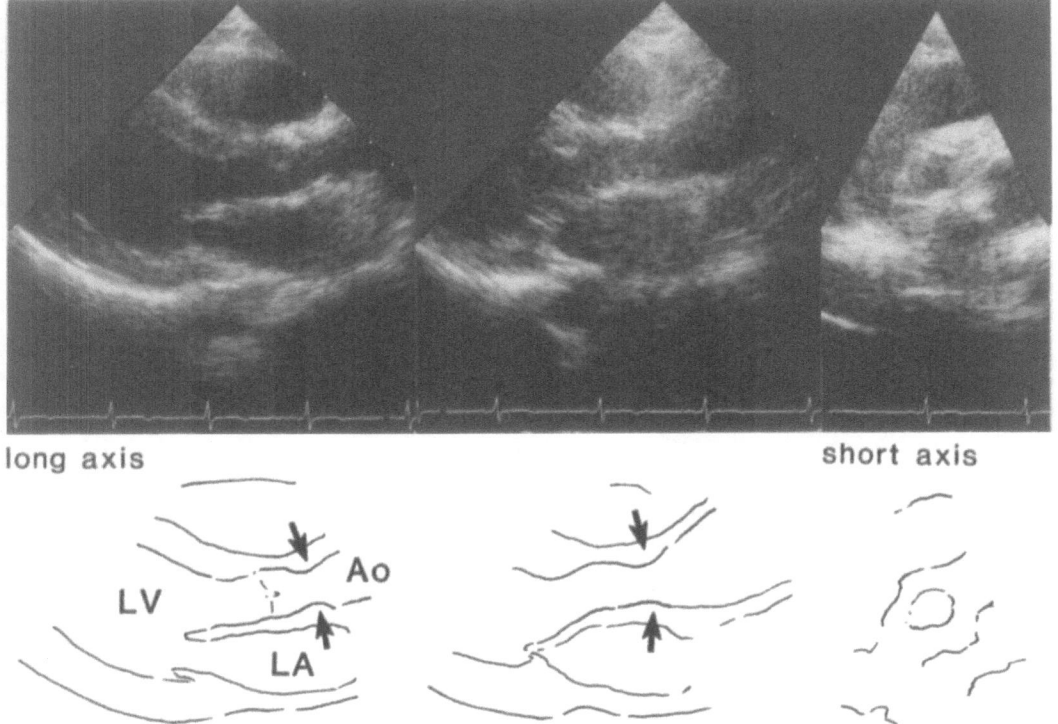

Figure 4.51.   Parasternal long and short axis view illustrating a mild stenotic area above the aortic valve (arrow), with post-stenotic dilatation in a patient with supravalvular aortic stenosis.

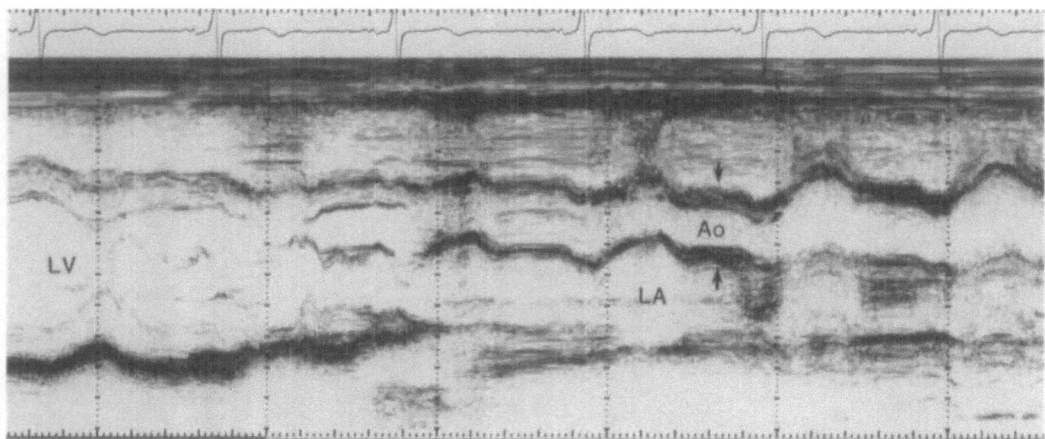

Figure 4.52. M-mode scan of a 16 year-old female with supravalvular aortic stenosis. A stenotic portion of the ascending aorta with increased echo intensity of its walls (arrow) and post-stenotic dilatation are clearly illustrated.

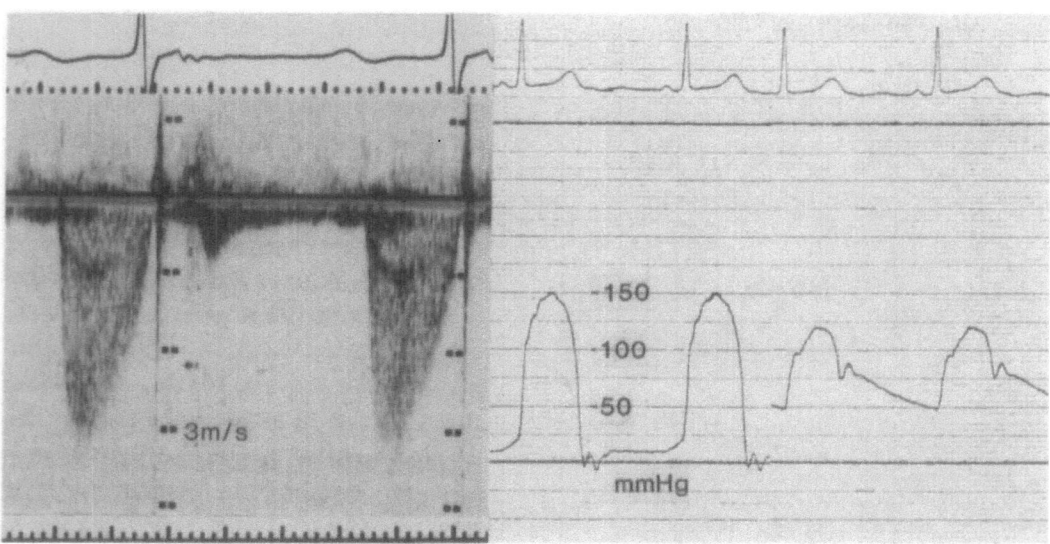

Figure 4.53. CW Doppler and pressure tracings obtained by cardiac catheterization in a patient with supravalvular aortic stenosis. CW Doppler shows an increased peak velocity of aortic flow (3 m/sec) and a systolic pressure gradient about 36 mm Hg by a simplified Bernoulli equation ($PG = 4V^2$). The pressure tracing shows a very similar systolic pressure gradient (about 30 mm Hg).

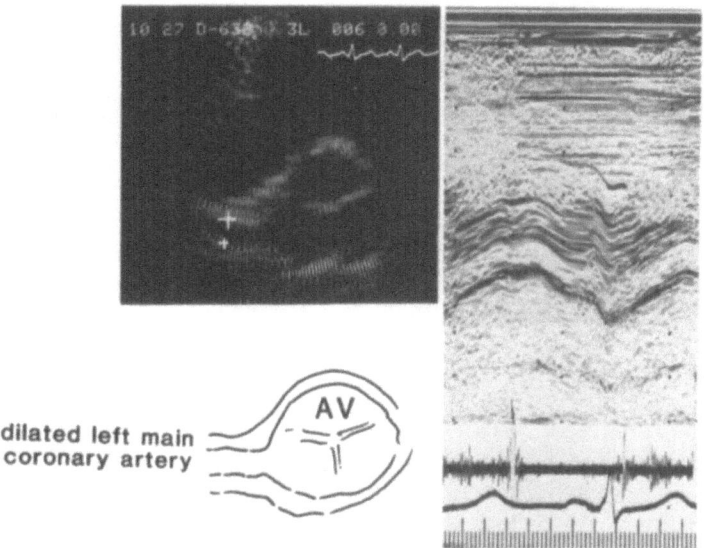

Figure 4.54. Parasternal short axis view and M-mode echocardiograms from a patient with a coronary artery fistula. A left main coronary artery dilatation is shown.

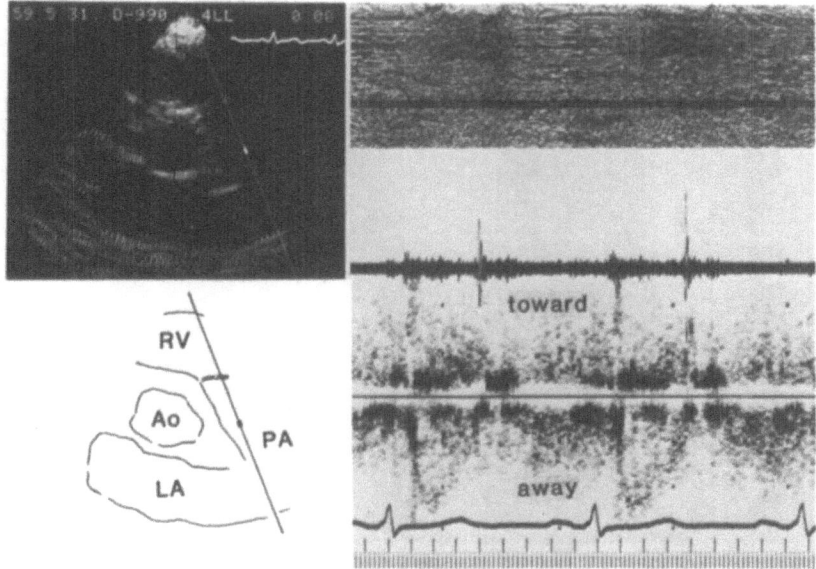

Figure 4.55. Pulsed Doppler echocardiogram of a patient with coronary artery fistula. A turbulent flow is demonstrated in the main pulmonary artery.

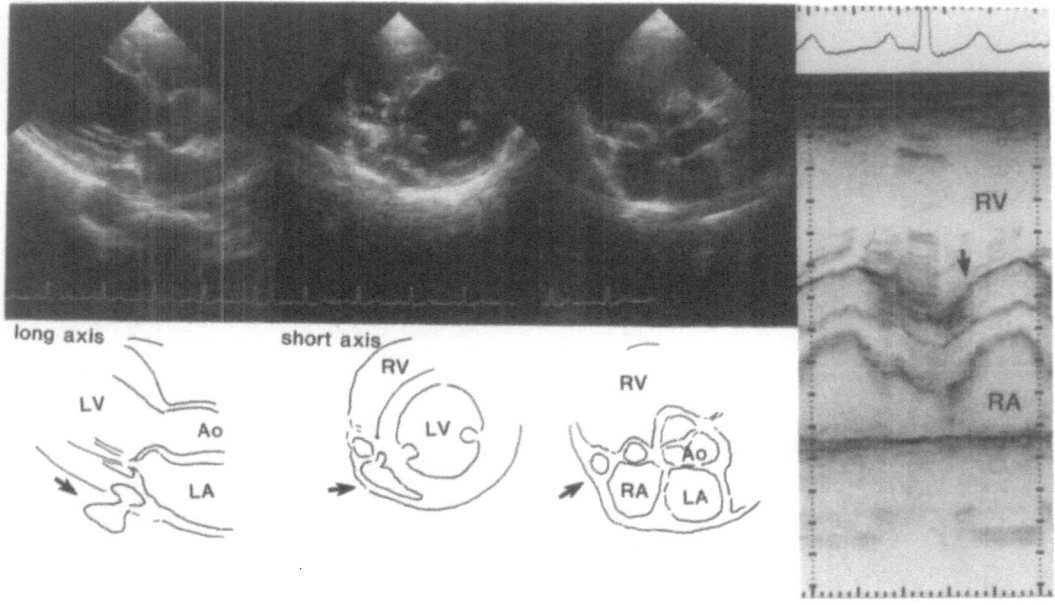

Figure 4.56. Parasternal long and short axis view and M-mode echocardiograms from a patient with a coronary artery fistula. Significantly dilated coronary arteries are demonstrated.

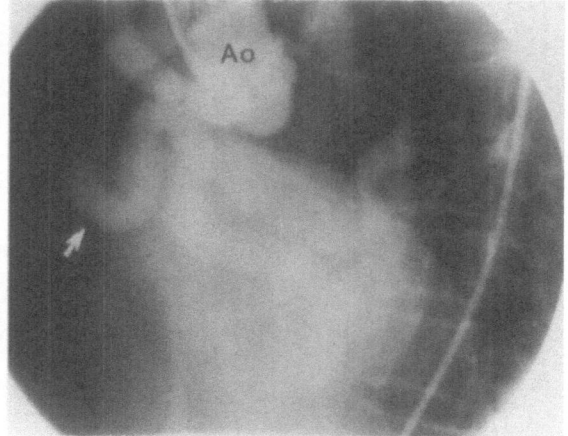

Figure 4.57. Right coronary angiogram of a patient with coronary artery fistula. A significantly dilated right coronary artery is opacified by cinéangiogram. This finding is compatible with the echocardiogram (Figure 4.56).

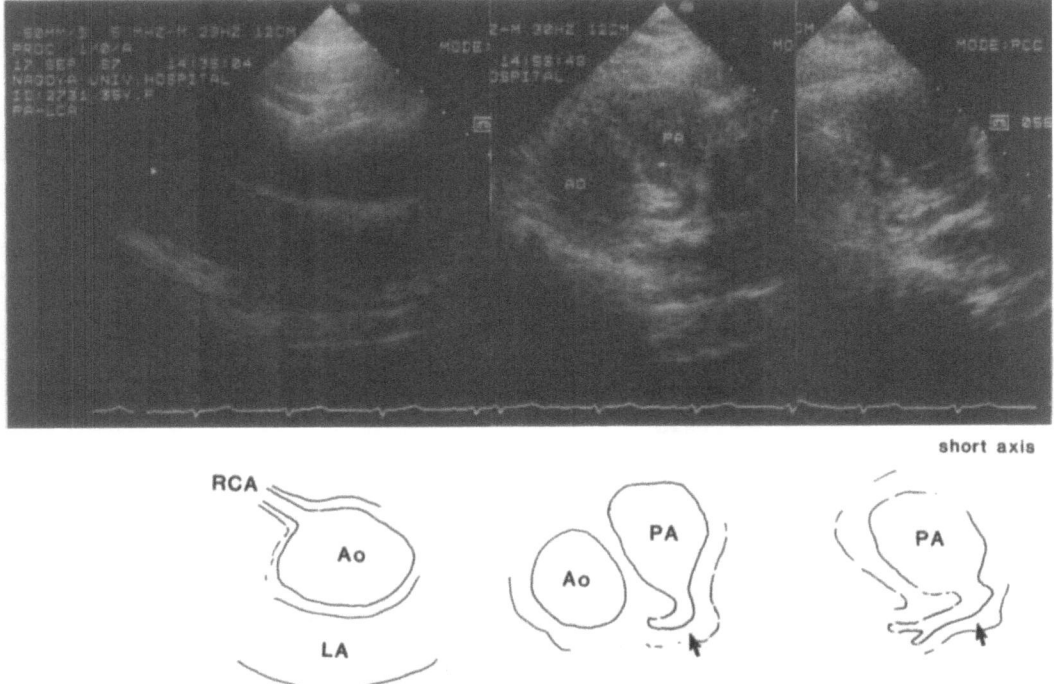

Figure 4.58. Parasternal short axis view from a patient with anomalous origin of the left coronary artery from the pulmonary artery. The left coronary artery arising from the pulmonary trunk can be observed. A dilated right coronary artery is also observed.

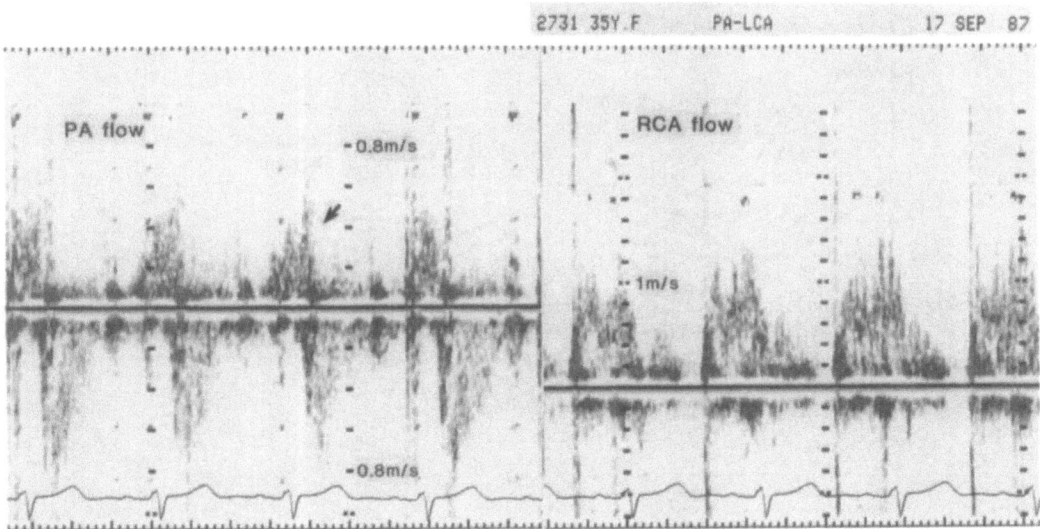

Figure 4.59. Pulsed Doppler echocardiogram from a patient with anomalous origin of the left coronary artery from the pulmonary artery. The pulsed Doppler echocardiogram recorded near the orifice of the left main coronary artery in the pulmonary trunk demonstrates the runoff from the anomalous left coronary artery as the retrograde flow during diastole (left panel). An increased flow in the right coronary artery is also observed (right panel)

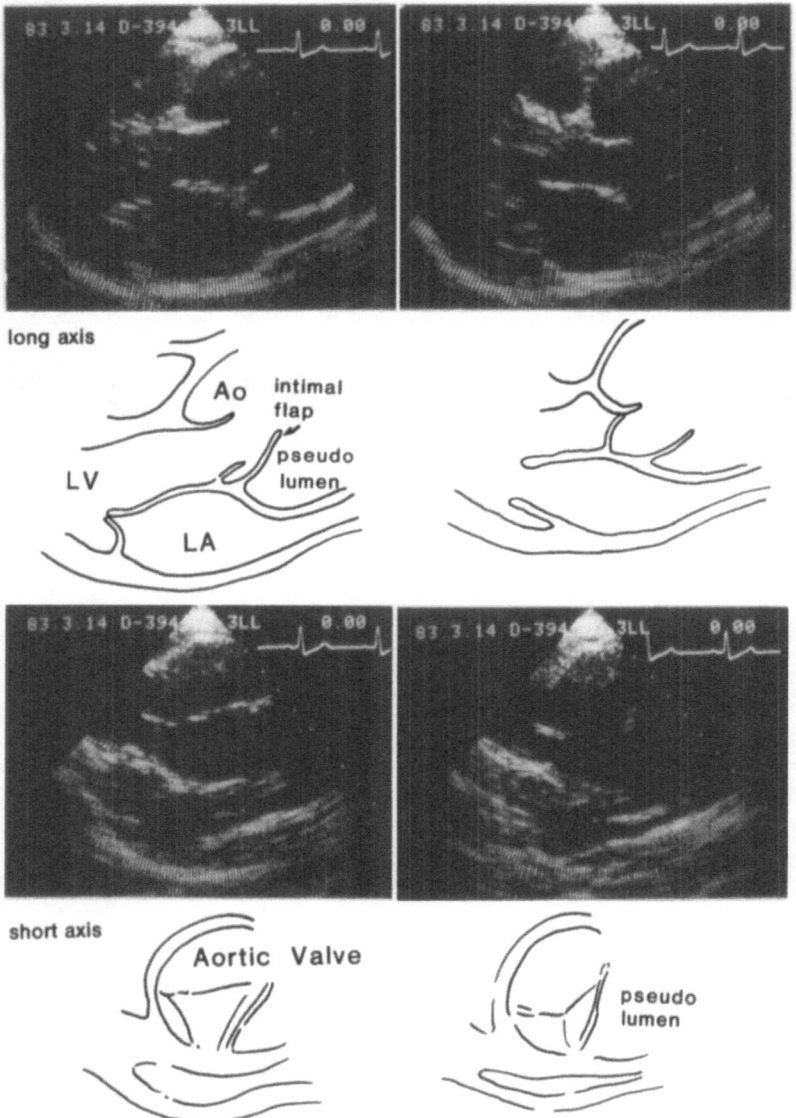

Figure 4.60.   Parasternal long and short axis views from a patient with Marfan's syndrome. A severe aortic dilatation with a dissecting aneurysm (pseudolumen) is demonstrated.

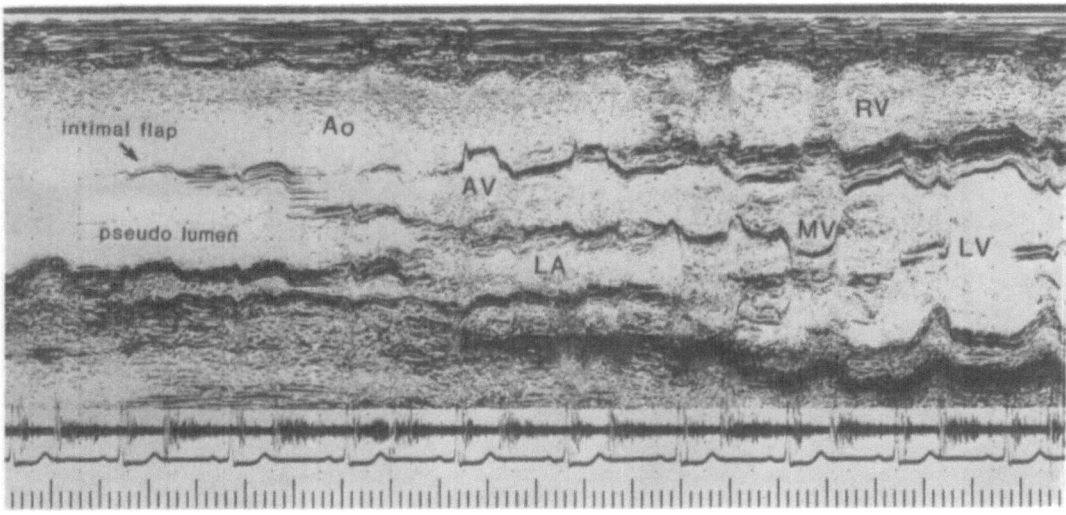

Figure 4.61. M-mode scan illustrating the intimal flap and pseudolumen of a dissecting aneurysm in a patient with Marfan's syndrome.

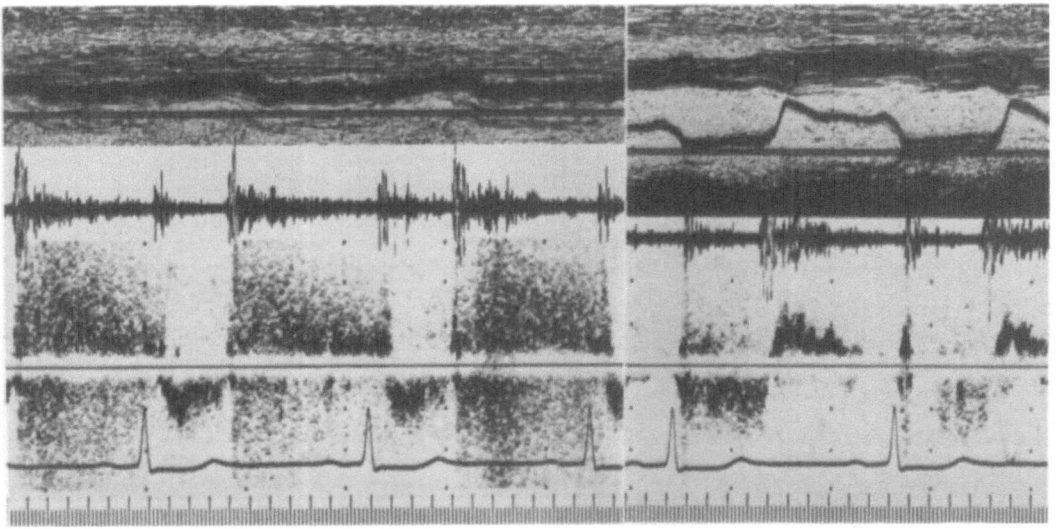

Figure 4.62. Pulsed Doppler echocardiogram of a patient with Marfan' syndrome. The left panel shows a diastolic turbulent flow in the left ventricular outflow tract (AR). The right panel shows a systolic turbulent flow in the left atrium (MR).

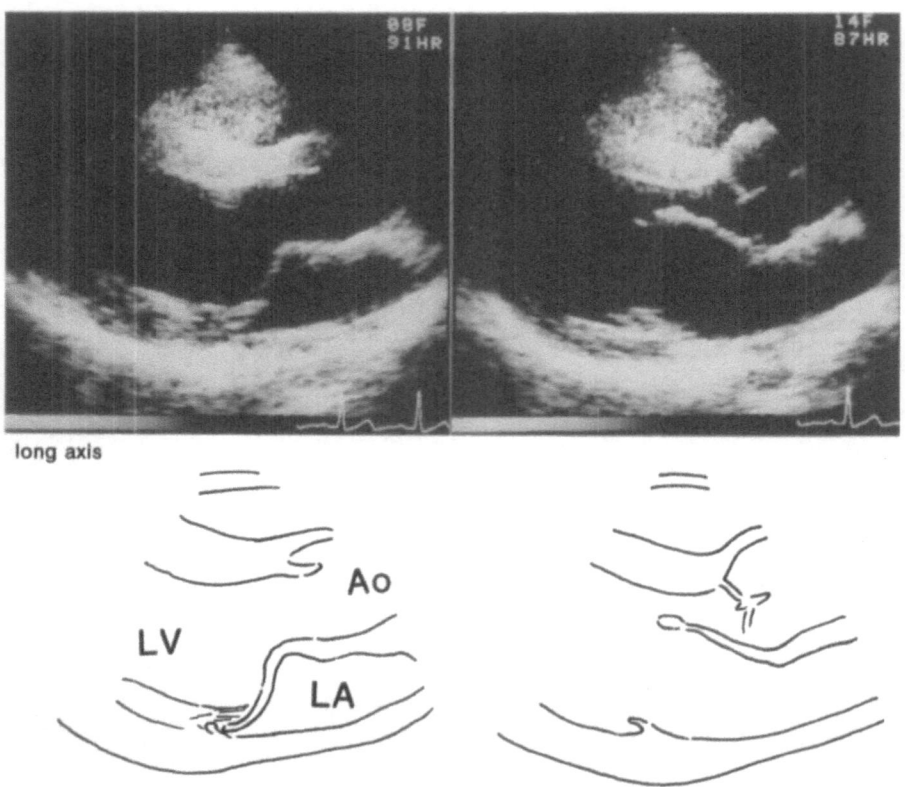

Figure 4.63. Parasternal long axis view of a patient with Marfan' syndrome. Prolapse of the anterior mitral valve leaflet (arrow) is clearly demonstrated without important annuloaortic ectasia.

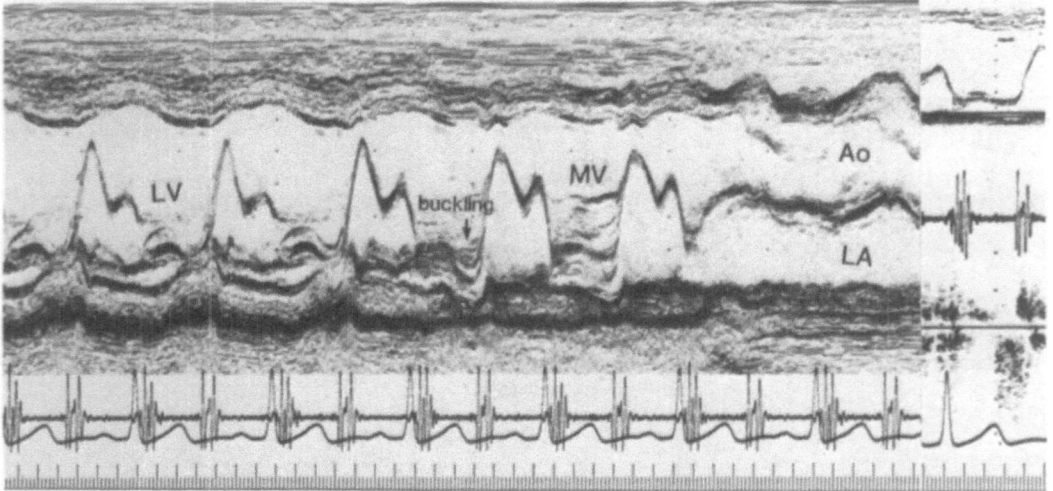

Figure 4.64. M-mode scan and pulsed Doppler echocardiogram illustrating a late systolic buckling of the mitral valve with systolic regurgitant flow due to prolapse in a patient with Marfan' syndrome.

18. Anomalous origin of the left main coronary artery from the pulmonary trunk

Anomalous origin of the left coronary artery from the pulmonary artery is a rare congenital cardiac anomaly. Using two-dimensional echocardiography, one can detect an anomalous left coronary artery arising from the pulmonary trunk (Figure 4.58). A dilated right coronary artery is another sign of this anomaly. This dilatation suggests the presence of collaterals supplying the left coronary from the right. Pulsed Doppler echocardiography can demonstrate the coronary-to-pulmonary artery shunt as the retrograde flow near the orifice of the left main coronary artery in the pulmonary trunk during diastole. An increased flow in the right coronary artery is also observed (Figure 4.59).

19. Marfan's syndrome

Marfan's syndrome is a systemic disease that also involves the cardiovascular system, such as annuloaortic ectasia (Figures 4.60, 61), and mitral valve prolapse (Figure 4.63, 64). These abnormalities may be detected by two-dimensional and M-mode echocardiography. Using Doppler techniques, the presence and severity of aortic and/or mitral regurgitation may be assessed (Figure 4.62). The annuloaortic ectasia is sometimes complicated by a dissecting aneurysm.

CHAPTER 5

Coronary artery disease

Echocardiography is an important tool for the assessment of patients with coronary artery disease (CAD). There are some limitations to its use related to the difficulty of obtaining optimal images. To understand the echocardiographic alterations due to coronary artery disease, it is necessary to have a good knowledge of the cardiac anatomy, especially the wall segments (Figure 5.1). Using echocardiography one can assess regional segments of the affected left ventricular wall in coronary artery disease. These segments fail to thicken during systole – in fact they thin – producing systolic bulging of the ischemic segment. Infarcted myocardium frequently shows an increased echo intensity. Two-dimensional echocardiography, sometimes in association with Doppler echocardiography, has been shown to be effective in diagnosing the mechanical complication of myocardial infarction, including ventricular septal rupture, ruptured papillary muscle, papillary muscle dysfunction, cardiac rupture, ventricular aneurysm, pseudoaneurysm and right ventricular infarction.

1. Wall motion abnormalities

Wall motion abnormalities represent an important indication of the presence of myocardial ischemia or infarction. M-mode is a limited method for evaluation of the global cardiac wall motion and two-dimensional examination is therefore preferable. Many of the sophisticated echocardiographic segmental classifications have been recommended. However, a simpler system of segmental division is more practical for clinical use. Thus, the short axis views at basal and midventricular level can be divided into four segment. The apex is considered as one segment (Figure 5.1). The severity of wall motion abnormalities is classified as Hypokinesis, Akinesis and Dyskinesis or Aneurysmal Bulging.

2. Wall thickening and echo intensity abnormalities

Sometimes the evaluation of wall motion abnormalities is complicated by the compensatory hyperkinetic motion of the adjacent normal cardiac muscle. Normally, the myocardium thickens during systole but, in the presence of ischemia, this does not occur. A more specific finding for detection of an infarcted area is abnormal wall thinning. Sometimes the increase in echo intensity of the myocardium can reflect the fibrosis of infarcted areas (Figures 5.2, 3). With recent improvement of echocardiographic equipment, myocardial tissue character-

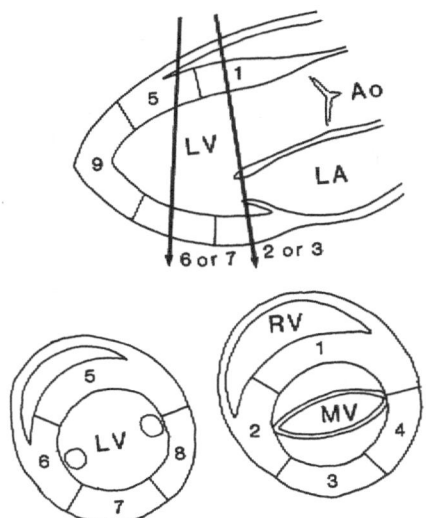

Figure 5.1. Schematic illustration of the left ventricular wall segments. (1) anteroseptal (basal), (2) inferior (basal), (3) posterior (basal), (4) lateral (basal), (5) anteroseptal (middle), (6) inferior (middle), (7) posterior (middle), (8) lateral (middle), (9) apical.

ization may become an important tool for the evaluation of patients with coronary artery disease. In this method, the phase, amplitude, and frequency of backscattered ultrasound from the myocardial tissue is used to characterize the fibrosis of infarcted areas.

3. Complications of myocardial infarction

A. Ventricular aneurysm

This complication frequently occurs in patients with extensive myocardial infarction. The detection of an aneurysm is easily carried out by two-dimensional echocardiography, which is the method of choice for clinical diagnosis. The most common site for aneurysm is the apical portion (Figures 5.4, 5), but it can occur in any part of the ventricle (Figures 5.6, 7). In this condition, the blood flow stasis near the aneurysm sometimes become echogenic and can be seen (Figure 5.4). Doppler echocardiography can explain the hemodynamic derangements secondary to aneurysm, for example, systolic reversal of flow into the aneurysmatic sac (Figure 5.8).

B. Mural thrombus of the left ventricle

This complication usually occurs during the acute phase of myocardial infarction. Commonly, the thrombus is located adjacent to a dyskinetic portion, especially in the apex (Figures 5.9, 10). Two-dimensional echocardiography plays an important role in the evaluation of patients with left ventricular thrombi because, in the chronic phase, the thrombus usually tends to disappear.

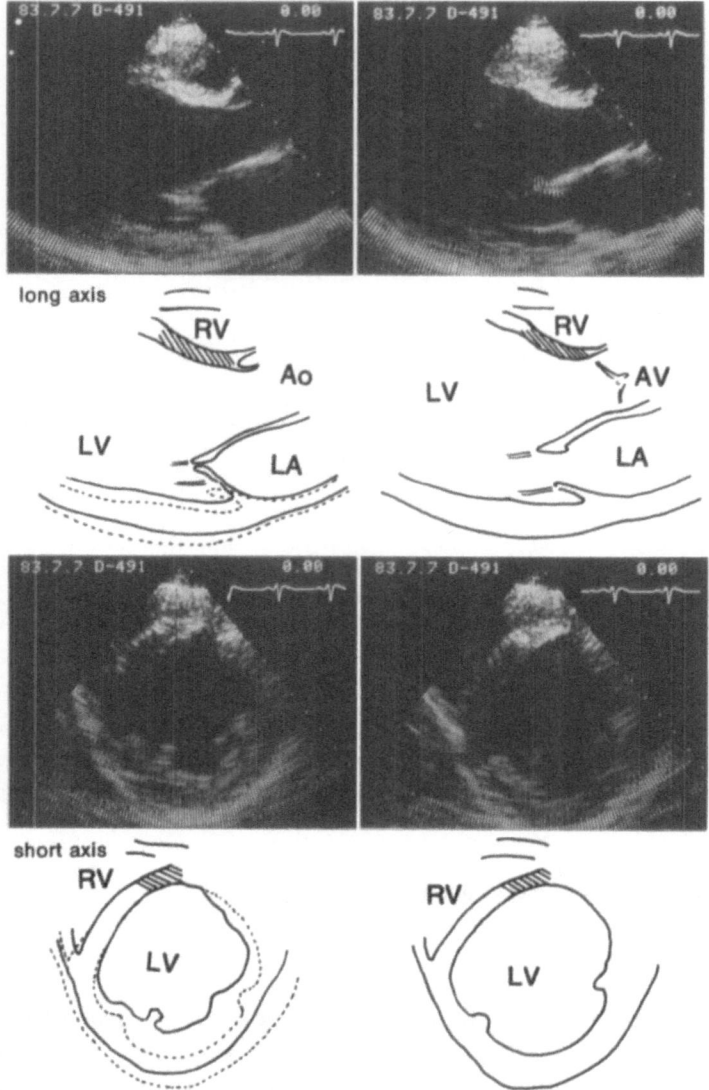

Figure 5.2.   Two-dimensional long and short axis view from a patient with an anteroseptal myocardial infarction. Akinesis, depressed systolic wall thickening and increased echo intensity of the anteroseptal wall are noted.

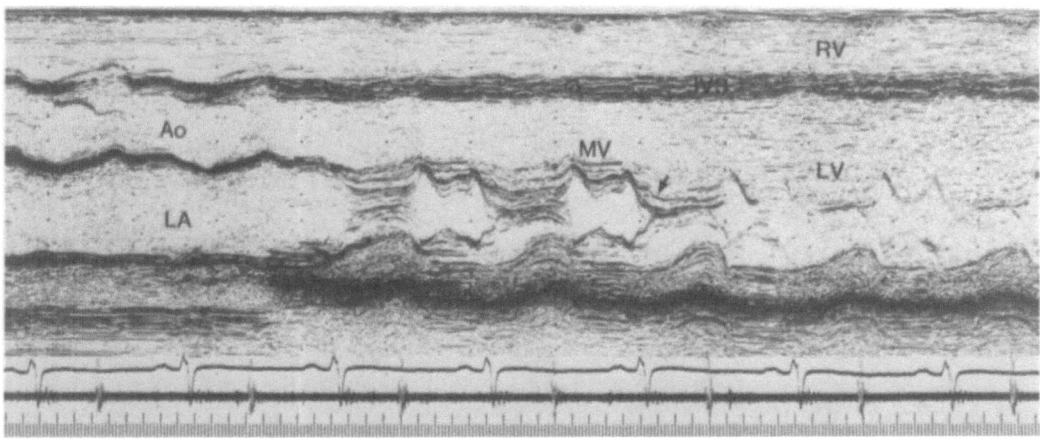

Figure 5.3. M-mode scan of a patient with an anteroseptal myocardial infarction. The interventricular septum (IVS) demonstrates akinesis, loss of systolic wall thickening and increased echo intensity.

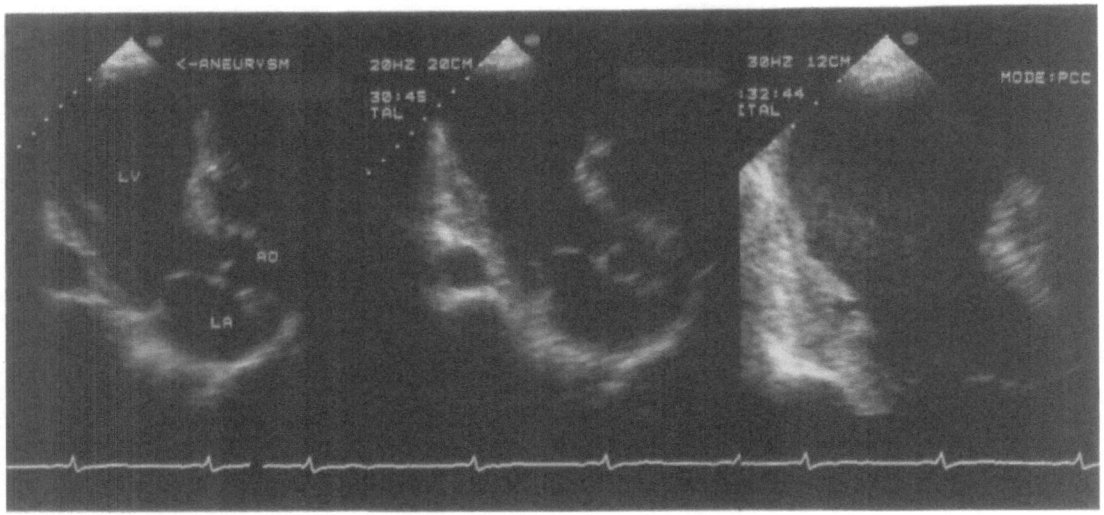

Figure 5.4. Apical long axis view of a patient with left ventricular aneurysm. This figure illustrates an apical aneurysm. In the left panel, systolic bulging of the aneurysmatic area is visible. Near the aneurysm, intra-ventricular smoke-like echoes are noted, due to flow stasis (right panel).

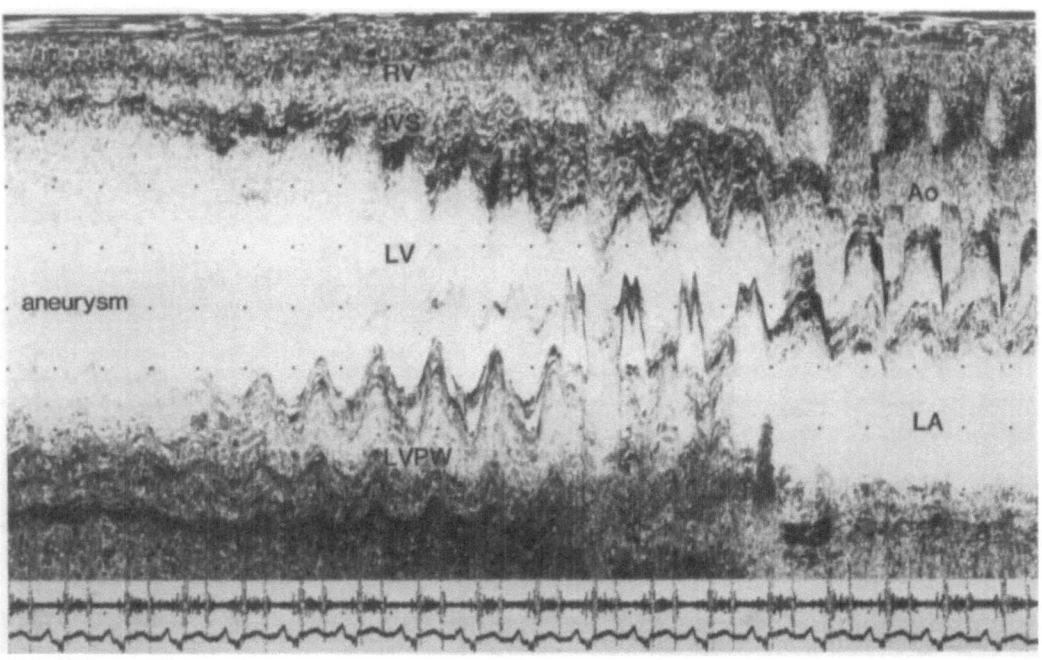

Figure 5.5. M-mode scan of a patient with left ventricular aneurysm. Severe dilatation of the apical area with compensatory hyperkinetic motion of the basal portions can be observed.

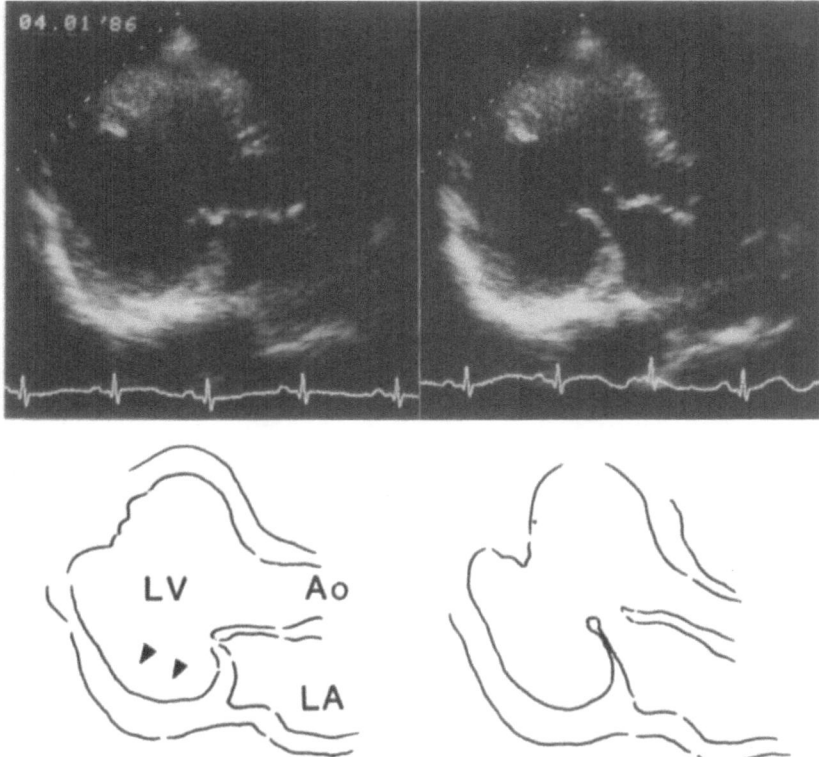

Figure 5.6. Parasternal long axis view demonstrating aneurysmatic bulging of the left ventricular posterior wall (arrow head) due to myocardial infarction.

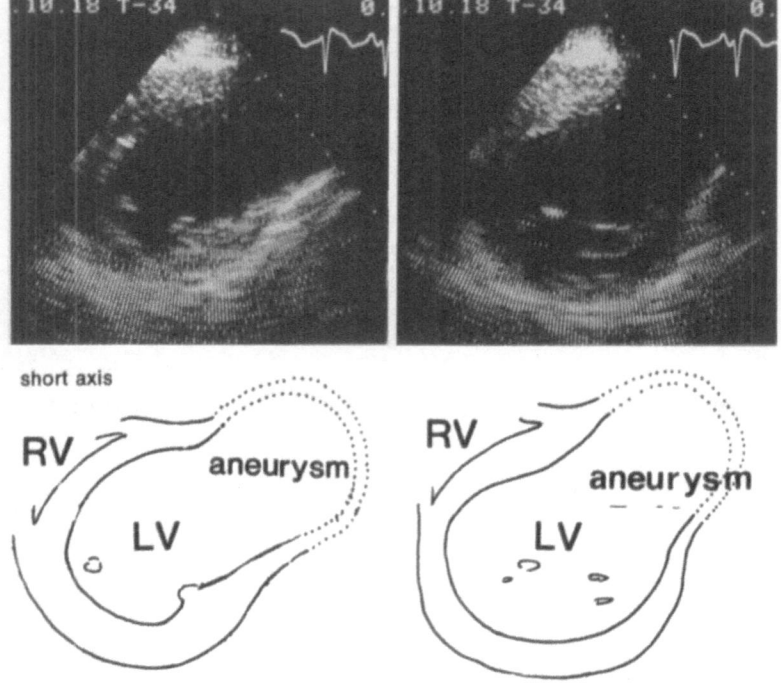

Figure 5.7.   Parasternal short axis view of a patient with left ventricular aneurysm of the lateral wall.

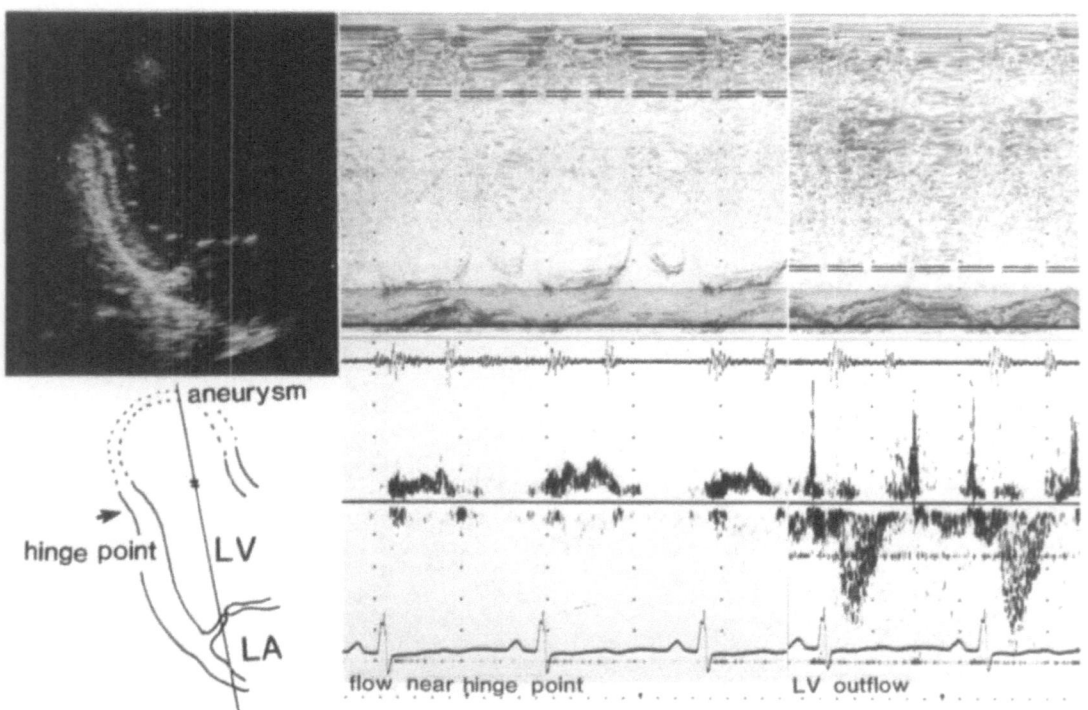

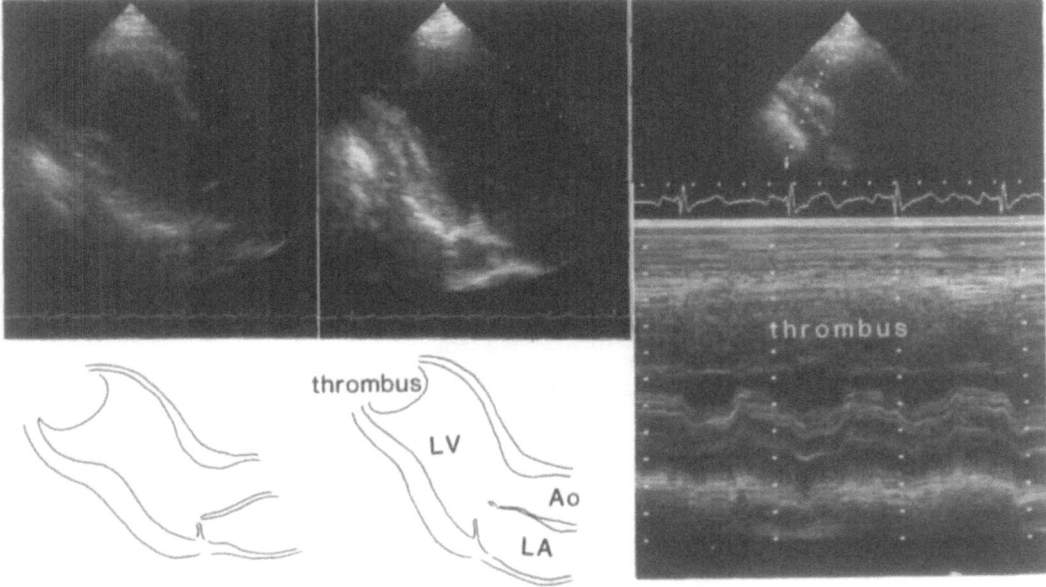

Figure 5.9. Two-dimensional and M-mode echocardiograms of a patient with a left ventricular apical thrombus in the acute phase. The M-mode shows a cloud of echoes from the thrombus in the anterior portion of apex and the posterior wall motion is dyskinetic. This thrombus disappeared in the chronic phase.

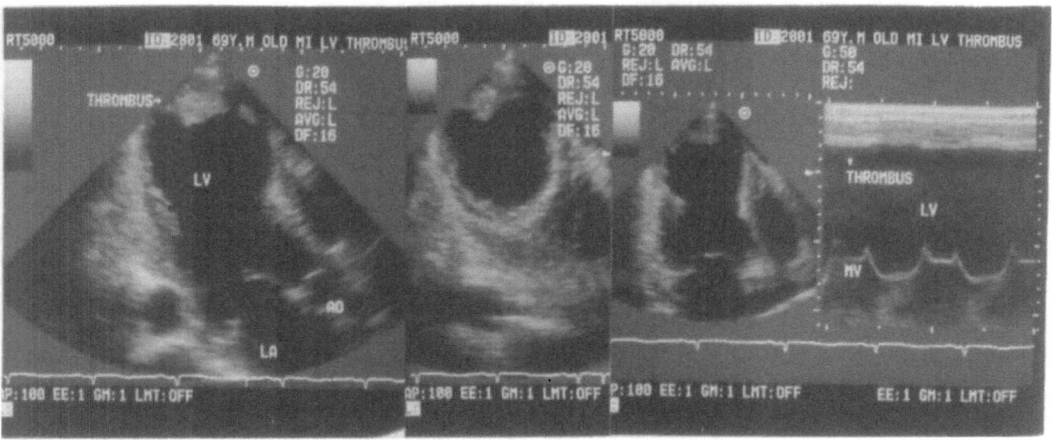

Figure 5.10. Two-dimensional and M-mode echocardiograms of a patient with a left ventricular apical thrombus in the chronic phase. In this case, the echogenicity of the thrombus is stronger than that in Figure 5.9.

Figure 5.8. Pulsed Doppler echocardiogram of a patient with an apical aneurysm. When the sample volume is positioned in the aneurysmatic area, a systolic reversal of flow is demonstrated (left panel). The right panel shows a normal systolic ejection flow in the basal portion.

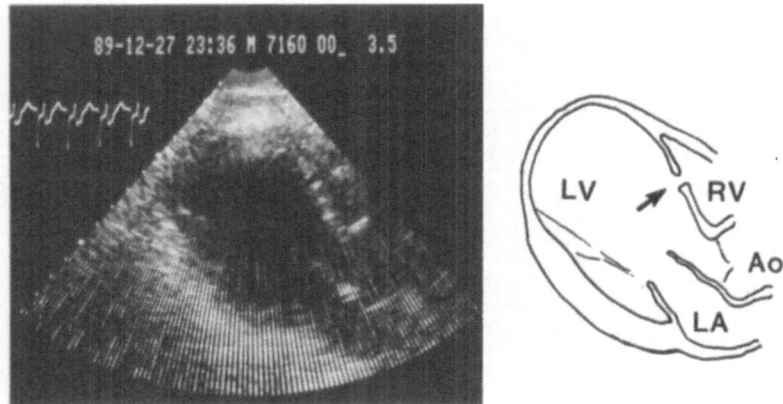

Figure 5.11. Apical long axis view demonstrating a ventricular septal rupture (arrow) in a patient with an acute myocardial infarction.

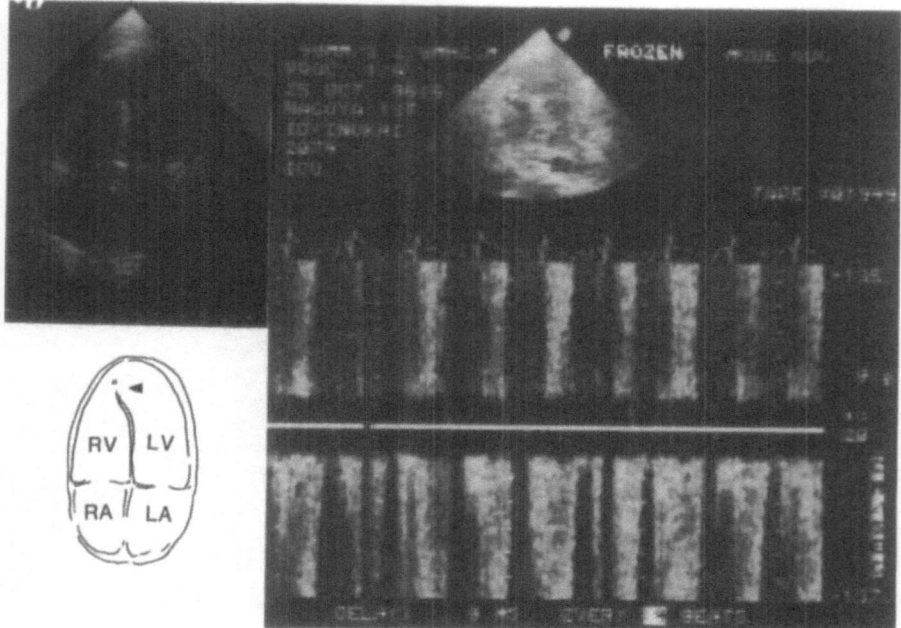

Figure 5.12. Apical four-chamber view and pulsed Doppler echocardiogram of a patient with a ventricular septal rupture. The rupture of the interventricular septum near the apex can be seen (arrow head). Pulsed Doppler shows systolic turbulent flow on the right ventricular side.

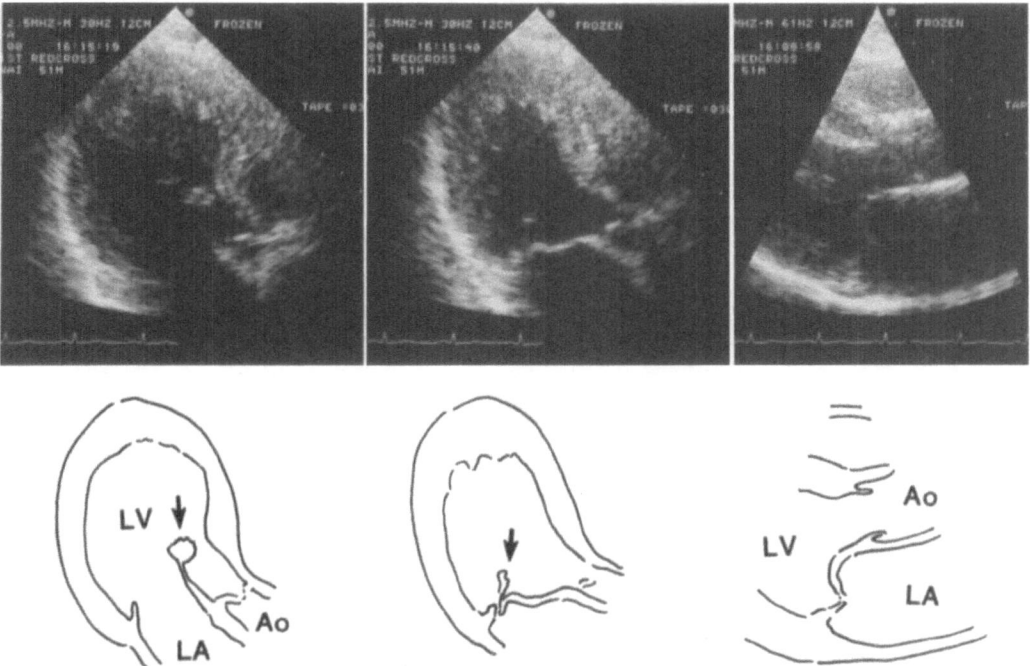

Figure 5.13.   Apical and parasternal long axis view of a patient with posterior papillary muscle rupture. One can see an abnormal echo attached to the anterior mitral leaflet, and irregular motion (arrow). Flail mitral valve leaflets (anterior and posterior) are also clearly observed.

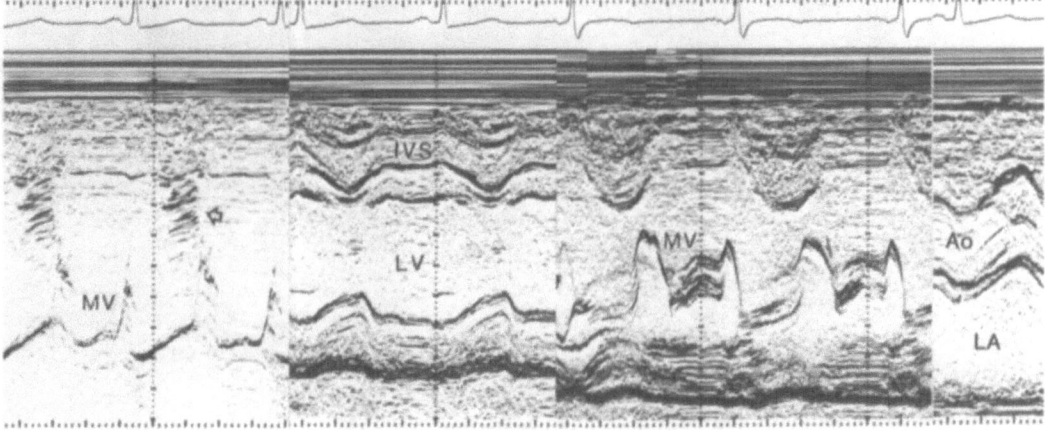

Figure 5.14.   M-mode echocardiogram of a patient with a posterior papillary muscle rupture. The left panel shows an abnormal echo in the left ventricle (arrow) obtained from the apical approach. In contrast, the ordinary parasternal approaches do not demonstrate this.

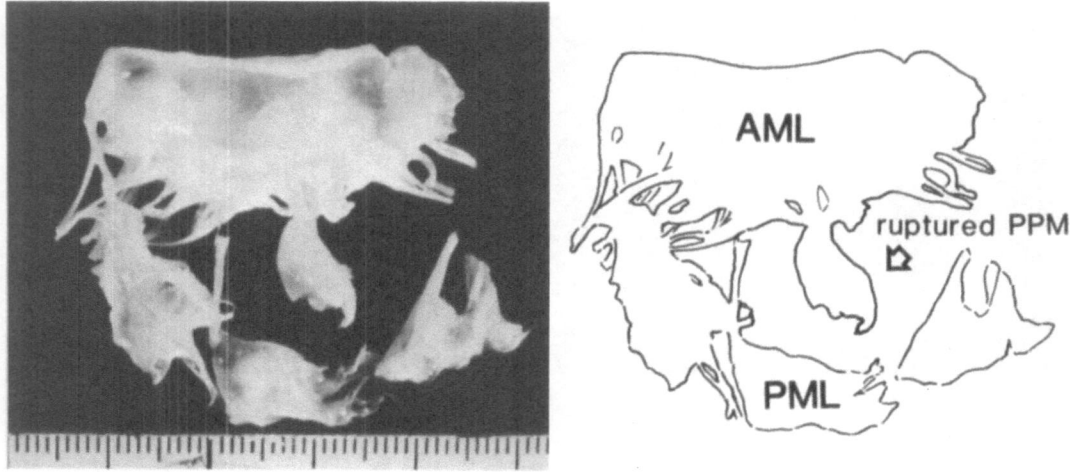

Figure 5.15.   Operatory specimen of mitral valve in a patient with posterior papillary muscle rupture. One can appreciate the ruptured posterior papillary muscle (PPM) attached to the anterior mitral leaflet (AML).

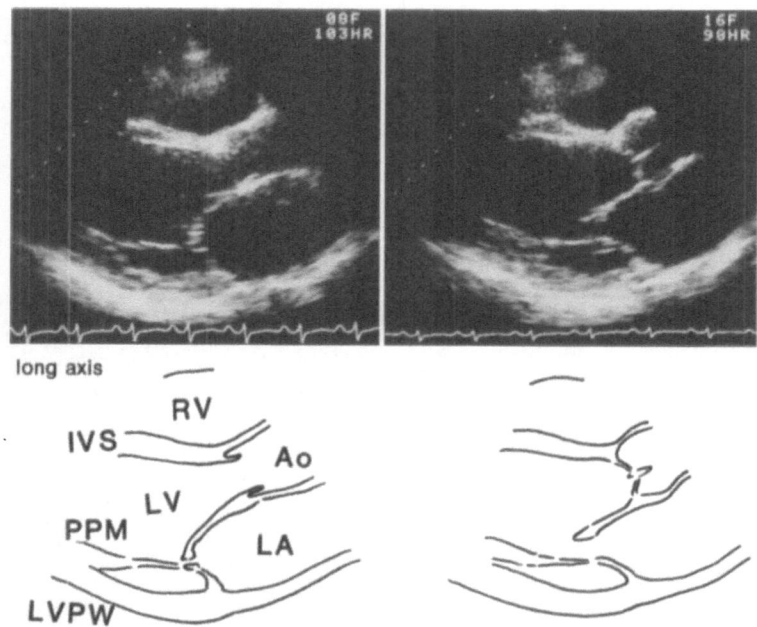

Figure 5.16.   The parasternal long axis view demonstrates a posterior mitral valve prolapse due to papillary muscle dysfunction in a patient with an inferior myocardial infarction.

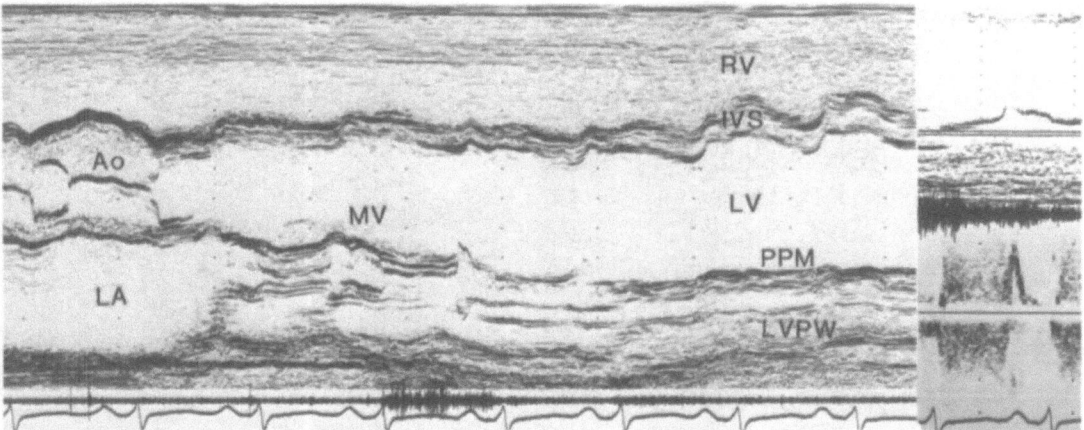

Figure 5.17. M-mode scan and pulsed Doppler echocardiogram of a patient with an inferior myocardial infarction and papillary muscle dysfunction. Left vaentricular posterior wall akinesis and increased echo intensity of the posterior papillary muscle (PPM) are clearly demonstrated. The right panel shows a systolic flow turbulent in the left atrium corresponding to mitral regurgitation.

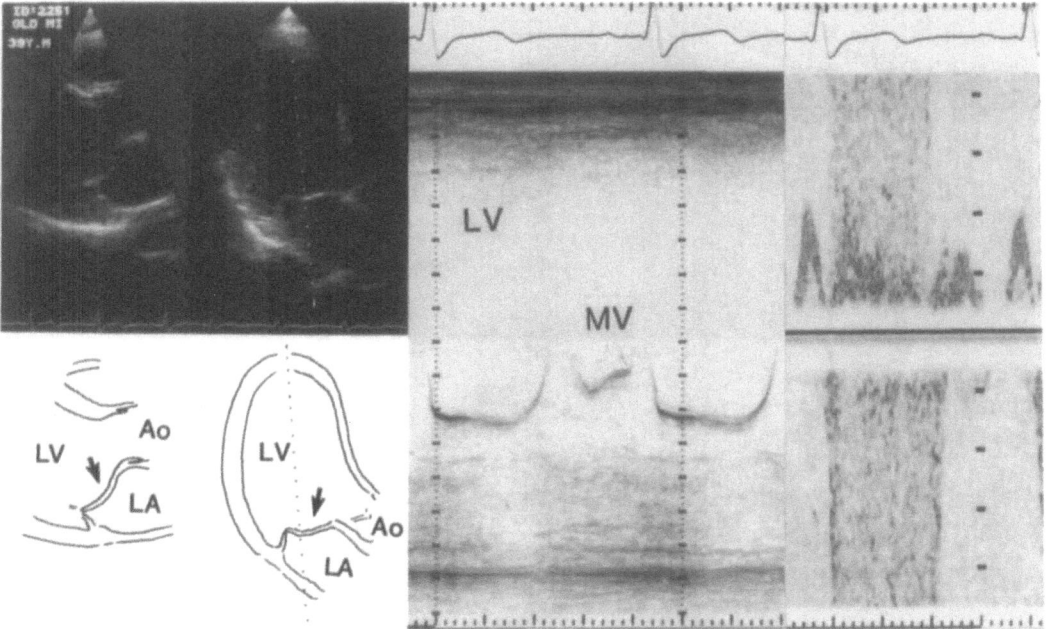

Figure 5.18. Parasternal and apical long axis view, M-mode and pulsed Doppler echocardiogram of a patient with an inferior myocardial infarction. Parasternal and apical long axis views show an anterior mitral valve prolapse (arrow). The M-mode echocardiogram obtained from the apical approach illustrates the posterior displacement of the anterior mitral leaflet. The pulsed Doppler echocardiogram demonstrates a systolic flow turbulence in the left atrium (mitral regurgitation).

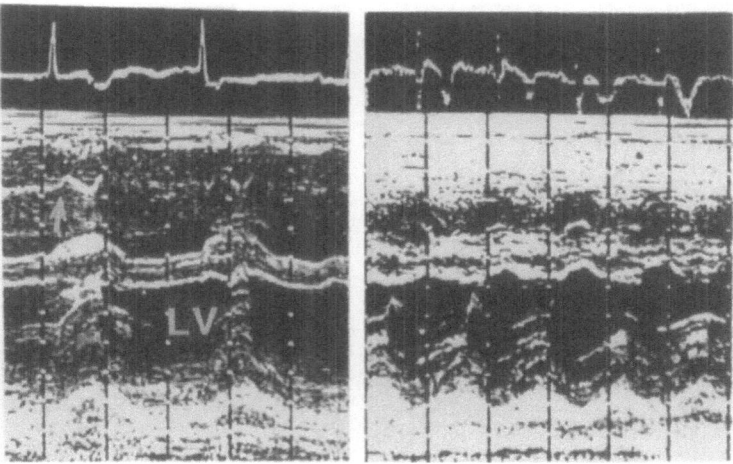

Figure 5.19. M-mode echocardiogram of a patient with a right ventricular myocardial infarction. The left panel illustrates right ventricular dilatation and systolic anterior motion of the interventricular septum. The increased systolic thickening of the interventricular septum suggests a compensatory motion due to right ventricular dysfunction. In the right ventricle, a Swan-Ganz catheter echo is indicated by an arrow. The right panel shows the echocardiogram of the same patient one month after the acute phase, with improvement of the interventricular septal motion and right ventricular dimensions.

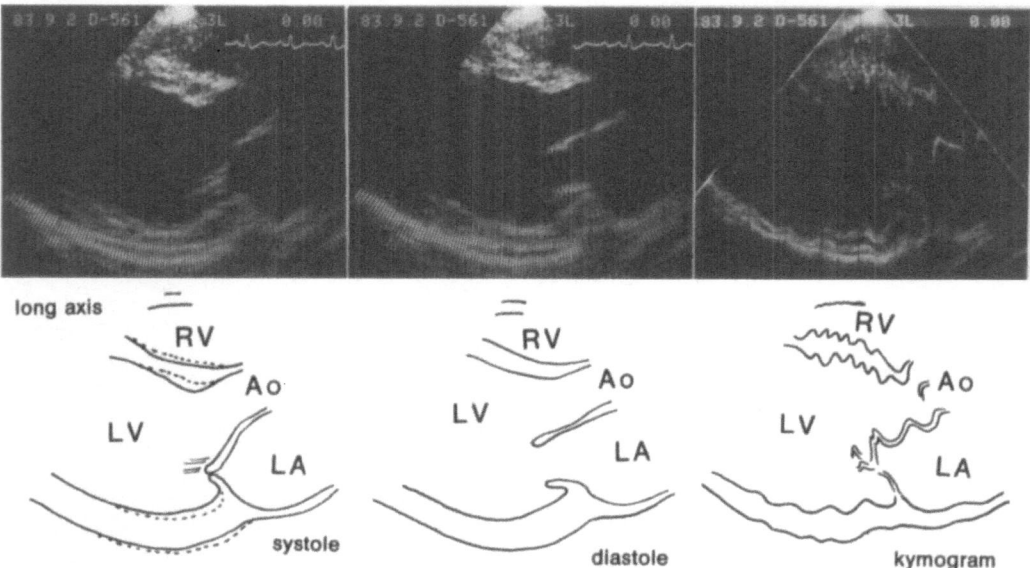

Figure 5.20. Parasternal long axis echocardiogram and kymogram of a patient with an ischemic cardiomyopathy. Left ventricular dilatation and severe hypokinesis are present. The right panel demonstrates the same findings by a kymographic image.

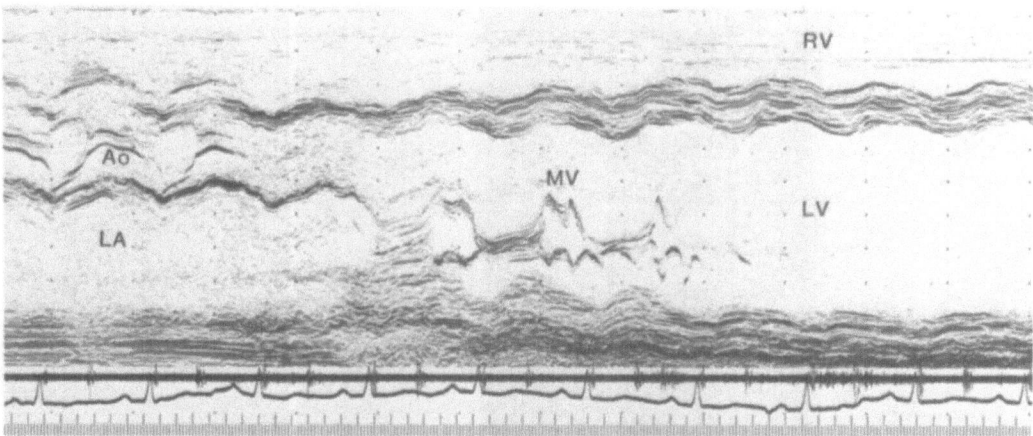

Figure 5.21. M-mode scan of a patient with an ischemic cardiomyopathy. One notes the left ventricular dilatation and severe hypokinesis, it is very difficult to differentiate ischemic from dilated cardiomyopathy.

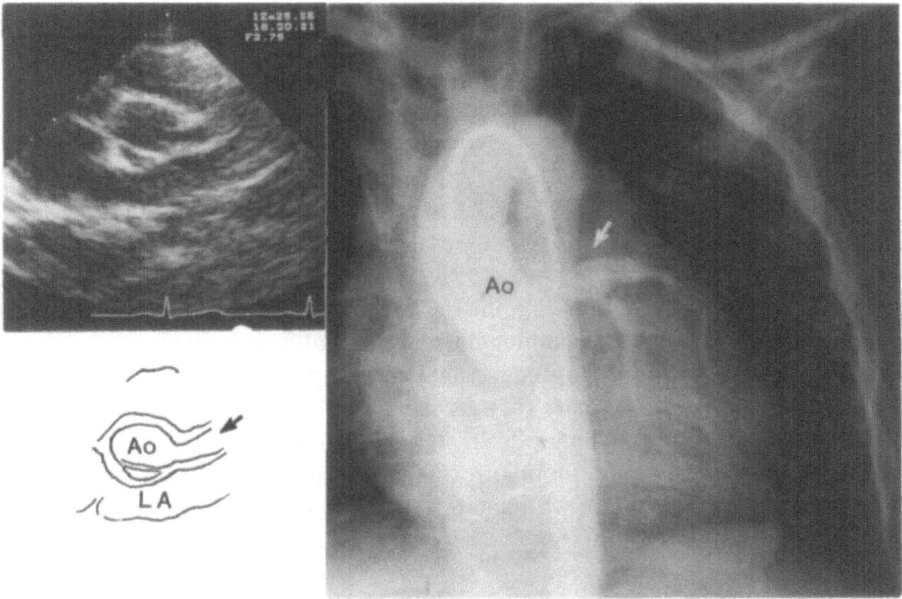

Figure 5.22. Parasternal short axis view and aortogram demonstrating aneurysmatic dilatation of the left main coronary artery (arrow) in a nine year old patient with Kawasaki's disease.

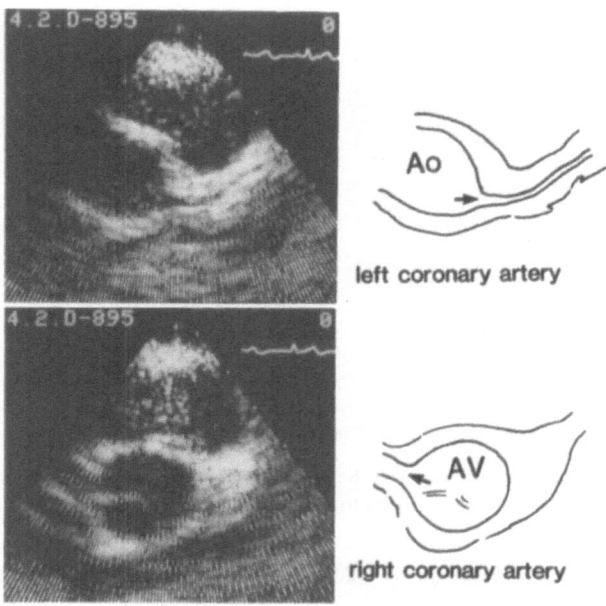

left coronary artery

right coronary artery

Figure 5.23.   Parasternal short axis view of a ten year-old patient with Kawasaki's disease. Increased echo intensity
of the left coronary artery (arrow) can be seen, in contrast, the right coronary artery is normal.

C. Rupture of the ventricular septum

Rupture of the ventricular septum complicates the course of a myocardial infarction, and
prompt detection is essential for planning correct medical management and in determining
the time of surgery. Recently, two-dimensional and Doppler echocardiography have been
shown to demonstrate the presence of ventricular septal rupture. Usually, the defect is
located near the apical portion (Figure 5.11). Visualization by two-dimensional echocardiography is sometimes difficult and Doppler echocardiography can discern an abnormal flow
across the interventricular septum with higher sensitivity and specificity (Figure 5.12).

D. Mitral regurgitation

Following an acute myocardial infarction, mitral regurgitation can occur due to rupture or
dysfunction of the papillary muscle. Using two-dimensional echocardiography, the ruptured
papillary muscle and flailing mitral valve can be demonstrated (Figures 5.13, 14, 15). Papillary
muscle dysfunction usually occurs in patients with inferior myocardial infarction. In this case,
we can appreciate the diminished systolic shortening and increased echo intensity of the
posterior papillary muscle (Figures 5.16, 17) and sometimes the presence of mitral valve
prolapse (Figure 5.18).

E. Right ventricular myocardial infarction

The right ventricle is also affected by coronary artery disease. In patients with inferior
myocardial infarction this complication frequently occurs. Echocardiographic findings in-

clude right ventricular dilatation with abnormal motion of right ventricular free wall and/or interventricular septum (Figure 5.19).

4. Ischemic cardiomyopathy

This condition is a chronic disease that is originated from myocardial ischemia. The echocardiographic findings of ischemic cardiomyopathy and dilated cardiomyopathy are very similar and sometimes coronary angiography is necessary to differentiate between the two (Figures 5.20, 21).

5. Examination of coronary arteries

Using two-dimensional echocardiography, one can evaluate the proximal portion of the left and right coronary arteries. Several diseases can be demonstrated, for example atherosclerotic plaques, coronary arterio-venous fistula and Kawasaki's disease. The echocardiographic findings consist of stenosis of the lumen, aneurysmatic dilatation (Figure 5.22) and increased echo intensity of the coronary artery walls reflecting an inflammatory process (Figure 5.23).

Myocardial diseases

1. Hypertrophic cardiomyopathy

Hypertrophic cardiomyopathy (HCM) is a disease that is characterized by a hypertrophied and non dilated left ventricle. This hypertrophy occurs mainly in the interventricular septum, and is usually called 'asymmetric septal hypertrophy' (ASH) (Figures 6.1, 2). Hemodynamically, this disease can be divided into hypertrophic obstructive cardiomyopathy (HOCM) and hypertrophic non-obstructive cardiomyopathy. HOCM has a systolic pressure gradient between the left ventricular cavity and left ventricular outflow tract. This hemodynamic alteration bears several names that emphasize its obstructive nature; muscular subaortic stenosis or idiopathic hypertrophic subaortic stenosis (IHSS). The characteristic echocardiographic findings of HOCM involve the systolic anterior motion (SAM) of the mitral valve or chordae tendineae and partial systolic closure of the aortic valve shown by M-mode (Figures 6.3, 4). The Doppler method can indicate the presence, localization, and severity of an intraventricular obstruction by showing alterations in the ejection flow. With the apical approach, the pulsed Doppler echocardiogram shows highly aliased left ventricular outflow velocity at the level of the narrowest flow trajectory, and continuous wave Doppler echocardiography should be utilized to measure the peak flow velocity through the narrowed outflow tract (Figure 6.5). This left ventricular outflow recording has a late systolic peak which is characteristic of a dynamic obstruction to flow. The faded appearance of the spectral flow pattern in late systole is caused by the reduced volume of blood through the obstructed outflow tract. This reduced flow volume can be also reflected as late systolic semi-closure of the aortic valve in M-mode echocardiogram (Figure 6.6). The optimally recorded peak velocity can be translated to the peak intraventricular pressure gradient using the modified Bernoulli equation. This measurement can also be applied to evaluate the effect of beta-blockade in decreasing the outflow obstruction (Figure 6.7). In non-obstructive cardiomyopathy, the peak ejection velocity shows up slightly higher than that in normal subjects, but does not exceed 2 m/sec (Figure 6.8). Pulsed Doppler findings can suggest impaired diastolic filling if the transmitral flow shows decreased peak velocity in the rapid filling phase and a compensatory increase due to atrial contraction (Figure 6.9). This disease is frequently accompanied by mitral regurgitation, possibly due to left ventricular geometrical distortion

$\longrightarrow$

Figure 6.1. Long and short axis two-dimensional echocardiogram of a patient with hypertrophic non-obstructive cardiomyopathy (HCM). Marked hypertrophy of the interventricular septum is noted.

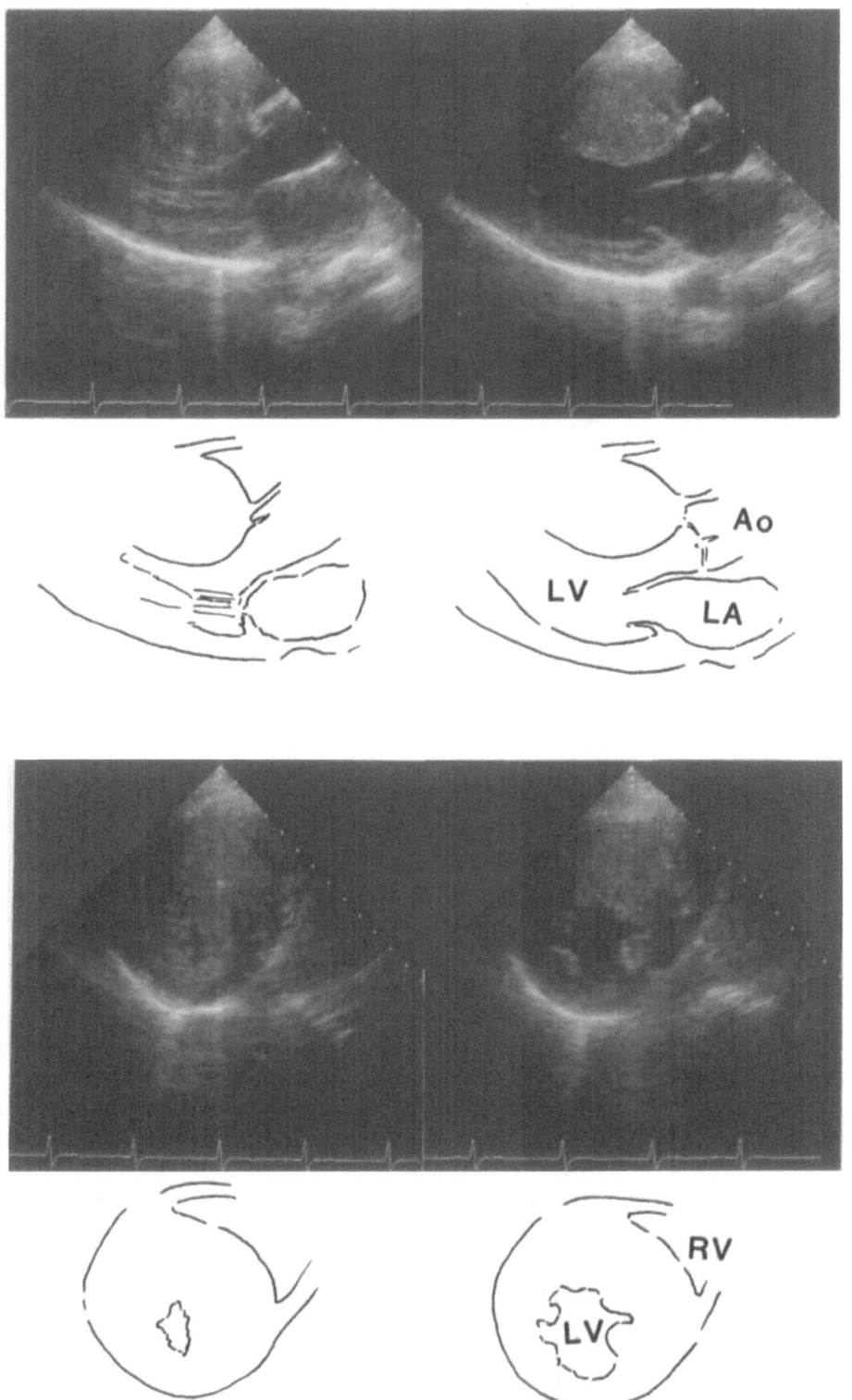

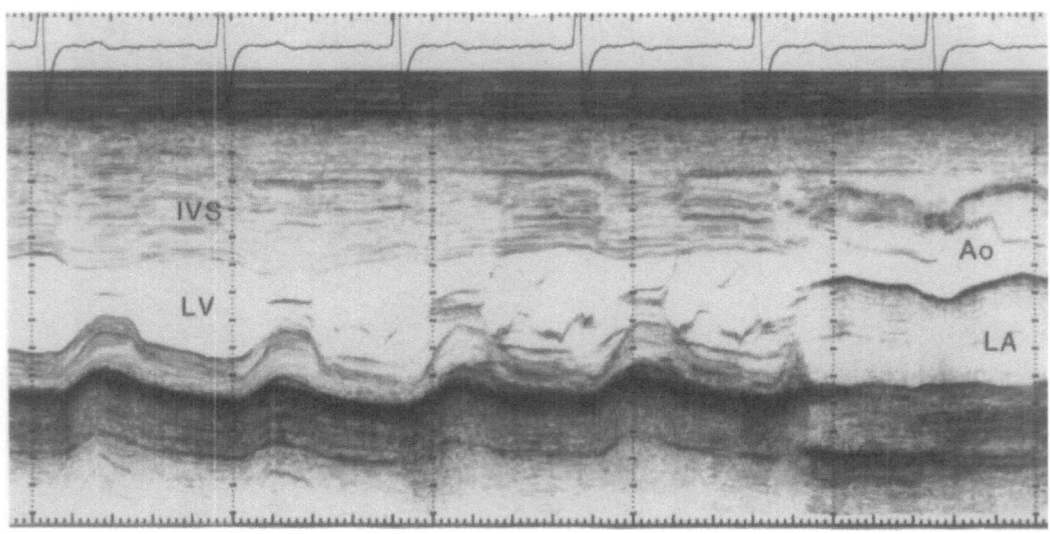

Figure 6.2.   M-mode scan of a patient with HCM. A markedly hypertrophied interventricular septum (IVS) is observed, without SAM of the mitral valve. Hypokinesis of IVS is also observed.

and/or mitral leaflet-septal contact (Figure 6.10). When this hypertrophy occurs only in the left ventricular apex, it is called 'Apical Hypertrophy' (Figures 6.11, 12). It may also occur in the posterior wall, lateral wall or, in rare cases, in the whole left ventricle (Figures 6.13, 14).

2. Dilated cardiomyopathy

Dilated cardiomyopathy (DCM) is also a primary myocardial disease that is manifested by left ventricular dilatation and poorly contracting left ventricular walls. The left ventricular walls tend to be thinner due to myocardial degenerative changes and the left ventricular cavity turns from ellipsoid to circular in shape (Figures 6.15, 17). In the M-mode, one can see the characteristic findings of dilated cardiomyopathy, such as poor anterior motion of the aorta, gradual closure of aortic valve and decreased mitral valve opening (Figure 6.16). The B-B' step of the anterior mitral leaflet is frequently seen, and might reflect elevated left ventricular end-diastolic pressure. Two-dimensional and Doppler method can demonstrate the mitral valve prolapse and regurgitation due to left ventricular geometrical distortion and papillary muscle dysfunction (Figure 6.18). The flow pattern in left ventricular outflow is usually normal in appearance, but the peak velocity may be lower than 0.6 m/sec and the flow velocity integral is small, whose findings represent the low cardiac output state (Figure 6.19). The development of a left ventricular intracavitary thrombus due to blood stasis sometimes occurs (Figure 6.20).

In rare cases right ventricular dysplasia can occur, in which the ventricular musculature is partially or totally replaced by fatty and fibrous tissue. In such patients, clinical manifestations are mainly due to arrhythmia and therefore this entity is termed 'arrhythmogenic right ventricular dysplasia' (ARVD). Echocardiographic findings consist of dilatation of the right ventricle with abnormal bulging (Figure 6.21). Interventricular septal motion can be affected without evidence of pulmonary artery dilatation or pulmonary hypertension (Figures 6.22, 23) which emphasize its idiopathic origin.

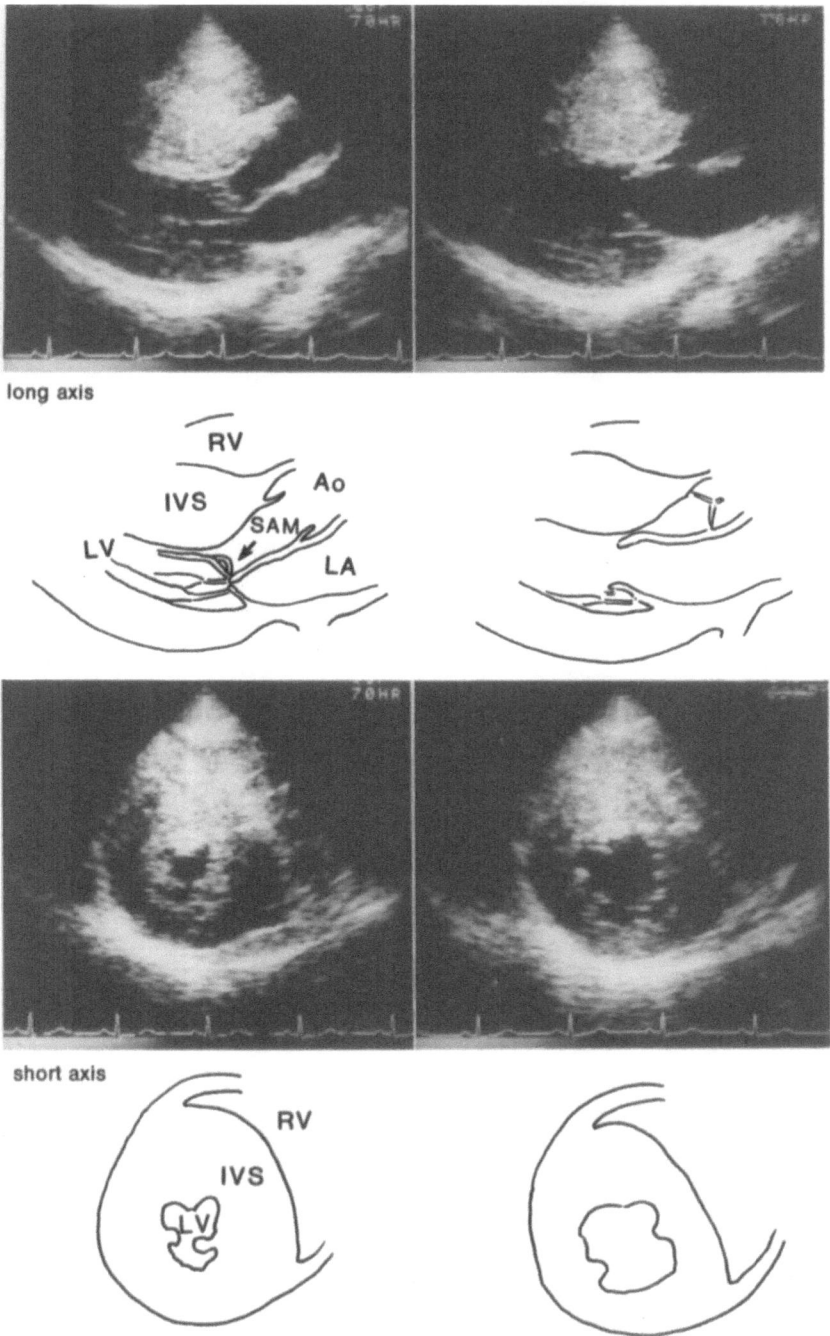

long axis

RV

IVS

Ao

SAM

LV

LA

short axis

RV

IVS

LV

Figure 6.3. Long and short axis two-dimensional echocardiogram of a patient with hypertrophic obstructive cardiomyopathy (HOCM). In the long axis view, the IVS is markedly hypertrophied and systolic anterior movement (SAM) of the chordae tendineae is demonstrated. Asymmetrical septal hypertrophy (ASH) can also be seen.

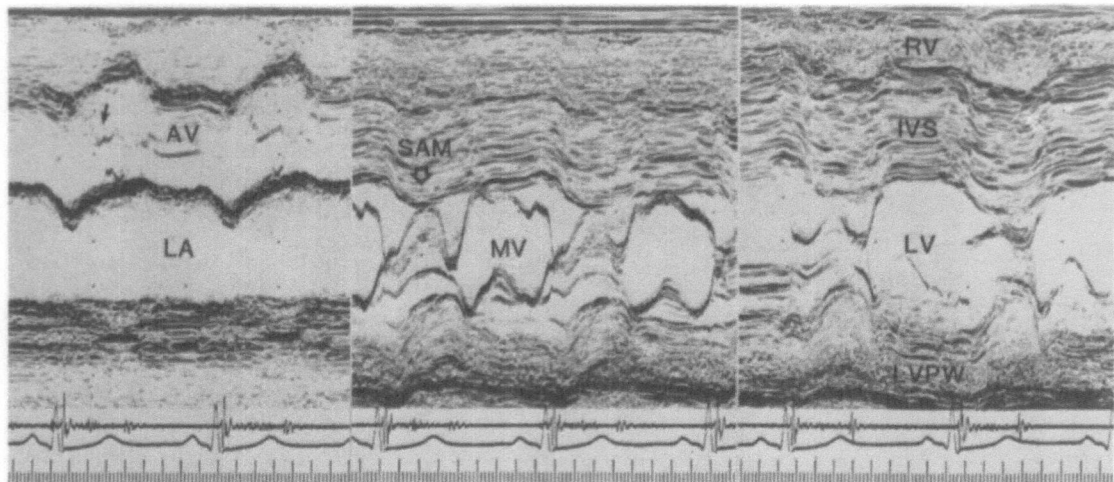

Figure 6.4. M-mode echocardiogram of a patient with HOCM. The aortic valve has a partial systolic closure and the mitral valve echo shows typical SAM.

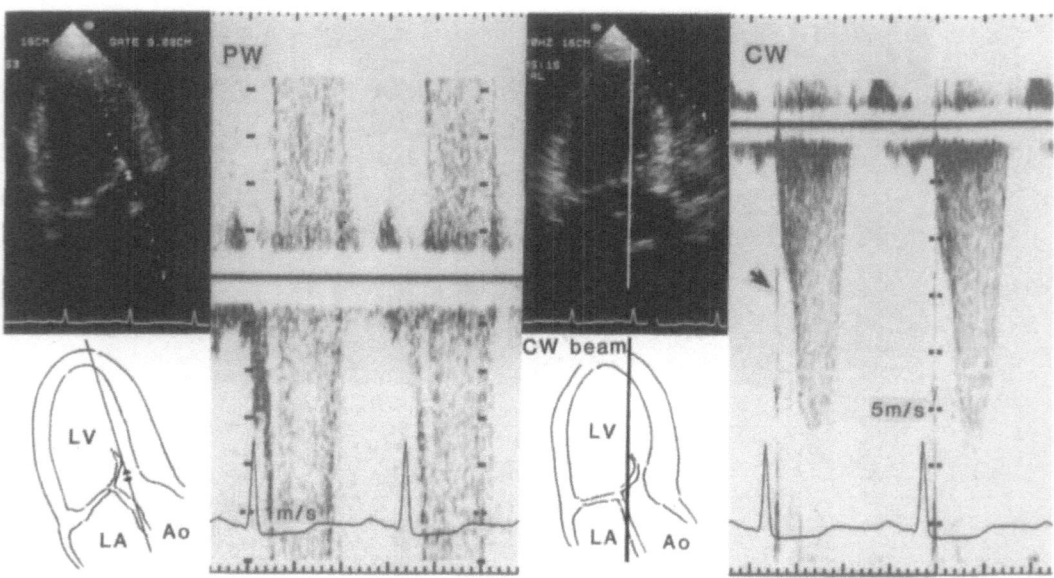

Figure 6.5. Pulsed and continuous wave Doppler echocardiogram in left ventricular outflow velocity of a patient with HOCM. The left ventricular ejection flow recorded by pulsed wave (PW) Doppler method at the site of outflow tract shows turbulence with multiple aliasing and its peak velocity cannot be assessed. Continuous wave (CW) Doppler echocardiogram of left ventricular outflow from the apical window shows the peaking of the flow velocity curve in late systole, whose finding is characteristic of a dynamic outflow obstruction (arrow). The maximal flow velocity of 5.5 m/sec indicates the existence of a peak pressure gradient of 121 mm Hg.

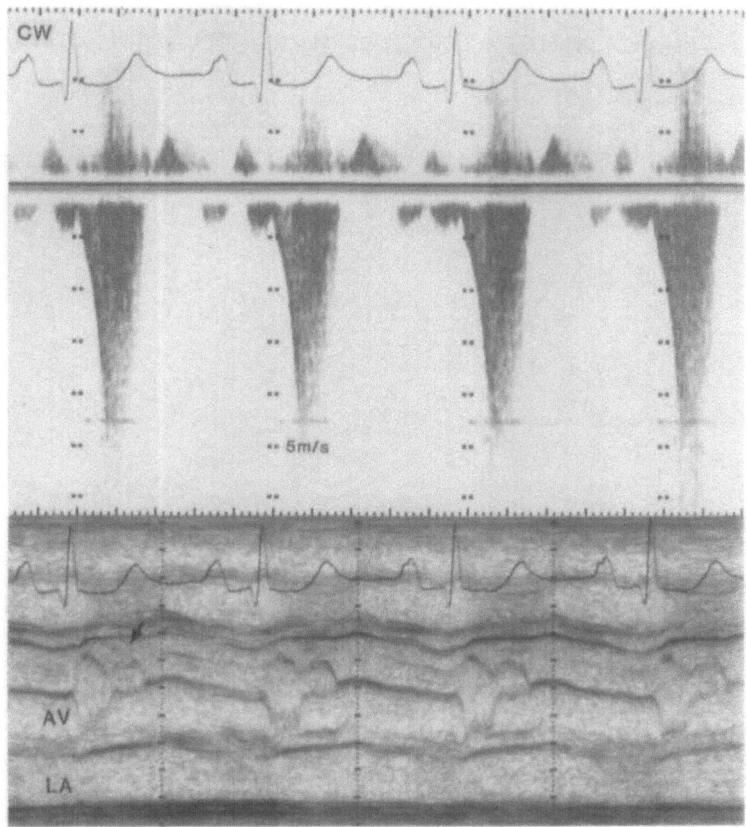

Figure 6.6. Continuous wave Doppler and M-mode echocardiogram of a patient with hypertrophic obstructive cardiomyopathy. Continuous wave Doppler echocardiogram of left ventricular outflow from apical window (upper panel) shows the peaking of the flow velocity curve in late systole, the discovery of which is characteristic of a dynamic outflow obstruction. The maximal flow velocity of 5.0 m/sec indicates the existence of a peak pressure gradient of 100 mm Hg. The M-mode recording of the aorta (lower panel) demonstrates partial closure of the aortic valve (AV), whose timing is very similar as late systolic peaking of outflow velocity.

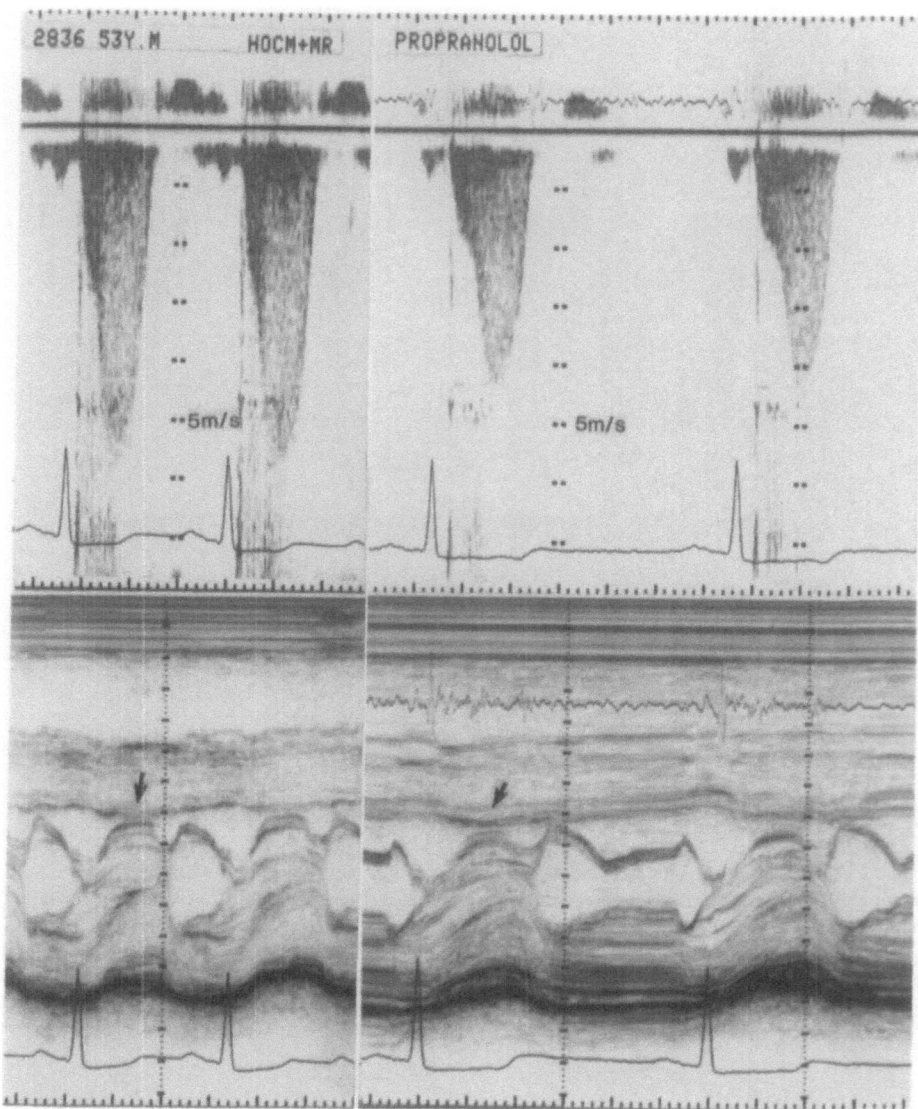

Figure 6.7. Continuous wave Doppler and M-mode echocardiogram of a patient with hypertrophic obstructive cardiomyopathy treated with beta-blockade. On the left, continuous wave Doppler echocardiogram of left ventricular outflow from apical window shows the peak flow velocity of 5.5 m/sec indicates the existence of a peak pressure gradient of 121 mm Hg. M-mode shows predominant SAM (arrow). After administration of propranolol, left ventricular outflow peak velocity decreases from 5.5 m/sec to 4.3 m/sec and also the degree of mitral-septal contact decreases.

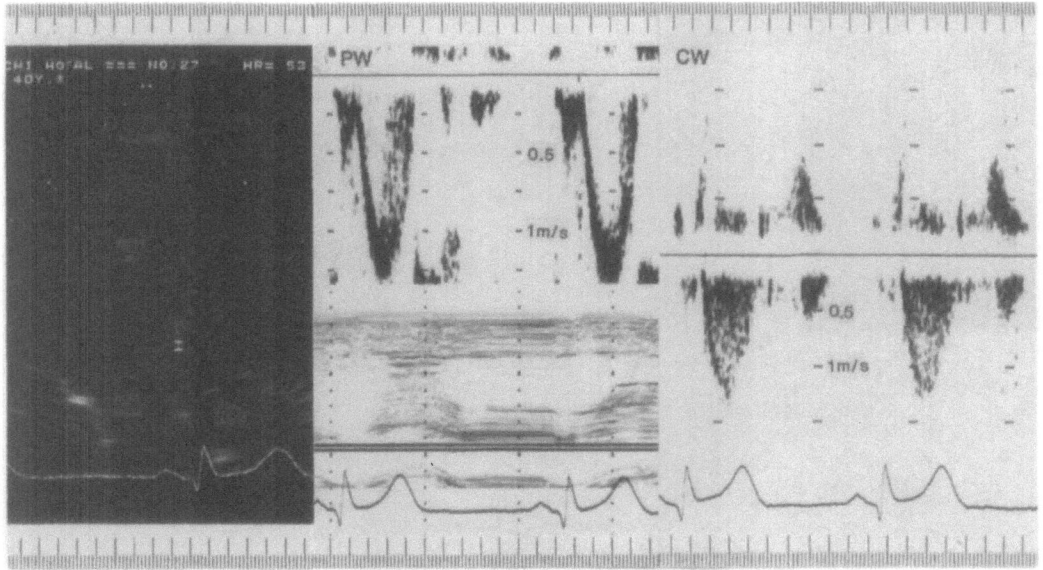

Figure 6.8. Pulsed and continuous wave Doppler echocardiogram of a patient with hypertrophic non-obstructive cardiomyopathy. Pulsed wave (PW) and continuous wave (CW) Doppler echocardiogram of left ventricular outflow from apical window shows the peaking of the flow velocity curve in mid systole. The maximal flow velocity of 1.2 m/sec does not indicate the existence of pressure gradient.

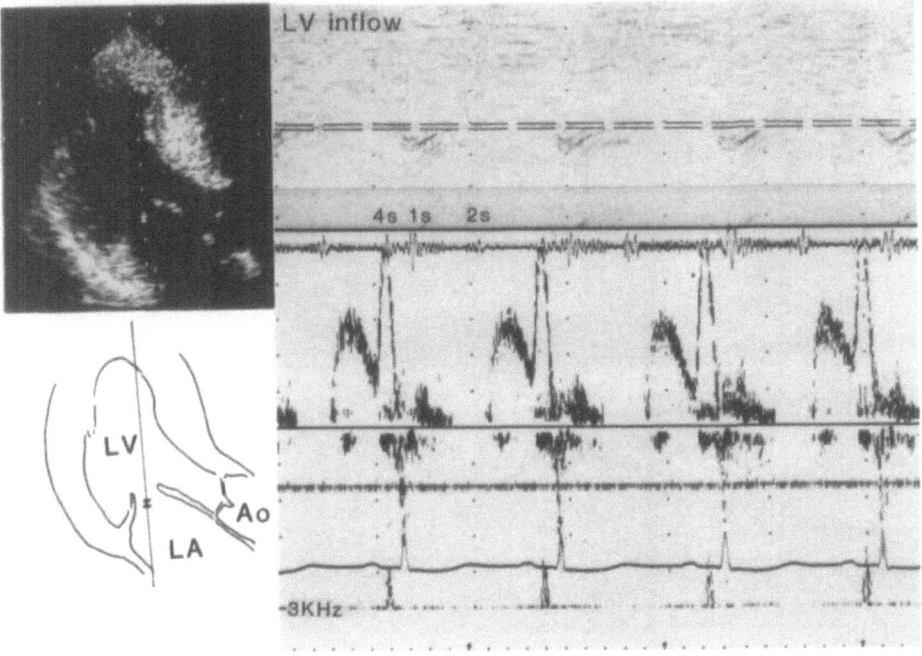

Figure 6.9. Pulsed Doppler echocardiogram of the left ventricular inflow velocity of a patient with hypertrophic obstructive cardiomyopathy. Transmitral flow shows decreased peak velocity in the rapid filling phase and exaggerated atrial systolic flow to the ventricle accompanied with a loud fourth sound (4S) in PCG.

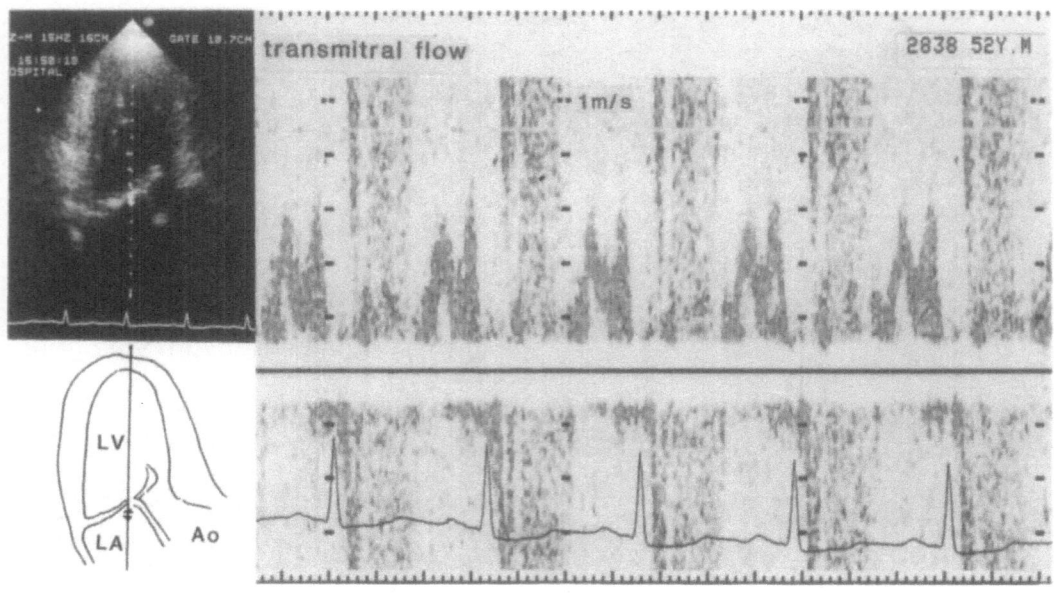

Figure 6.10. Pulsed Doppler echocardiogram of mitral regurgitation in a patient with hypertrophic obstructive cardiomyopathy. When the sample volume is placed in the left atrial cavity, a systolic turbulent flow is evident.

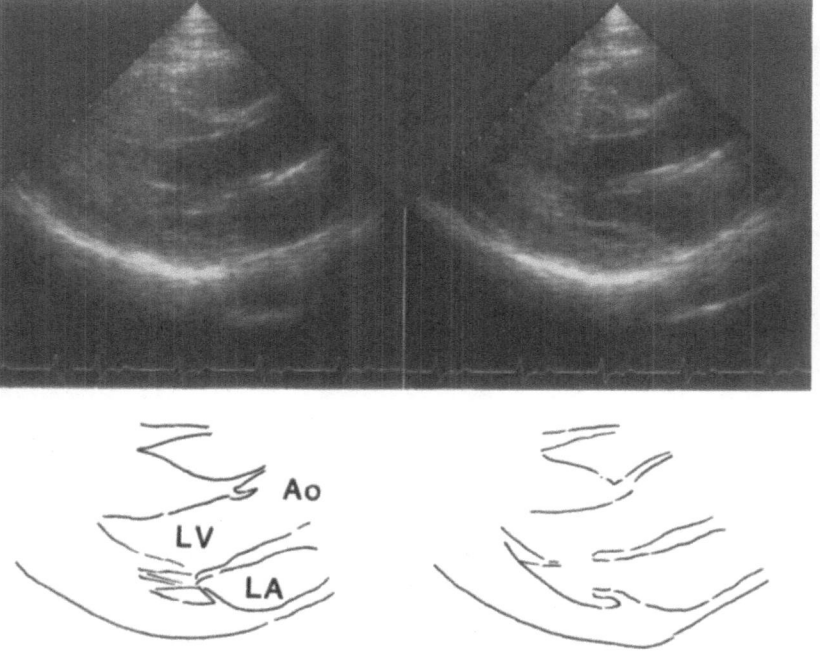

Figure 6.11. Long axis two-dimensional echocardiogram of a patient with apical hypertrophy.

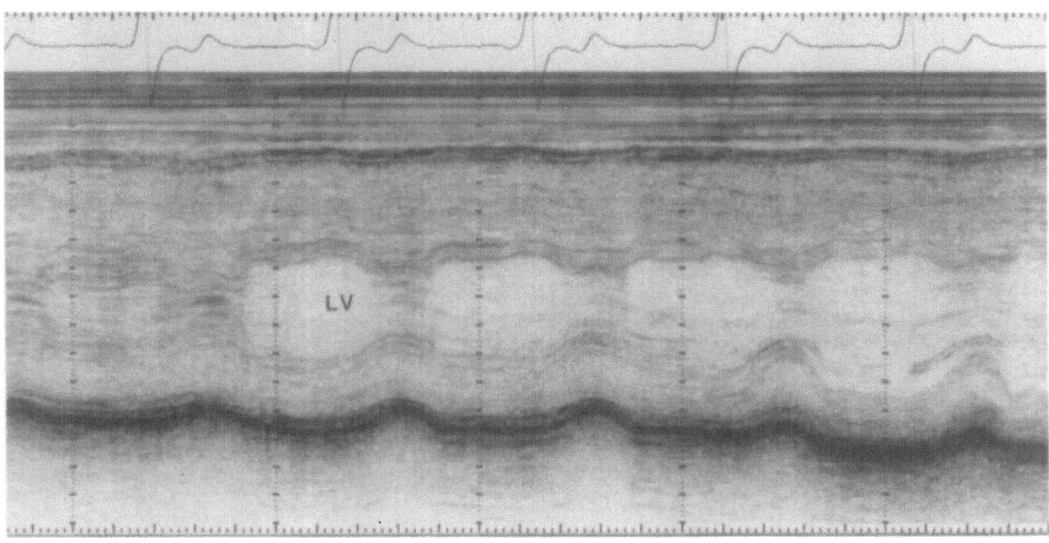

Figure 6.12. M-mode scan of a patient with apical hypertrophy. It is possible to appreciate progressive hypertrophy in the apical portion of left ventricle.

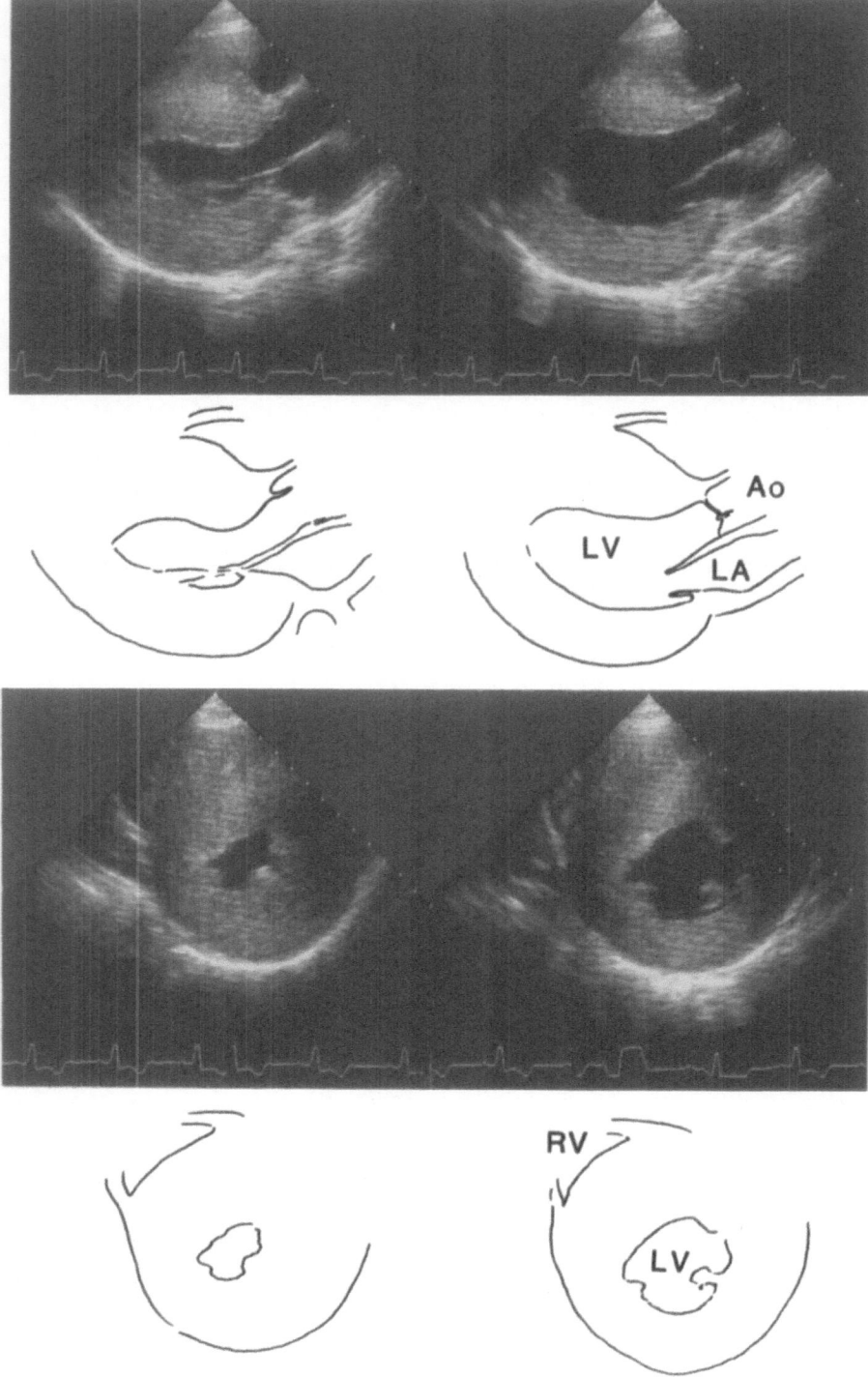

Figure 6.13. Long and short axis two-dimensional echocardiograms of a patient with a diffuse hypertrophic cardiomyopathy.

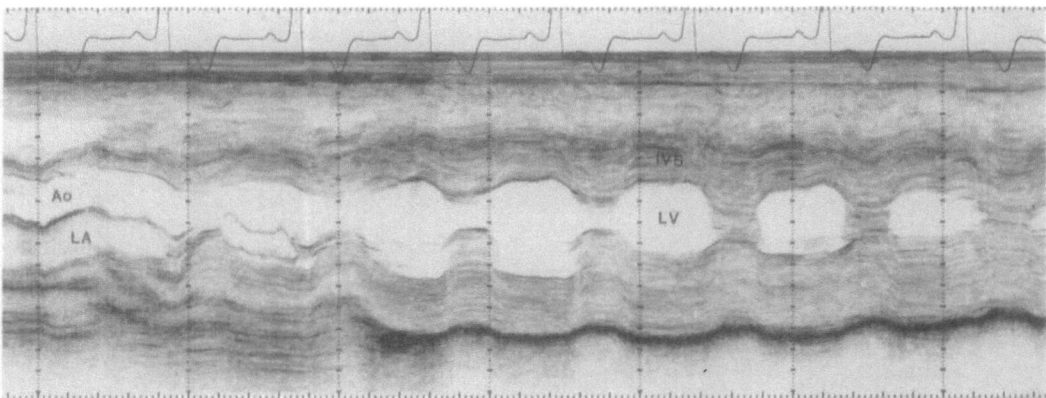

Figure 6.14. M-mode scan of a patient with a diffuse hypertrophic cardiomyopathy. This echocardiogram is compatible with the non-obstructive type because the aortic valve motion is normal and SAM is not appreciated.

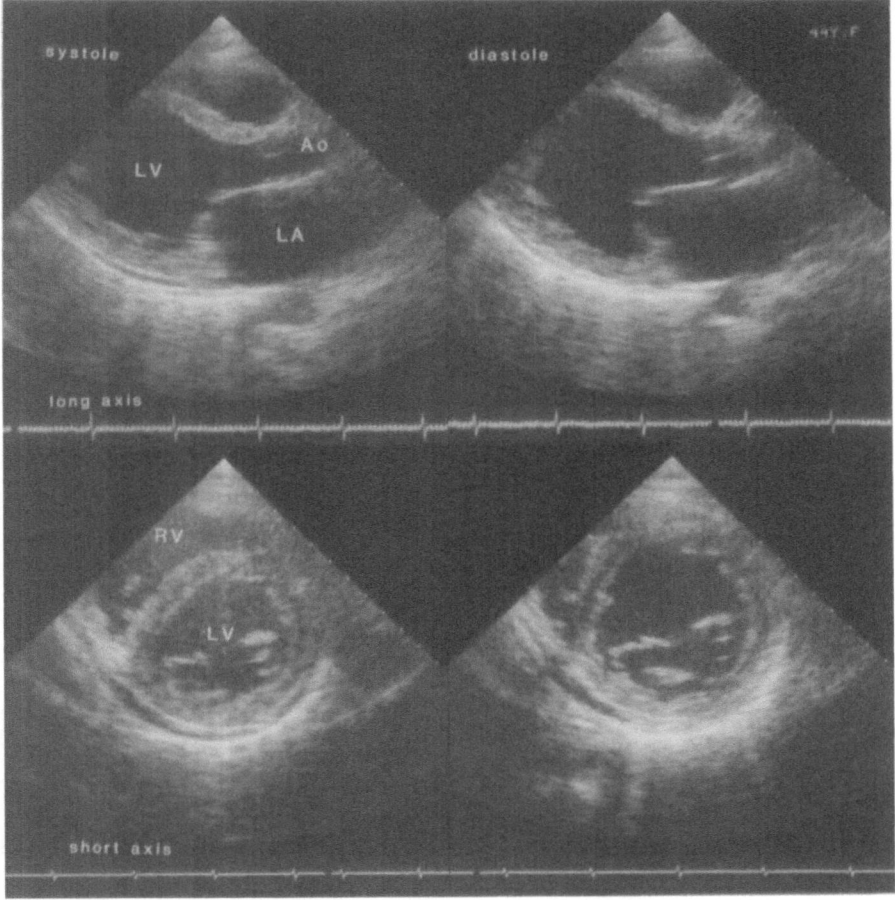

Figure 6.15. Long and short axis view of a patient with DCM. The left ventricle has a severe dilatation with diffuse hypokinesis.

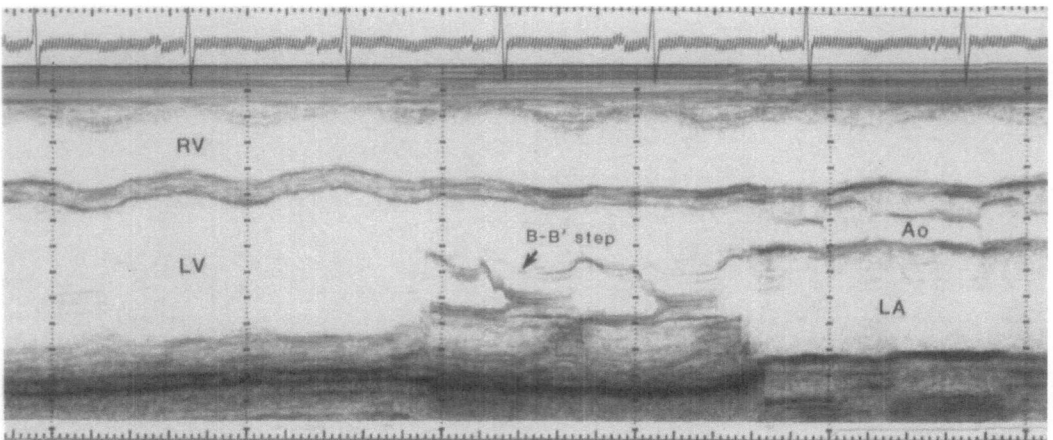

Figure 6.16. M-mode scan of a patient with DCM. The left ventricle is dilated and poorly contracted. The mitral valve shows a B-B' step. The aorta (Ao) shows reduced anterior motion.

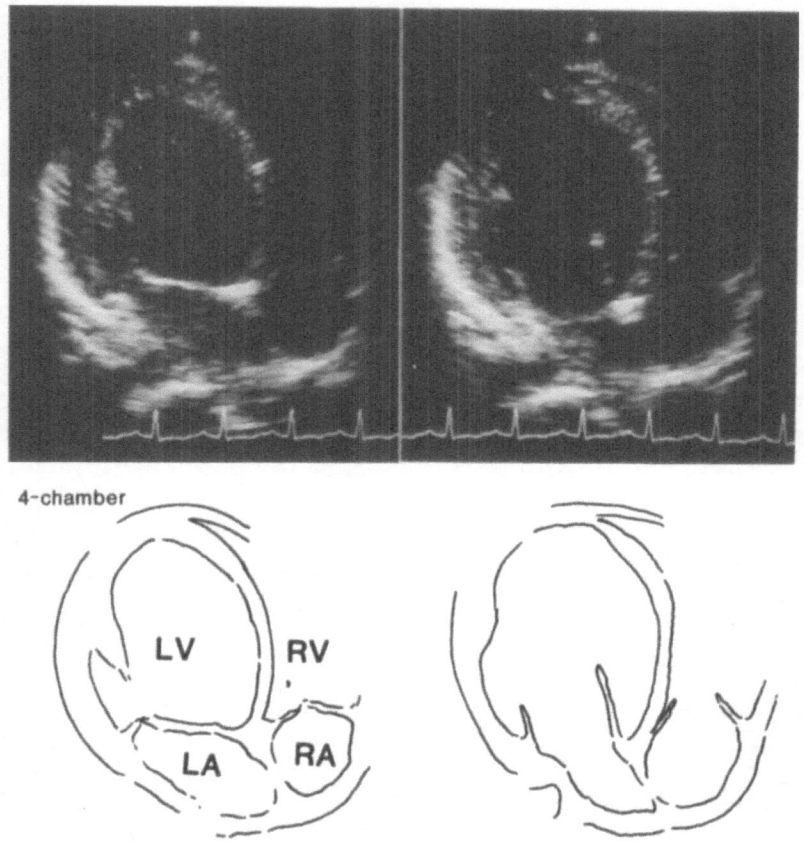

Figure 6.17. Apical four-chamber view of a patient with DCM. The configuration of the left ventricle tends to be circular.

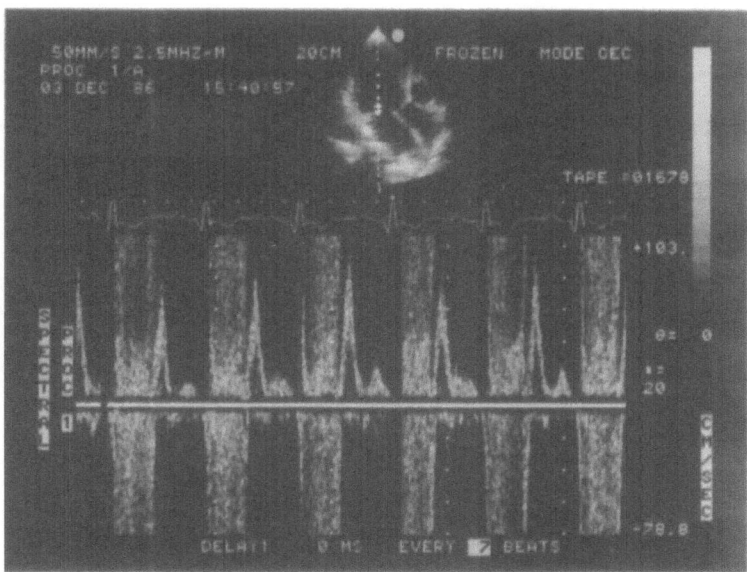

Figure 6.18. Pulsed Doppler echocardiogram of transmitral flow in a patient with DCM. When the sample volume is placed in the mitral annulus, a systolic turbulent flow (mitral regurgitation) is evident. In diastole, transmitral flow demonstrates an increased peak velocity in the rapid filling phase and decreased peak velocity in the atrial contraction phase. These findings suggest increased left ventricular end-diastolic pressure in patients with depressed left ventricular systolic function (see Figure 8.22).

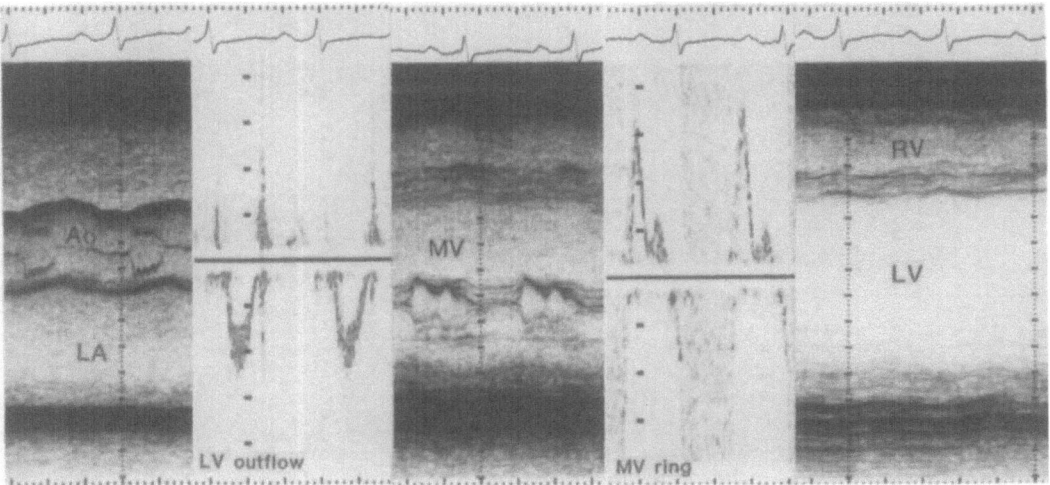

Figure 6.19. Pulsed Doppler echocardiogram of left ventricular ejection flow and inflow and M-mode of a patient with DCM. When the sample volume is placed in the left ventricular outflow, the peak velocity is approximately 0.5 m/sec and the small systolic velocity integral is observed. Transmitral flow demonstrates systolic mitral regurgitant flow and diastolic peaking flow in the rapid filling phase and decreased flow in the atrial contraction phase.

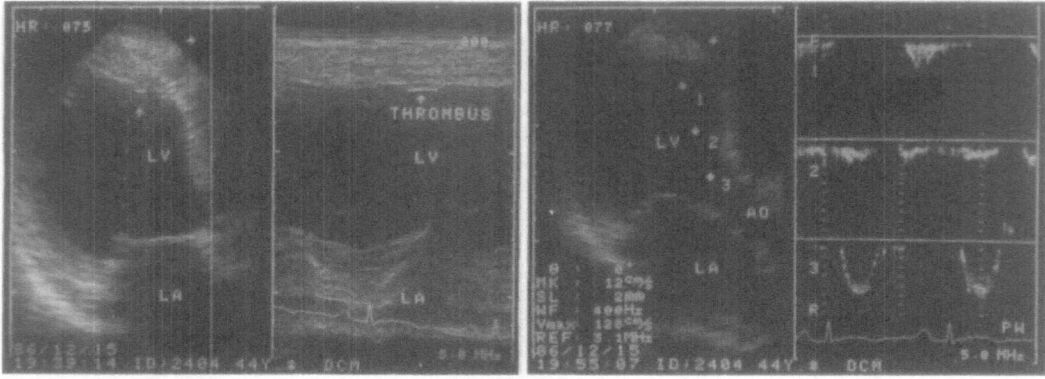

Figure 6.20. Two-dimensional, M-mode and multi-gated pulsed Doppler echocardiogram of a patient with DCM and mural thrombus. The left image shows an apical long axis view with left ventricular dilatation and apical mural thrombus (arrow). On the right, the multigated pulsed Doppler is implemented at three different points in the left ventricle (1: apical, 2: middle and 3: basal). In the apical portion, systolic flow is absent, in the middle portion one can see small ejection flow and in the basal portion the ejection flow is almost normal.

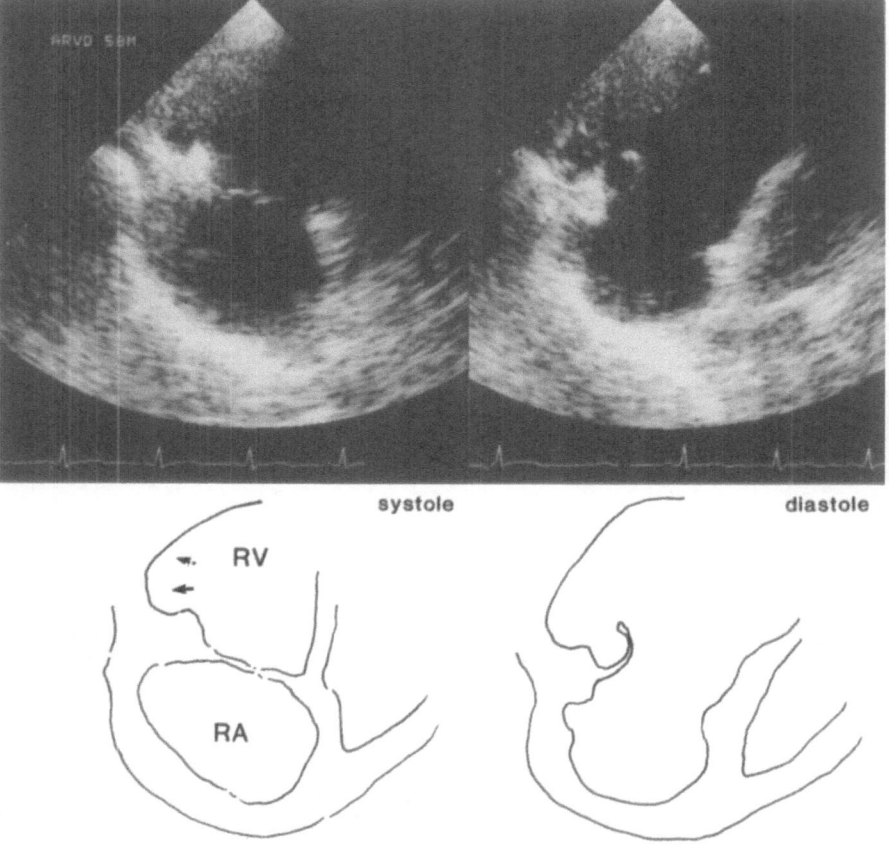

Figure 6.21. Parasternal right ventricular inflow view of a patient with arrhythmogenic right ventricular dysplasia. The right ventricular dilatation with an aneurysmatic portion (arrow) can be seen.

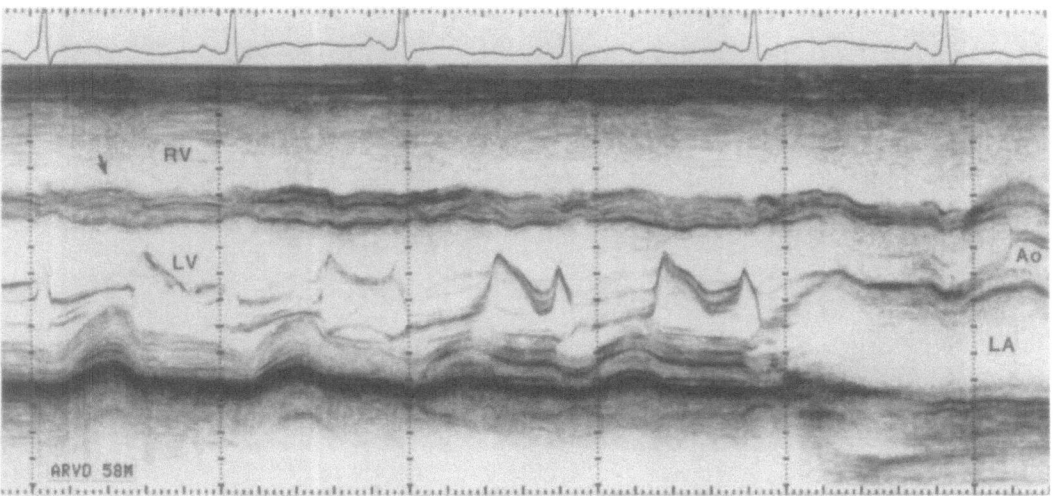

Figure 6.22. M-mode scan of a patient with arrhythmogenic right ventricular dysplasia. This figure shows right ventricular (RV) dilatation with systolic anterior motion and thickening of the interventricular septum (arrow).

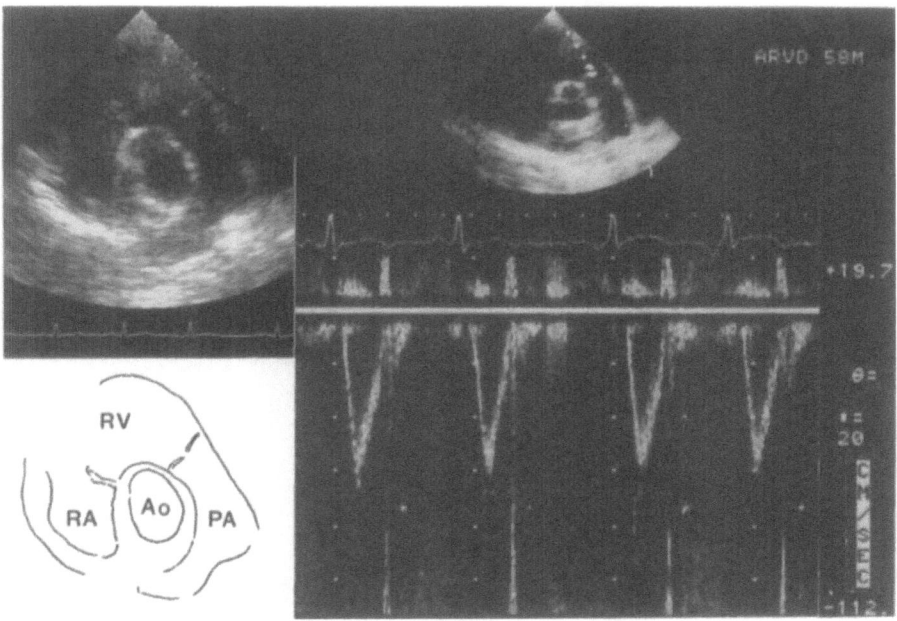

Figure 6.23. Two-dimensional parasternal right ventricular outflow view and pulmonary artery flow from a patient with arrhythmogenic right ventricular dysplasia. Normal dimensions of the pulmonary artery (PA) and normal flow profile are evident.

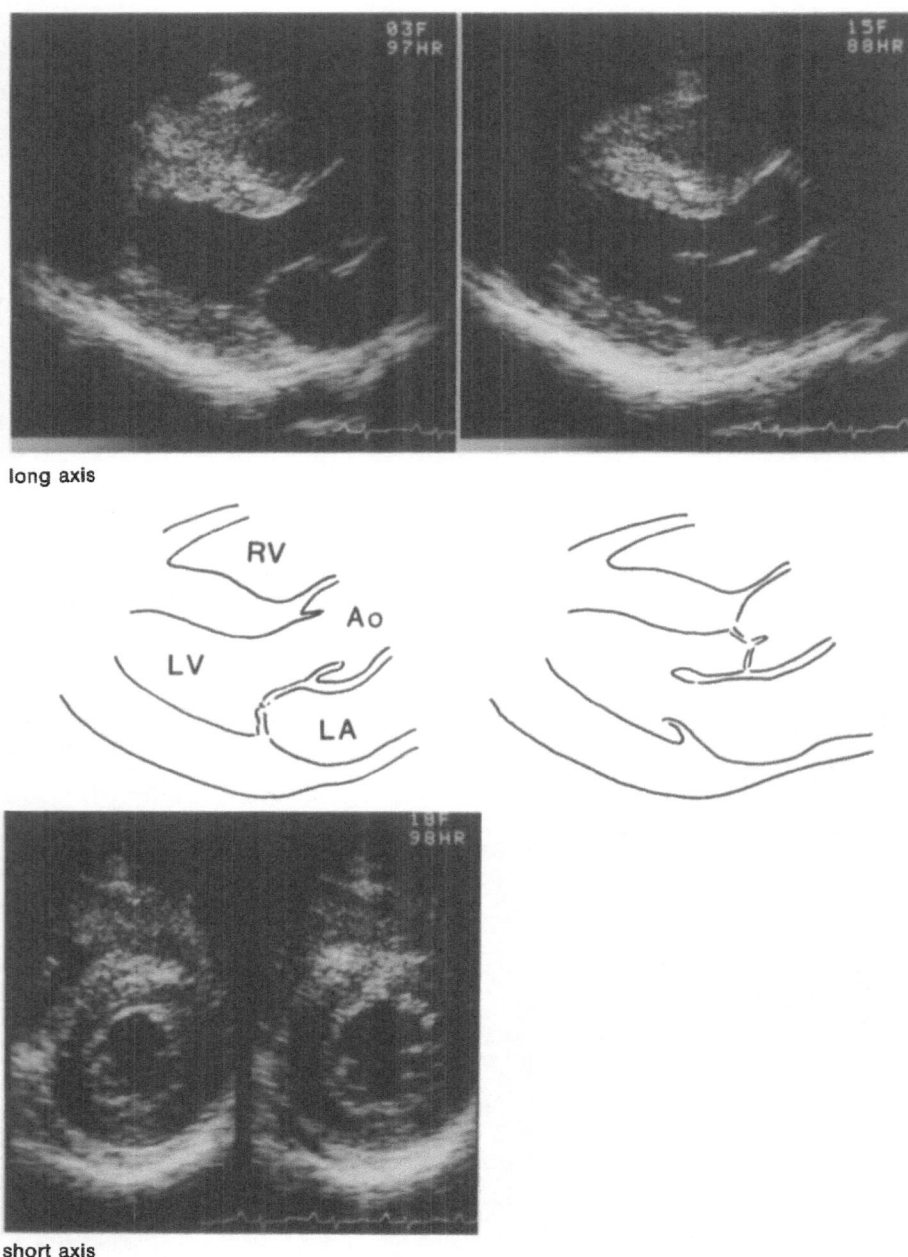

long axis

short axis

Figure 6.24. Long and short axis view of a patient with amyloidosis. It is possible to appreciate left ventricular hypertrophy without dilatation. The myocardium exhibits a characteristic 'granular sparkling texture'.

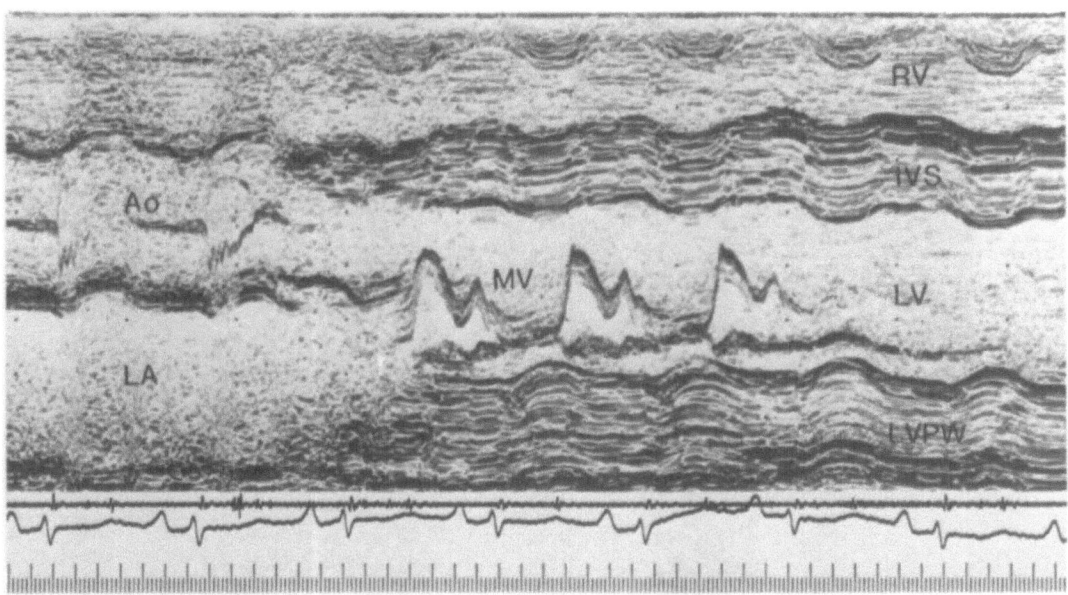

Figure 6.25.   M-mode scan of a patient with amyloidosis. The hypertrophied interventricular septum (IVS) and left
ventricular posterior wall (LVPW) can be observed. Left ventricular hypokinesis is also present.

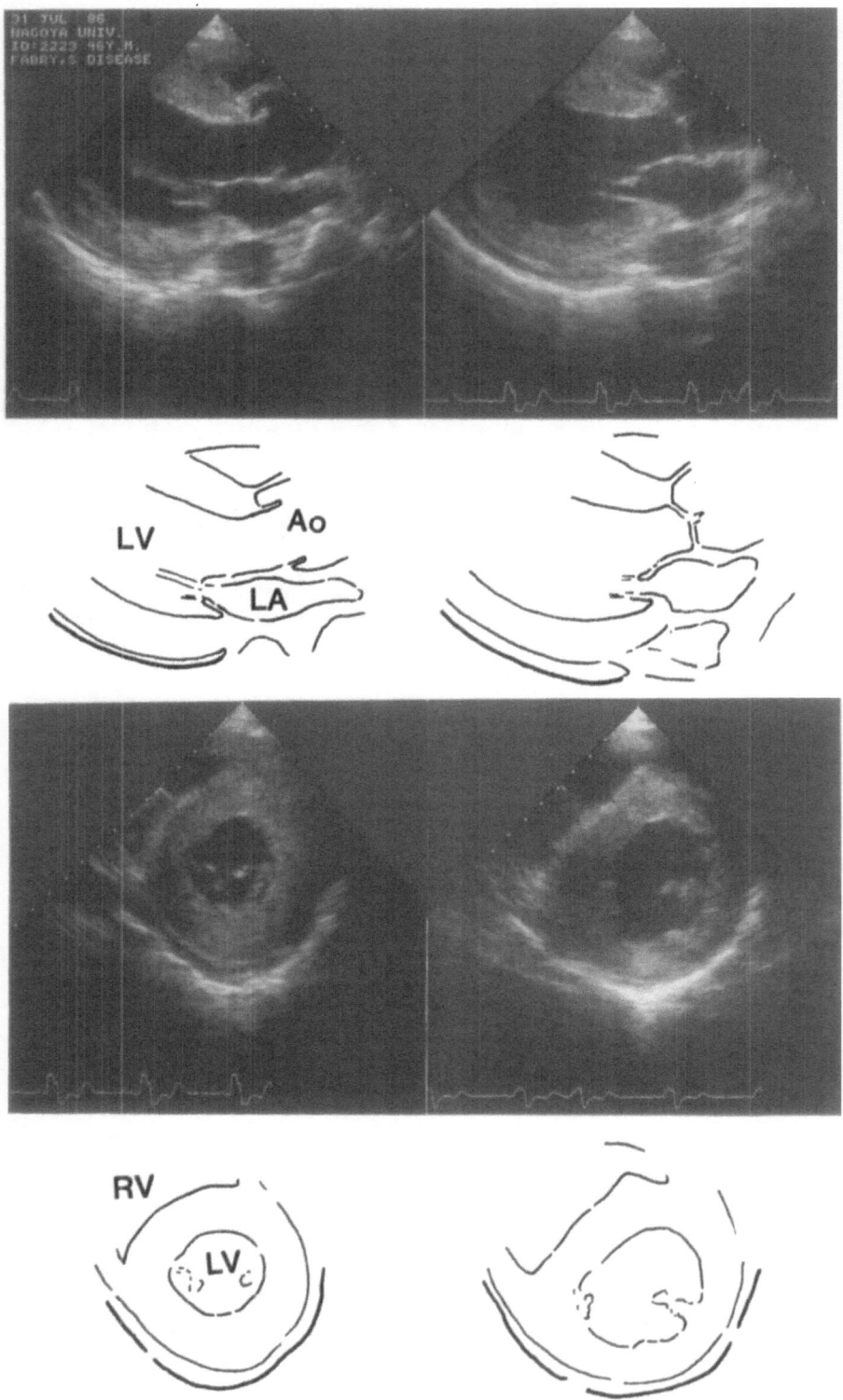

Figure 6.26.   Long and short axis view of a patient with Fabry's disease. One can see left ventricular hypertrophy and the myocardial echo demonstrates fine granular texture.

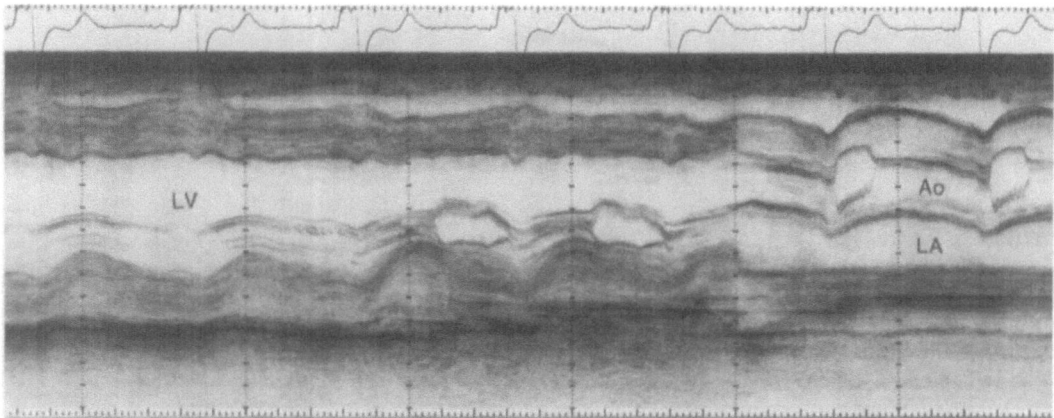

Figure 6.27. M-mode scan of a patient with Fabry's disease. Left ventricular hypertrophy with hypokinetic wall motion is detected. Aortic regurgitation was present in this patient as was suggested by a diastolic mitral valve fluttering.

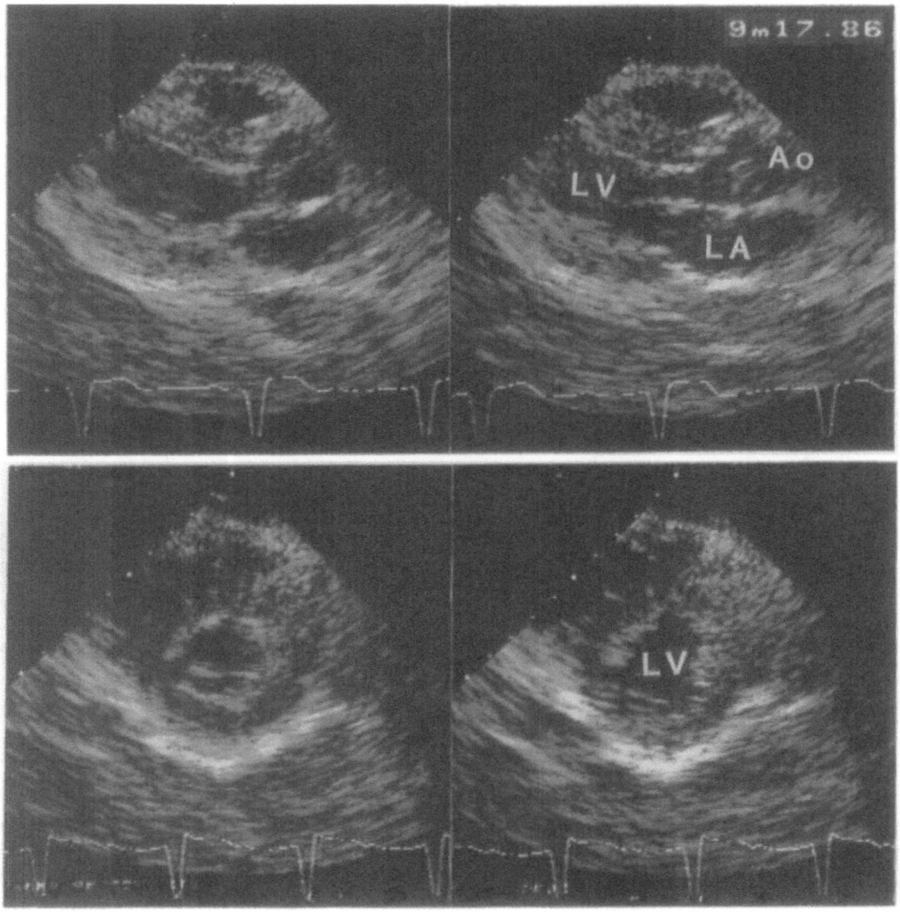

Figure 6.28. Long and short axis view from a patient with acute myocarditis. The left ventricular hypertrophy and abnormal wall motion (hypokinesis) is evident.

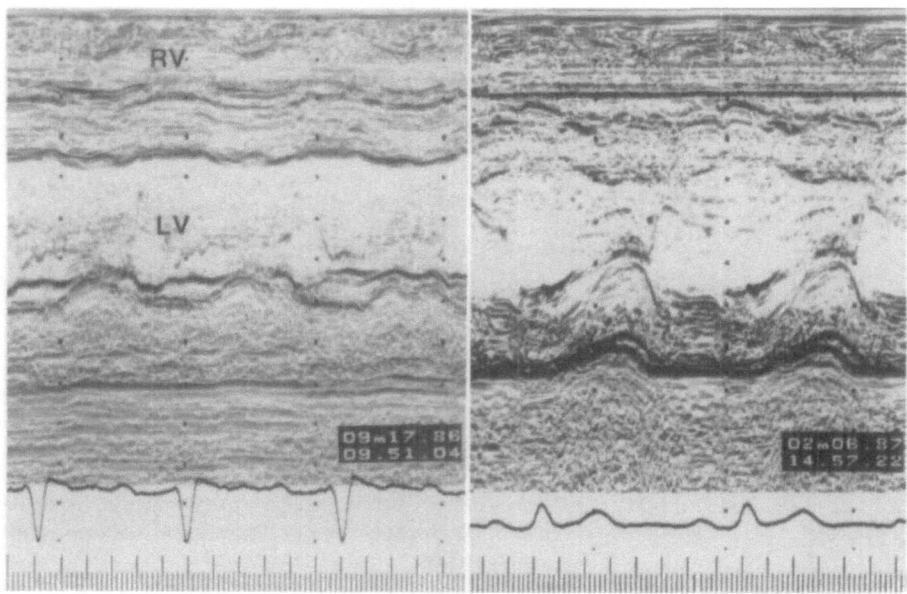

Figure 6.29. M-mode echocardiogram from a patient with myocarditis during the acute and chronic phases. The left ventricular hypertrophy and abnormal wall motion (hypokinesis) are evident in the acute phase (left panel). These abnormalities have almost completely disappeared in the chronic phase (right panel).

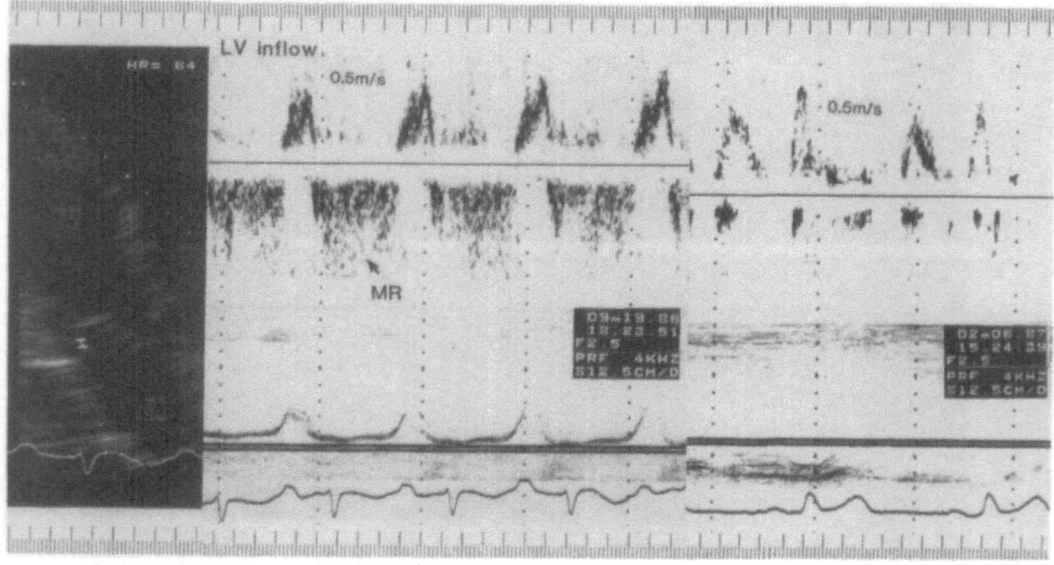

Figure 6.30. Pulsed Doppler echocardiogram from a patient with myocarditis during the acute and chronic phases. In the acute phase, left ventricular inflow shows mitral regurgitant flow (MR) and increased atrial contribution to left ventricular filling (left panel). These abnormalities have almost completely disappeared in the chronic phase (right panel).

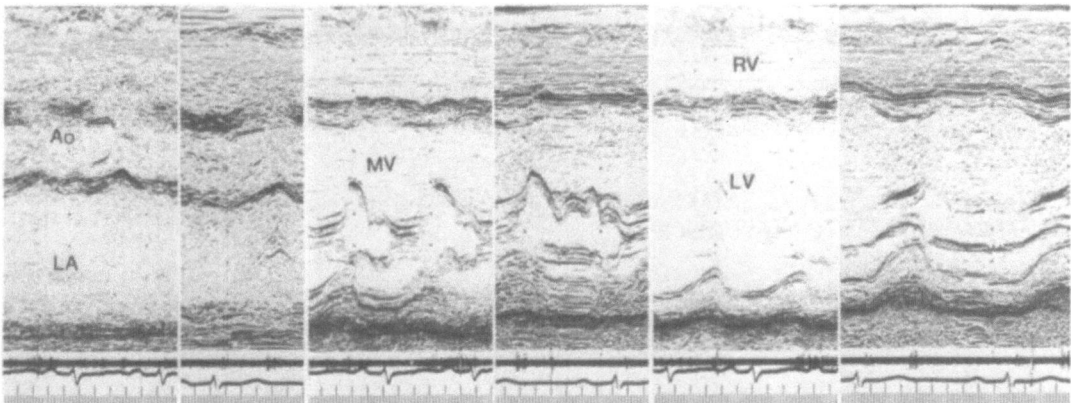

Figure 6.31. M-mode echocardiogram from a patient with leukemia during and after the treatment with doxorubi-cin. This figure illustrates the abnormal left ventricular function due to cardiac toxicity during chemotherapy (left panel). These alterations were reversible after cessation of the toxic agent in this patient (right panel).

3. Secondary cardiomyopathy

Secondary cardiomyopathy is a disease in which the cardiac muscle is secondarily affected by some other disorder. The common disorders which can produce myocardial changes include amyloidosis, hemochromatosis, sarcoidosis, Pompe's disease, and Fabry's disease. The most frequent type of secondary cardiomyopathy is amyloid heart disease. The characteristic findings of these diseases are diffusely hypertrophied and non-dilated left ventricle with decreased contractile motion. In the case of amyloidosis, the characteristic echoes that return from the myocardium have been described as 'granular sparkling' texture which would reflect the amyloid infiltration in the cardiac muscle (Figures 6.24, 25). When this finding is present, one can differentiate amyloidosis from other types of secondary cardiomyopathy, for example Fabry's disease (Figures 6.26, 27).

4. Inflammatory process of the myocardium

The myocardium is sometimes involved by inflammatory process. The most frequent origin is viral infection. Echocardiography can show the morphological and functional alterations due to myocardial inflammation. Characteristic findings consist of wall motion abnormalities (segmental or diffuse) and myocardial hypertrophy (Figure 6.28). In severe cases, left ventricular dilatation can occur. In some patients, mitral regurgitation is demonstrated by Doppler examination. These abnormalities present in the acute phase tend to disappear in a short time in many patients (Figures 6.29, 30).

5. Myocardial abnormality due to toxic agents

Some kinds of drugs used for the treatment of patients with malignancies can affect the myocardium. Doxorubicin has been reported to have an important cardiac toxicity. Echocardiography is useful in this situation because it can demonstrate left ventricular systolic dysfunction (Figure 6.31).

CHAPTER 7

Other cardiac diseases

1. Left atrial myxoma

Diagnosis of a left atrial (LA) myxoma is relatively easy by echocardiography, and especially by two-dimensional echocardiography. This method is useful for diagnosis of not only the presence of a myxoma, but also for the evaluation of its characteristics, including size, the site of attachment, consistency (fragile or not) and motility. Echocardiography is the method of choice for its clinical diagnosis and also has replaced angiocardiography for routine preoperative evaluation. The most usual appearance of a left atrial myxoma is that of a pedunculated large mass with well defined structure. The mass usually prolapses into the mitral orifice during diastole, and this can produce left ventricular inflow obstruction (Figures 7.1, 5). In systole, the tumor thrusts back into the left atrial cavity. Sometimes, myxoma has no stalk and does not prolapse to the mitral orifice (Figures 7.8, 9) or is so small that the mitral valve motion and the transmitral flow is not disturbed (Figures 7.10, 11). The hemodynamic alterations of left ventricular filling when a myxoma is present depend on its size and whether it prolapses into the left ventricle or not. Doppler echocardiography can provide information about hemodynamic alteration due to left atrial myxoma, consisting of disturbance of left ventricular filling (Figures 7.3, 4, 7) and sometimes mitral regurgitation (Figure 7.12). In the M-mode, one can see a cloud of tumor echoes in the left atrium and frequently tumor echoes are recorded behind the anterior leaflet of the mitral valve (Figures 7.2, 6, 9, 11). The E-F slope may be decreased, reflecting disturbance of left ventricular filling.

2. Right atrial myxoma

Cardiac myxoma sometimes occurs in the right atrium which is the second most common location. As in a left atrial myxoma, a right atrial myxoma usually pedunculates on the atrial septum and prolapses into the tricuspid orifice to produce right ventricular inflow disturbance, like tricuspid stenosis (Figures 7.13, 14).

3. Intracardiac rhabdomyoma

Cardiac rhabdomyoma, although uncommon, is the most frequent primary cardiac tumor found in infants and children. Rhabdomyoma is usually observed as discrete areas of in-

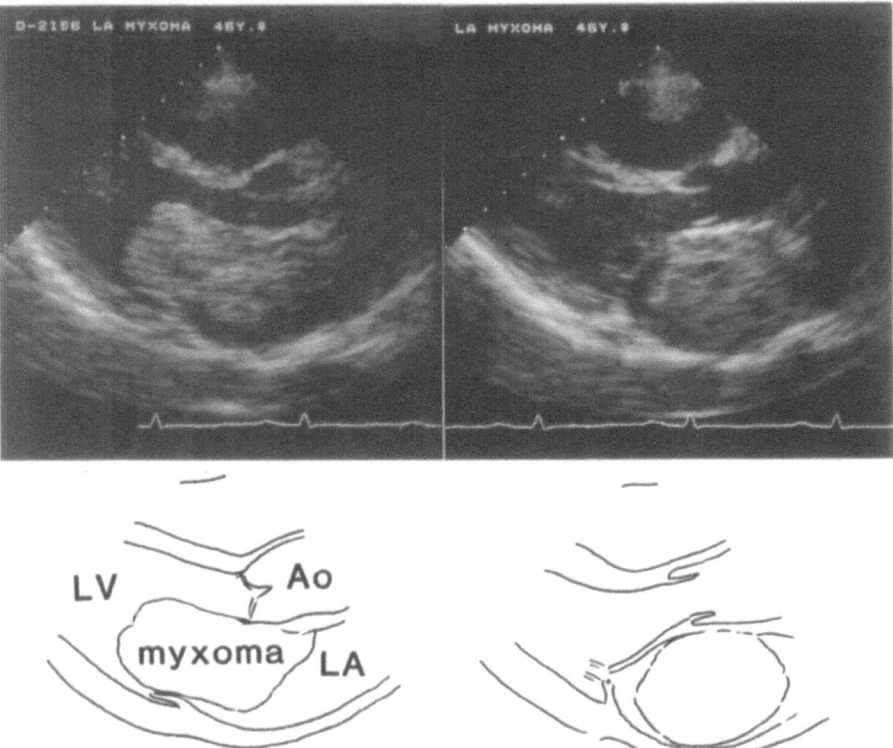

Figure 7.1. Long axis view of a patient with a large and prolapsing left atrial myxoma. A large myxoma prolapses into the mitral valve orifice and occludes the mitral annulus in mid diastole. This finding suggests the complete obstruction of the mitral orifice in mid diastole. In systole the myxoma thrusts back to occupy most of the left atrial cavity.

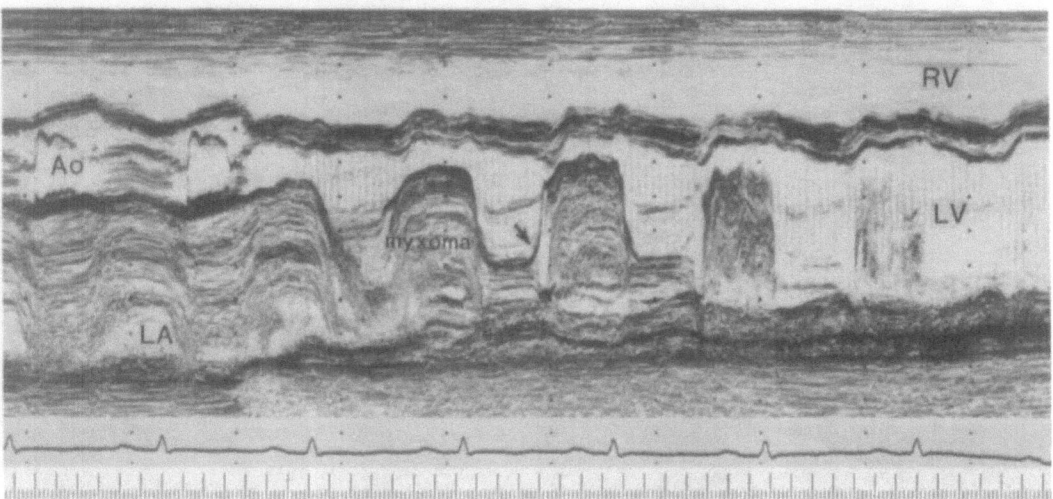

Figure 7.2. M-mode scan of a patient with large and prolapsing left atrial myxoma. The smoke-like echoes from the tumor are visible behind the anterior leaflet of the mitral valve during diastole. In early diastole, one can see the time interval between the mitral valve opening and the thrusting of the myxoma (arrow). The diastolic slope of the anterior mitral leaflet (E-F-slope) is reduced, as in mitral stenosis.

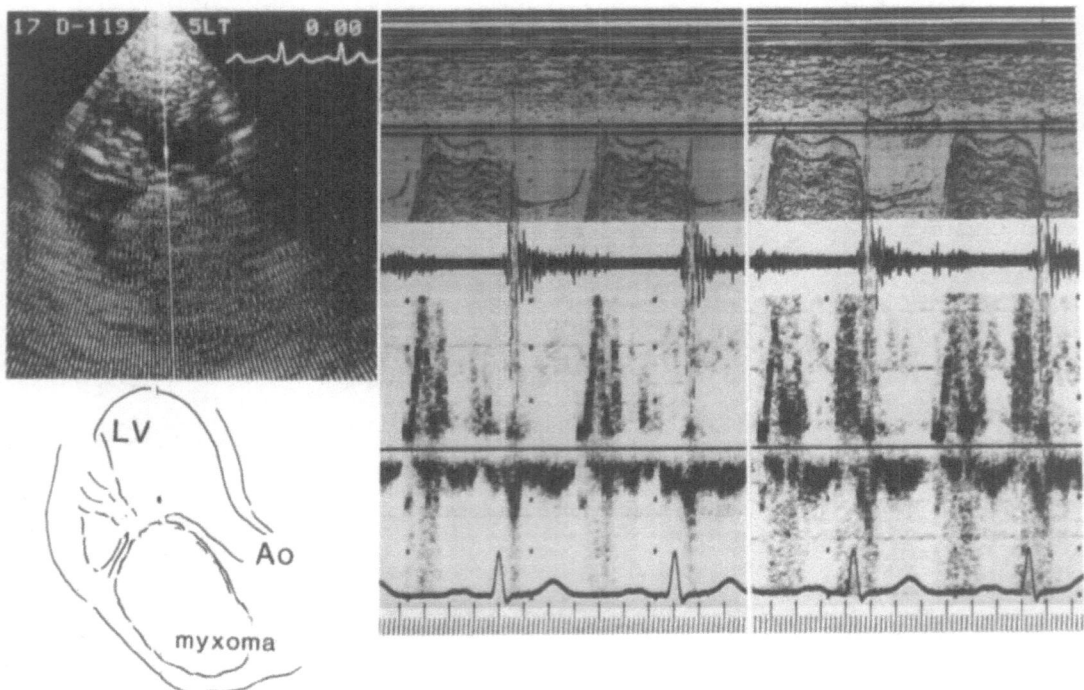

Figure 7.3. Pulsed Doppler recordings of a patient with a large and prolapsing left atrial myxoma. A high velocity of left ventricular inflow with short duration is observed just before the prolapse of the myxoma into the mitral orifice. After the myxoma prolapses into the mitral orifice, left ventricular inflow disappears almost completely. During the left atrial ejection phase, the left ventricular inflow can be seen in some of the sampling site.

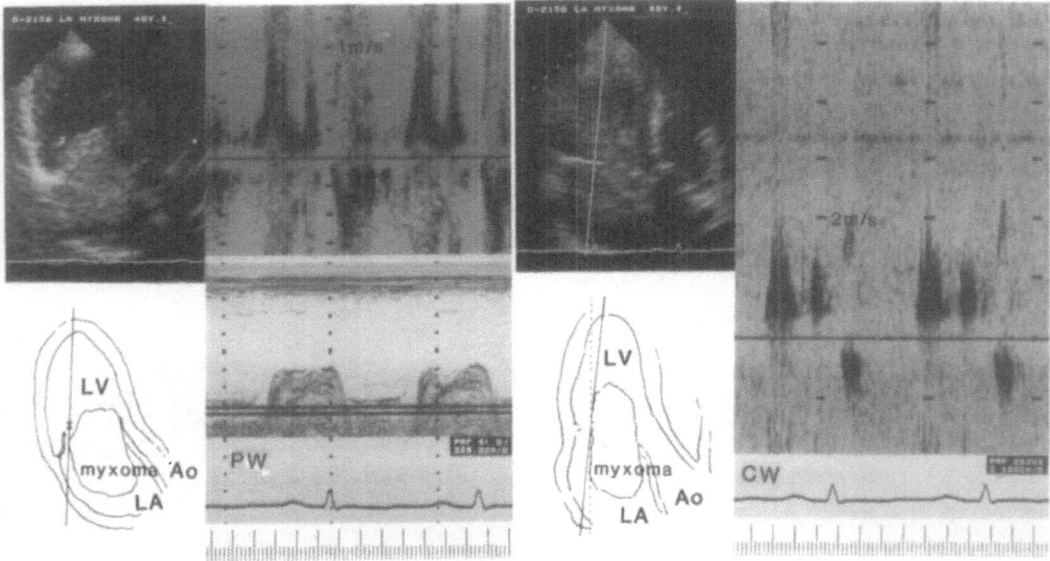

Figure 7.4. Pulsed wave (PW) and continuous wave (CW) Doppler recordings from a patient with a large and prolapsing left atrial myxoma. A high velocity (about 2 m/s) left ventricular inflow of a short duration is observed just before the prolapse of the myxoma into the mitral orifice. After the myxoma prolapses into the mitral orifice, the left ventricular inflow disappears almost completely. During the left atrial ejection phase, the left ventricular inflow can be seen. These findings are almost similar in both pulsed and CW Doppler recordings.

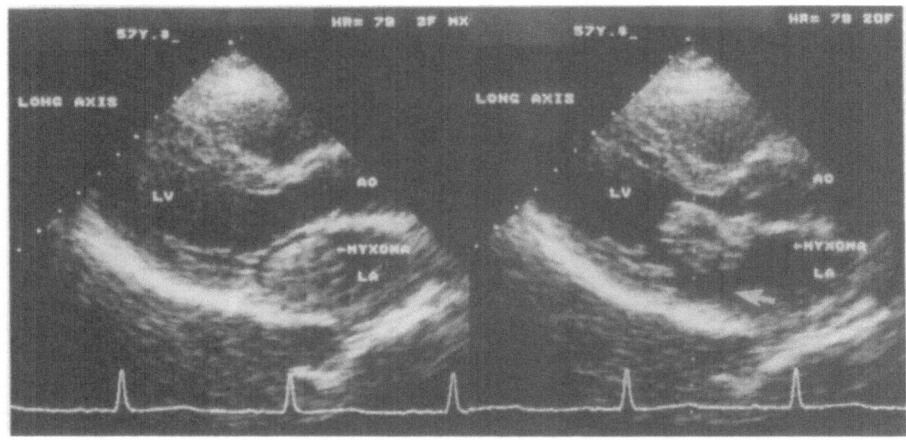

Figure 7.5. Long and short axis views of a patient with a medium-sized prolapsing left atrial myxoma. The myxoma prolapses into the mitral orifice, but a small space is visible between the myxoma and the mitral orifice (arrow), since the myxoma is smaller than the mitral orifice.

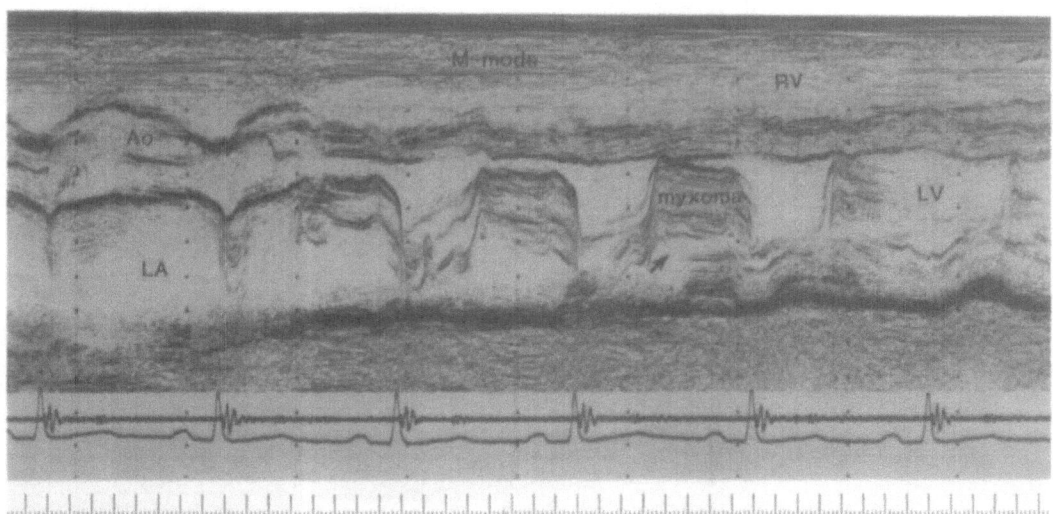

Figure 7.6. M-mode scan of a patient with a medium-sized prolapsing left atrial myxoma. The cloud of echoes from the tumor is observed behind the anterior mitral valve and the aortic root. The small space between the tumor and posterior mitral leaflet is observed in the M-mode echocardiogram.

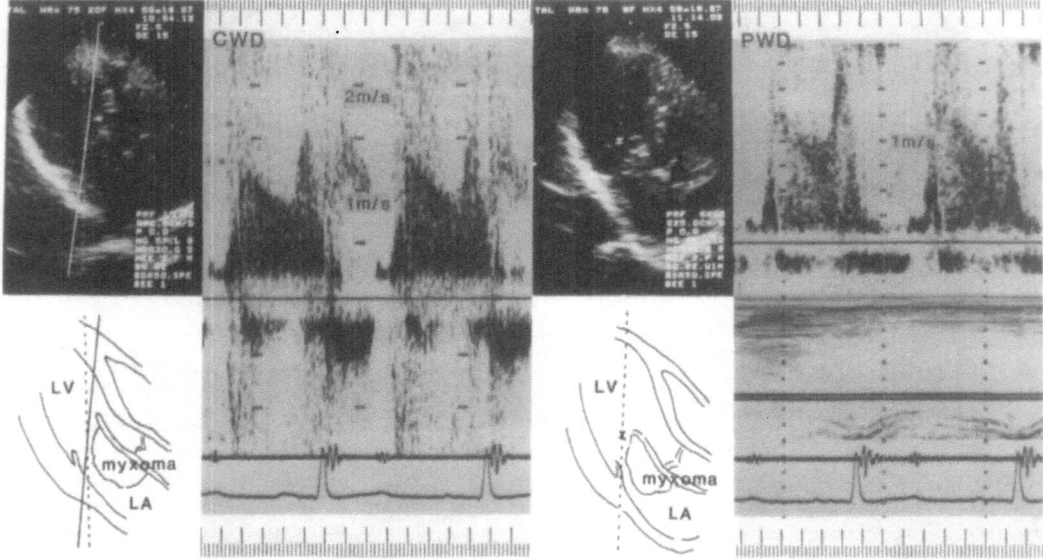

Figure 7.7. Pulsed and CW Doppler recording of a patient with a medium-sized and prolapsing left atrial myxoma. The early left ventricular inflow with short duration is observed just before the prolapse of the myxoma into the mitral orifice. After the myxoma prolapses into the mitral orifice, the left ventricular inflow shows increased peak velocity and prolonged pressure-half time, which is indistinguishable from those of patients with mitral stenosis.

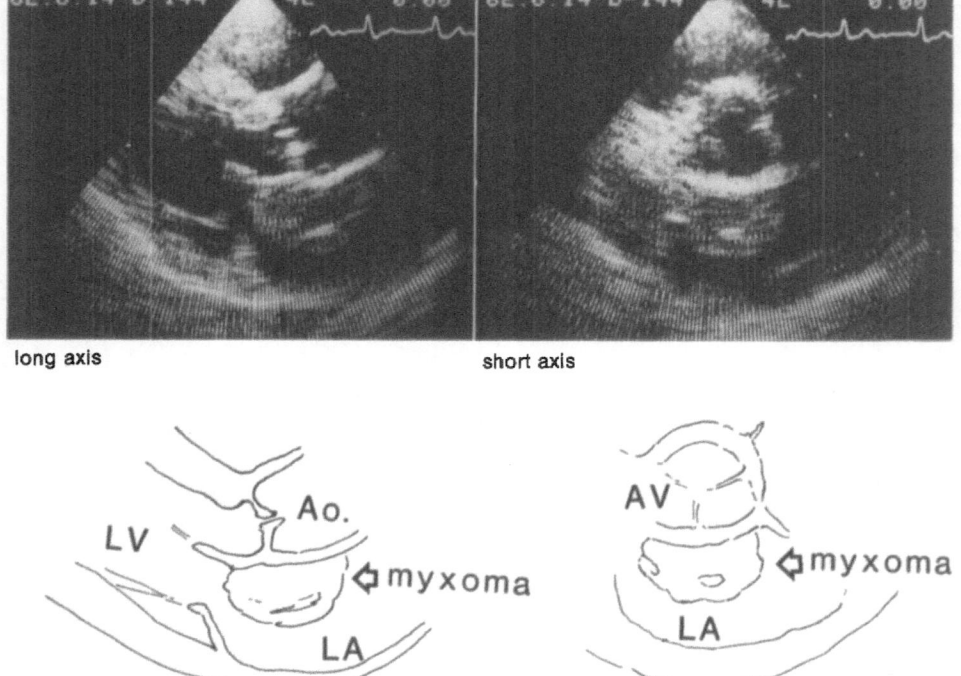

Figure 7.8. Long and short axis views of a patient with a moderate-sized fixed left atrial myxoma. A moderate-sized myxoma is shown on the anterior wall of the left atrium without a stalk and without movement during the entire cardiac cycle.

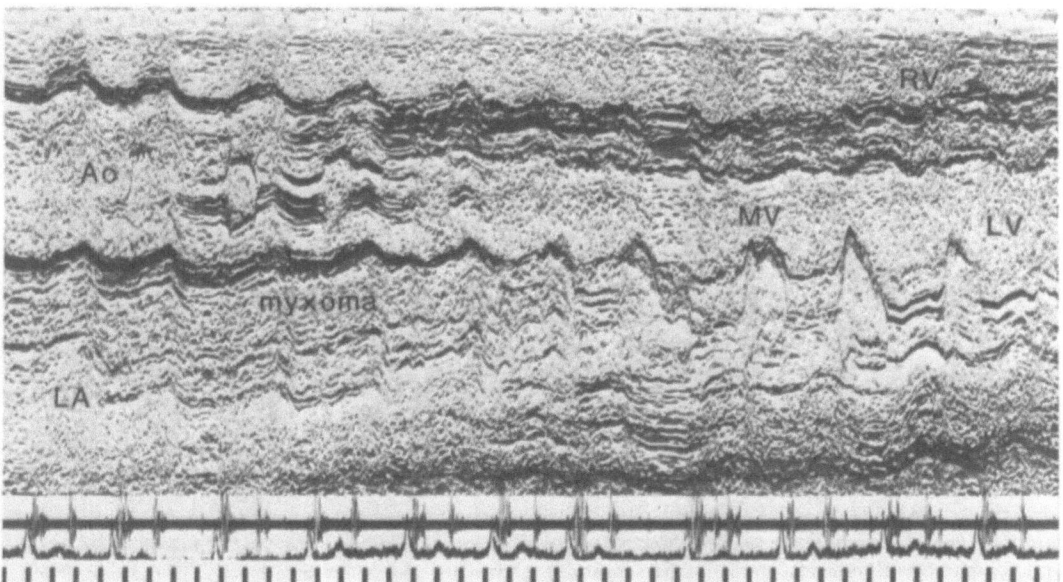

Figure 7.9. M-mode scan of a patient with a moderate-sized fixed left atrial myxoma. The tumor echoes are visible behind the posterior aortic wall throughout the cardiac cycle, but not behind the anterior leaflet of the mitral valve during diastole. The movement of the mitral valve leaflet is almost normal.

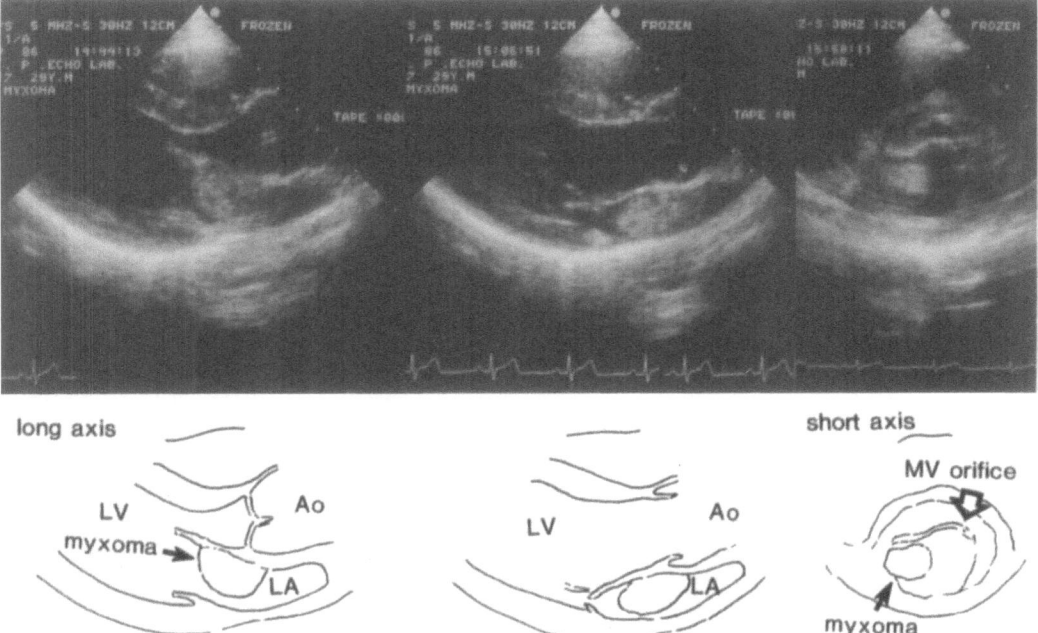

Figure 7.10. Long and short axis views from a patient with a small prolapsing left atrial myxoma. A small myxoma prolapses into the mitral orifice, but the mitral orifice is only partially occluded because of the small size of the tumor.

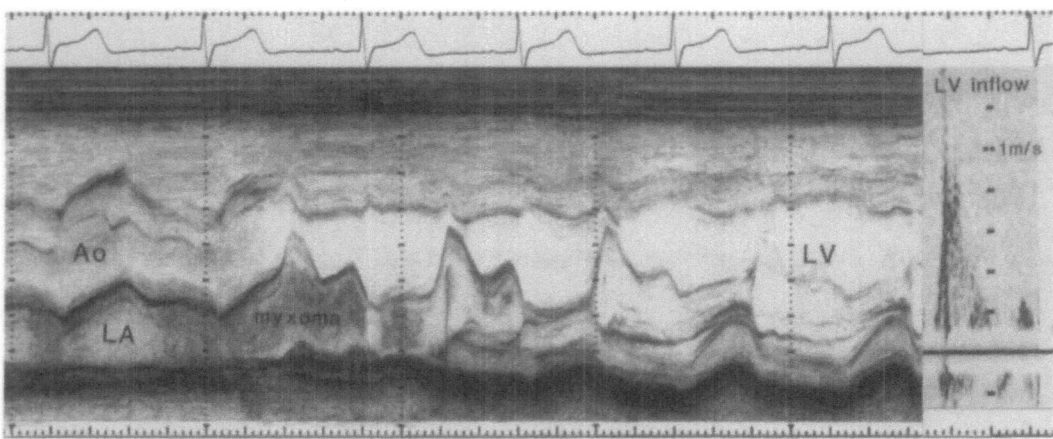

Figure 7.11. M-mode scan and pulsed Doppler echocardiogram of a patient with a small prolapsing left atrial myxoma. The tumor echoes are visible behind the anterior leaflet of the mitral valve, but the diastolic slope of the anterior mitral leaflet is almost normal, which suggests little left ventricular inflow disturbance. The transmitral flow shows no abnormalities.

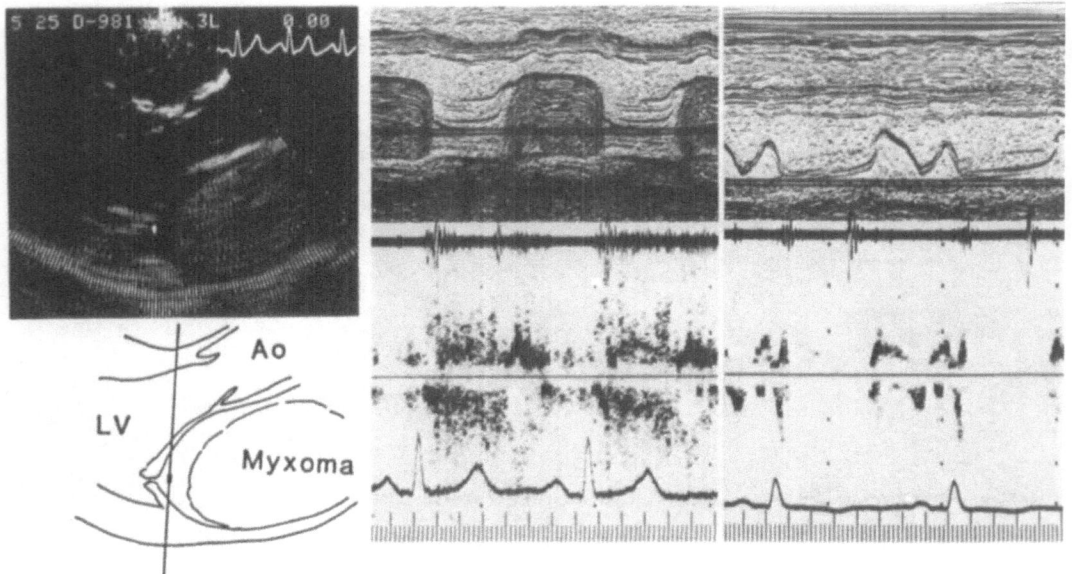

Figure 7.12. Pre and post surgical pulsed Doppler recording of a patient with left atrial myxoma and with mitral regurgitation. It is possible to appreciate the systolic turbulent flow in the left atrium. After surgical resection of left atrial myxoma, the mitral valve movement became normal and the mitral regurgitant signal disappeared.

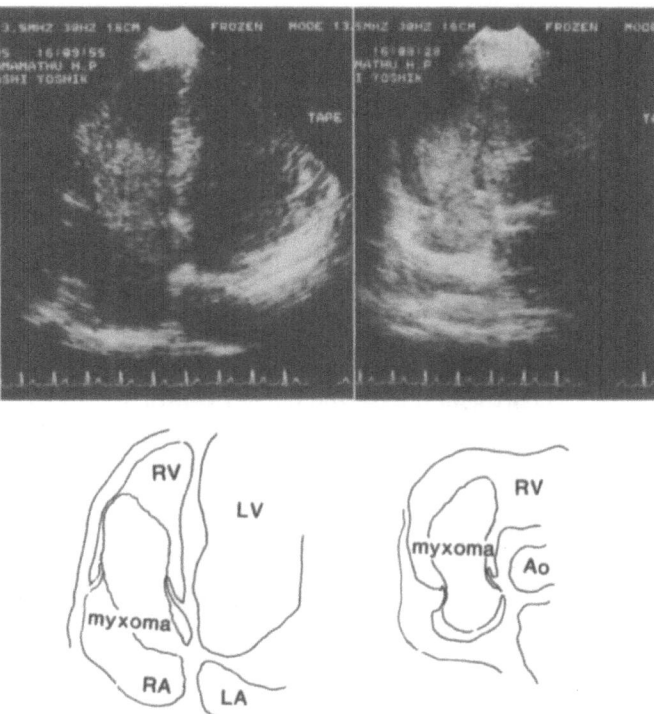

Figure 7.13. Four-chamber and right ventricular inflow view of a patient with a right atrial myxoma. The large myxoma prolapses into the tricuspid valve orifice during diastole.

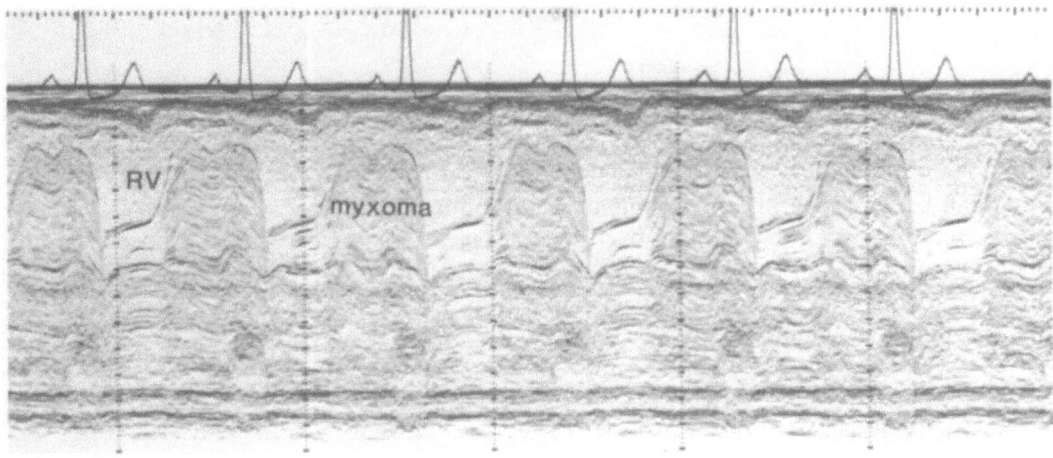

Figure 7.14. M-mode echocardiogram of a patient with a right atrial myxoma. The cloud of echoes from the tumor is visible behind the anterior leaflet of the tricuspid valve during diastole. The diastolic slope of the anterior tricuspid leaflet is also reduced.

creased acoustic density in the two-dimensional echocardiogram (Figure 7.15). M-mode echocardiography also demonstrates increased echogenic mass (Figure 7.16). The tumor is intracavitary and/or intramyocardial, often multiple and occurs more frequently in the left ventricle. Cardiac signs and symptoms in a patient with an intracardiac rhabdomyoma may result from obstruction to blood flow by an intracavitary tumor, diminished compliance or contractility by replacement of the myocardium, or disturbances of cardiac rhythm.

4. Left ventricular fibroma

The second most frequent cardiac tumor in children is a fibroma. A fibroma is a non-capsulated tumor that is usually generated from the left ventricular free wall or the IVS. If it protrudes into the left ventricular outflow tract, the hemodynamic alteration mimics subaortic stenosis. When it originates from the apical portion, no hemodynamic derangement occurs and electrocardiographic abnormalities such as ventricular arrhythmia and/or non-specific ST-T changes are the only clinical findings. It is sometimes possible to identify the abnormal tumor echoes in the myocardial tissue with relatively clear borders and calcified areas (Figure 7.17). It is quite important to diagnose the fibroma, since this tumor can be completely resected with a relatively simple surgical procedure (Figure 7.18).

5. Malignant primary cardiac tumor

Primary malignant cardiac tumors are mainly sarcoma. The incidence of primary malignant cardiac tumor is very low, therefore its typical echocardiographic signs remain unclear. In Figures 7.19, 20 and 21, the sarcoma originates from the postero-basal portion of left atrium with involvement of the mitral valve causing stenosis and regurgitation.

6. Secondary tumors of the heart

In the heart, the metastases of malignant tumors are more frequent than primary tumors. Lung and breast cancer are predominant in this entity (Figure 7.22). Ordinarily, the pericardium is the most affected area and several degrees of pericardial effusion can occur. Metastasis in the right cardiac cavities are more usual than in the left cavities. Malignant tumors sometimes directly extend through the inferior vena cava and can mechanically affect the tricuspid flow (Figure 7.23).

7. Pericardial effusion

The pericardial sac is normally a virtual space and usually cannot be identified by echocardiography. However, in the presence of pericardial effusion, this space can be appreciated as an echo-free space between the posterior left ventricular wall and posterior pericardium, and sometimes between the anterior pericardium and anterior right ventricular wall. Two-dimensional echocardiography can show not only the presence of pericardial effusion, but also the hemodynamic repercussion such as abnormal cardiac motion and right ventricular anterior wall compression or collapse in early diastole (Figure 7.24). In M-mode, the anterior and posterior cardiac walls are moving in similar directions in the presence of a large pericardial effusion (Figures 7.25, 26). In this condition, one cannot evaluate left ventricular function using M-mode; the pulsed Doppler method should be used instead (Figure 7.27). Sometimes, intrapericardial hemorrhage produces pericardial effusion and hematoma, which can be identified as an echogenic mass (Figure 7.28).

8. Pleural effusion

Pleural effusion can occasionally occur together with pericardial effusion, but this situation does not constitute a clinical diagnostic problem. Echocardiographically, it is possible to differentiate them, since pericardial echo can be identified between the two echo-free spaces (Figure 7.29).

9. Constrictive pericarditis

Chronic pericarditis can sometimes progress to constrictive pericarditis, due to fibrosis and/or calcification of the pericardium. Two-dimensional echocardiography provides information about the characteristics of the pericardium (Figure 7.30). M-mode has an important role in the evaluation of hemodynamic derangements. The most important finding is an abnormal IVS motion, which consists of early diastolic posterior movement followed by abrupt anterior displacement. This finding may reflect the restrictive condition of the left ventricle (Figure 7.31).

10. Pericardial defect

Pericardial defect is a rare congenital heart disease that is not usually accompanied by clinical problems. The most common type of this abnormality is the absence of a left pericardium. In this case, the heart shifts to the left and the right ventricle can be more visible in parasternal view (Figure 7.32). The exaggerated cardiac motion can simulate right ventricular dilatation accompanied by IVS paradoxical motion. These findings are sometimes indistinguishable from those of right ventricular volume overload such as ASD, especially in M-mode (Figure 7.33). In order to differentiate between these two conditions, the Doppler method plays an important role, since one can evaluate the relationship between right and left ventricular stroke volume (Figure 7.34).

11. False tendon

False tendon is a congenital variant, which can sometimes be seen in the left ventricle, without any certain clinical significance (Figure 7.35).

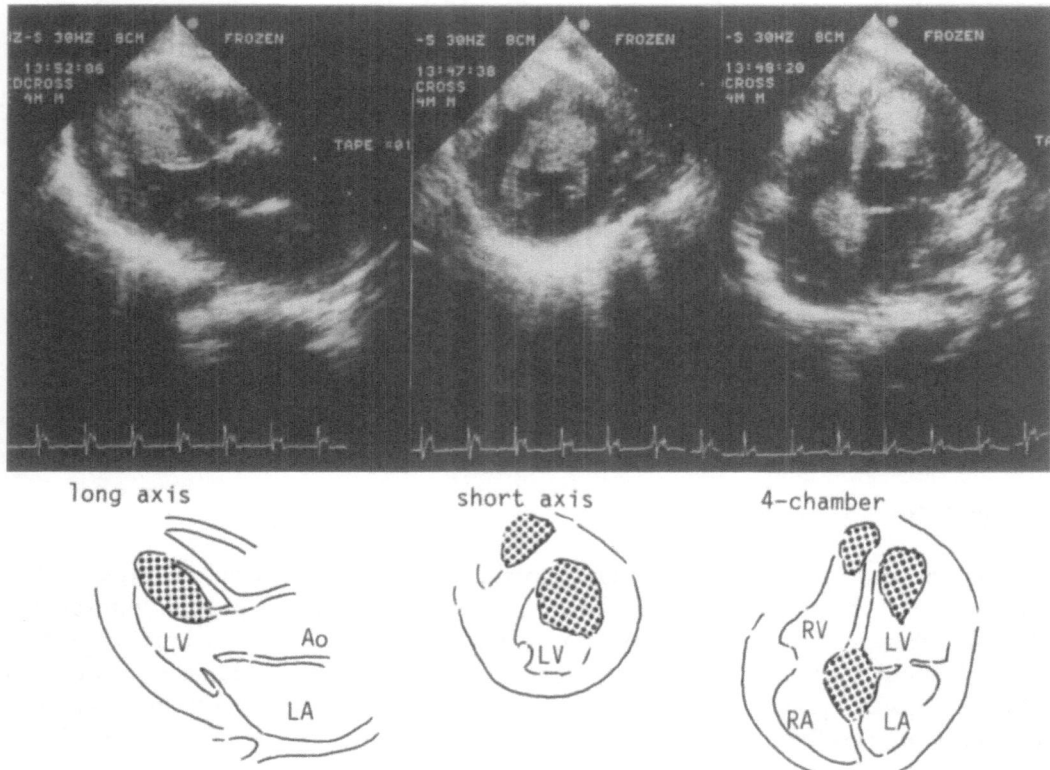

Figure 7.15. Two-dimensional echocardiogram of a 4 month-old patient with a cardiac rhabdomyoma. An increased echogenic mass (dotted area) protrudes into the left ventricular cavity in long and short axis view. The four-chamber view shows the echogenic mass located in the interatrial septum.

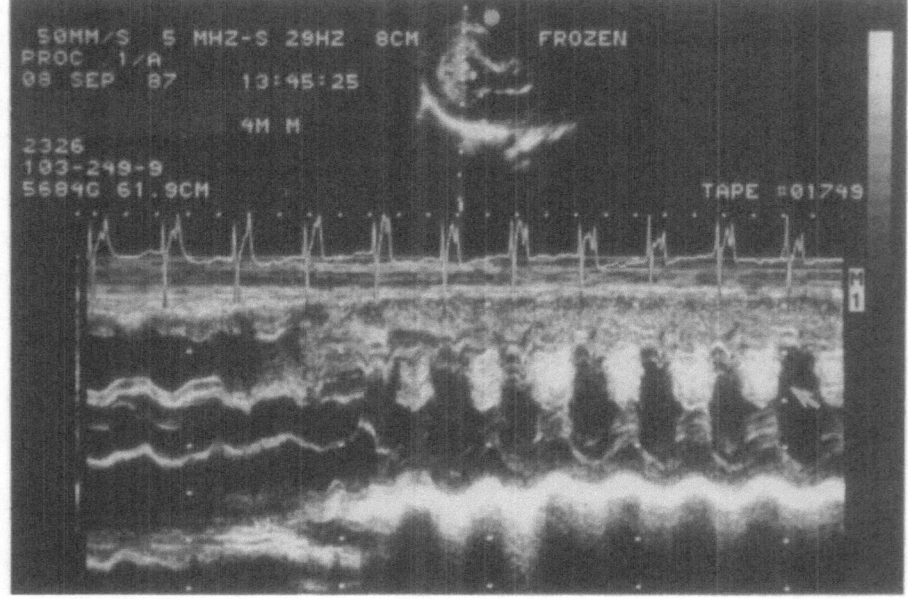

Figure 7.16. M-mode scan of a patient with a cardiac rhabdomyoma. Increased echogenic mass (arrow) protrudes into the left ventricular cavity during systole.

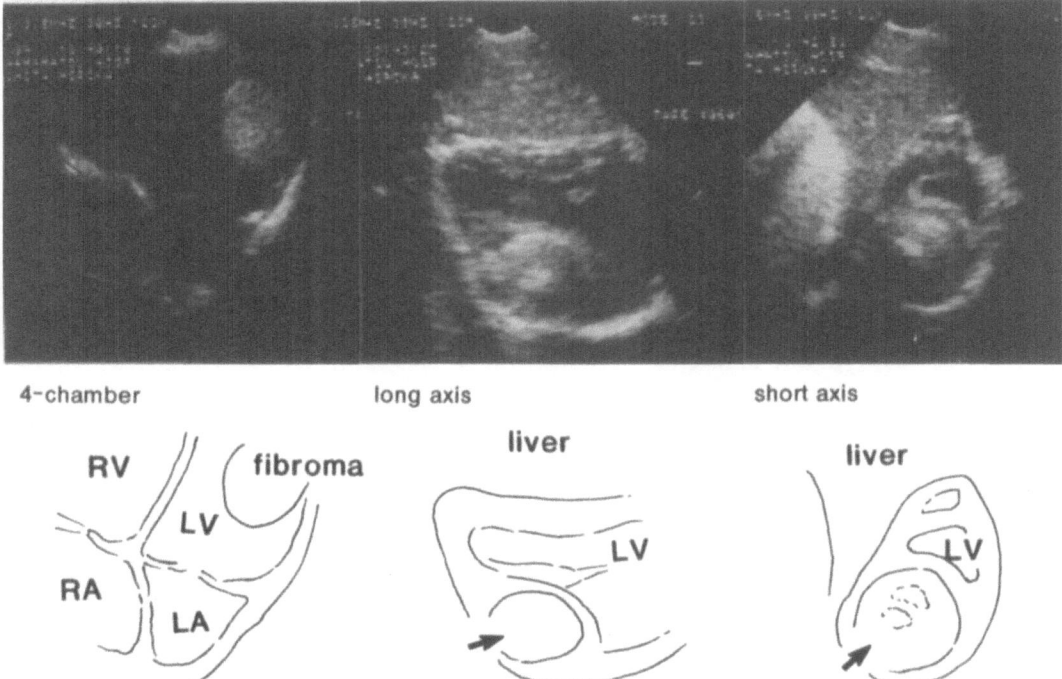

Figure 7.17. Two-dimensional echocardiogram of a patient with a left ventricular fibroma. In the apical four-chamber view, the tumor compresses the left ventricular cavity. Using the subcostal approach, one can distinguish the tumor echoes from the myocardial echoes. Calcified areas within the tumor are also visualized.

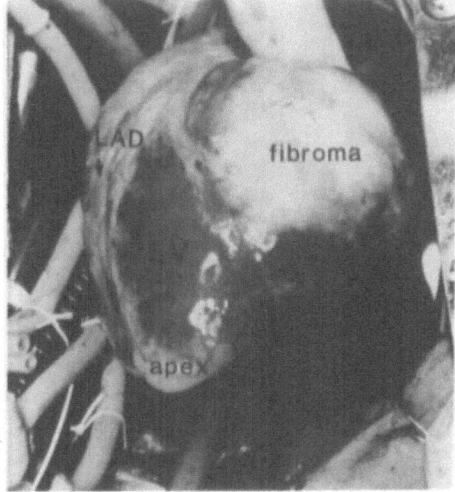

Figure 7.18. Operatory finding of left ventricular fibroma. One can see the fibroma existing on the left ventricular lateral free wall. In this case, the fibroma was easily resected.

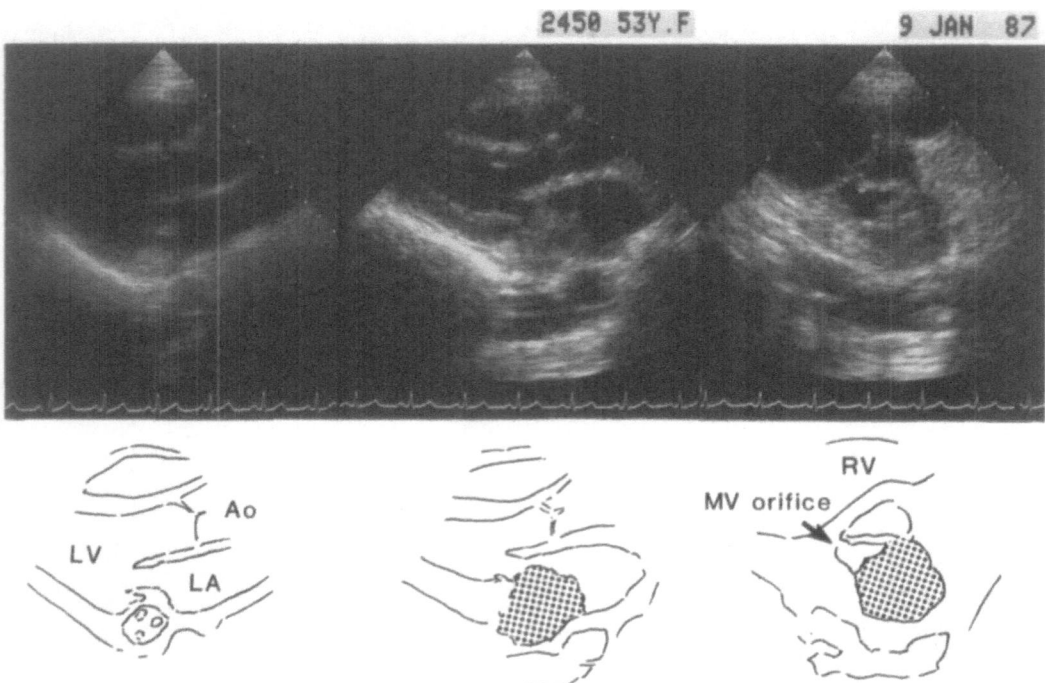

Figure 7.19. Parasternal long and short axis view of a patient with primary cardiac sarcoma. In the long axis view, the tumor is located on the posterior left atrial wall, mainly in the anterolateral side (dotted area). In short axis view, the mitral valve orifice shows stenosis due to tumor invasion.

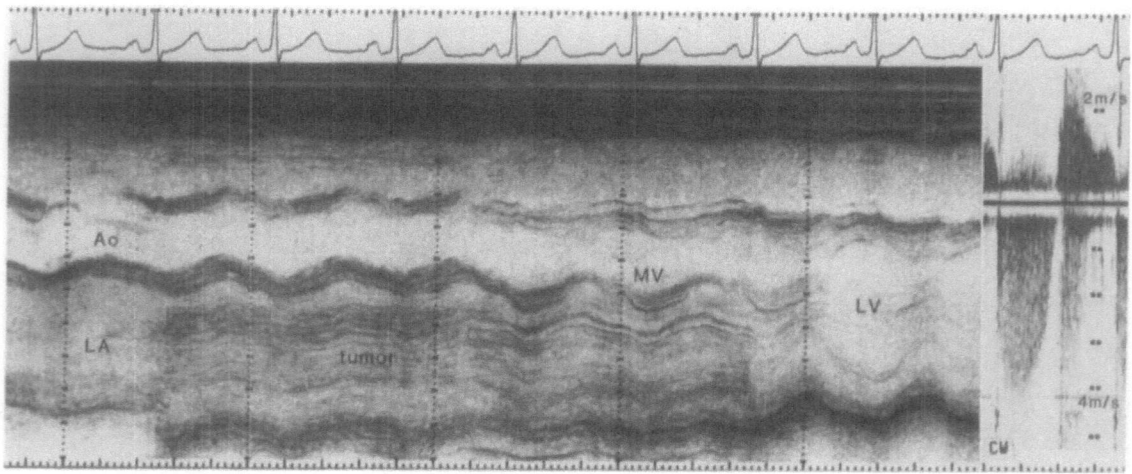

Figure 7.20. M-mode scan and CW Doppler echocardiogram of a patient with cardiac sarcoma. A cloud of echoes in the left atrial cavity and behind the anterior mitral leaflet is observed. CW Doppler shows an increased peak velocity of transmitral flow during diastole which indicates the presence of an obstruction. Mitral regurgitant flow is also illustrated.

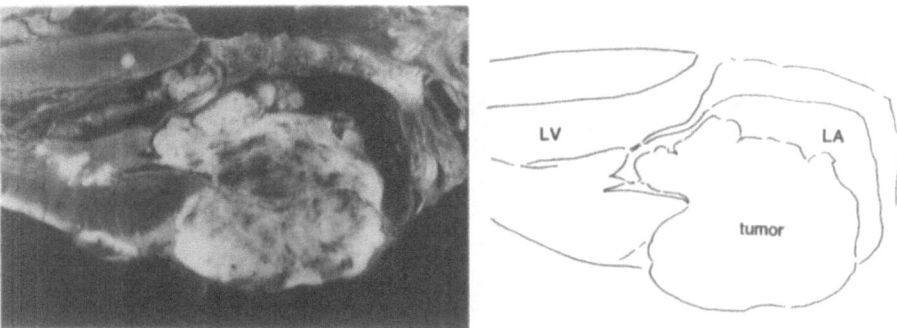

Figure 7.21. Autopsy specimen of a patient with primary cardiac sarcoma. This specimen was obtained 2 months after echocardiographic recordings (Figures 7.19, 20). The tumor is located on the posterior left atrial wall and invades the posterior mitral valve.

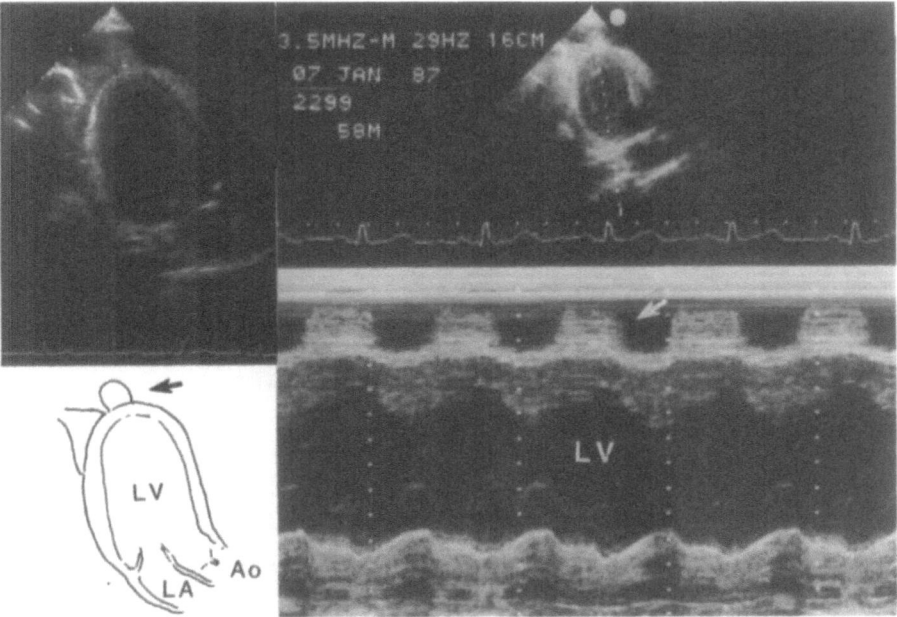

Figure 7.22. Apical long axis view of a patient with lung cancer. A tumor echo is clearly observed on the apical portion of left ventricle (black arrow). M-mode also illustrates the same finding (white arrow).

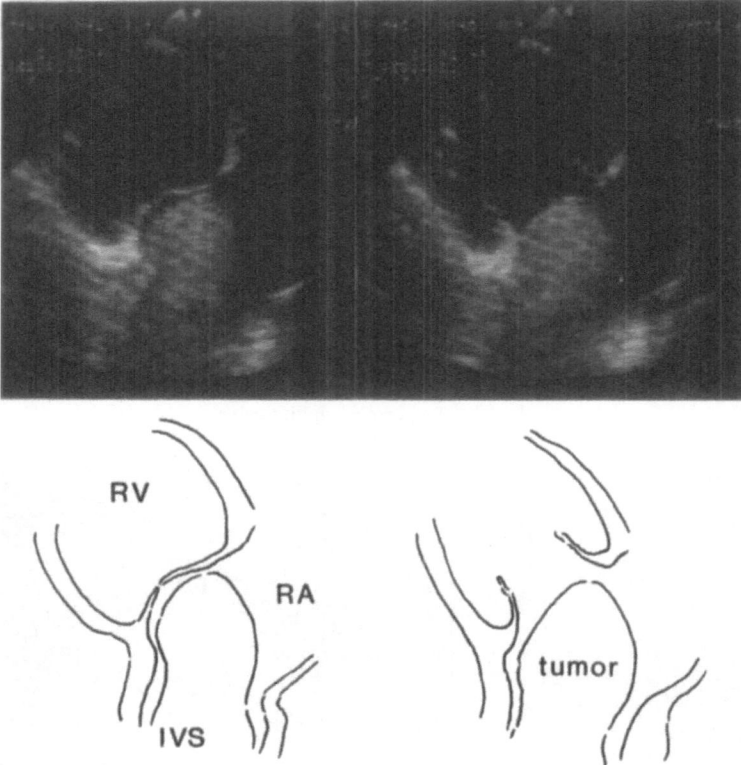

Figure 7.23.   Parasternal right ventricular inflow view of a 7 year-old patient with Wilms tumor. A large tumor in the
right atrium through the inferior vena cava is visible.

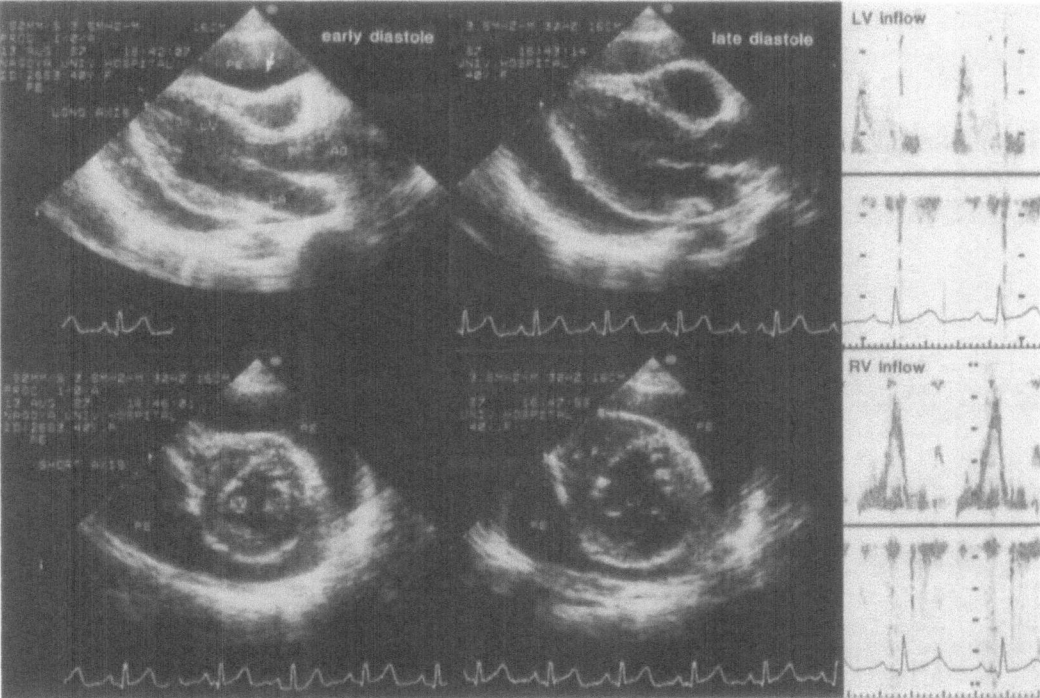

Figure 7.24.   Long and short axis views and pulsed Doppler echocardiograms of a patient with large pericardial effusion (PE). A large echo-free space is present around the heart. In real time, the pendular motion of the heart can be seen in the long axis view and the counter-clockwise rotation of the heart is recorded in the short axis view. During early diastole, the right ventricular collapse (arrow) can be observed. In late diastole and systole, the right ventricular free wall has a normal shape. The RV inflow demonstrates the depressed rapid filling and augmented atrial contribution due to this RV collapse. The LV inflow shows almost normal profile with low velocity.

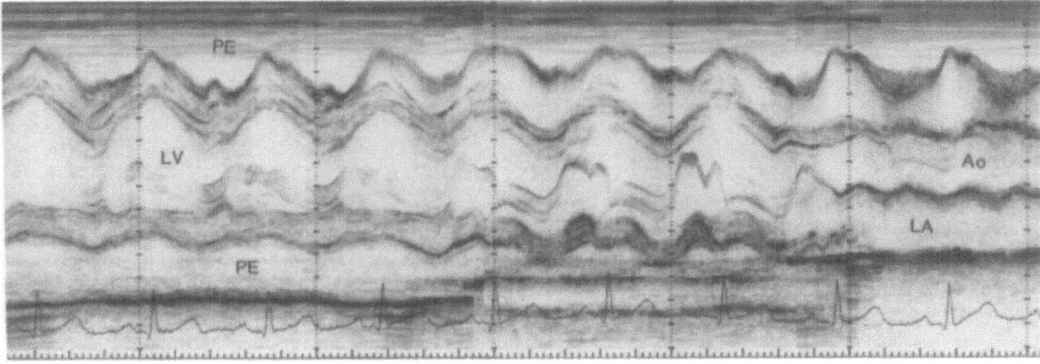

Figure 7.25.   M-mode scan of a patient with large pericardial effusion (a same case as in Figure 7.24). An anterior and posterior echo-free space is evident. The right ventricular cavity collapses mainly in early diastole.

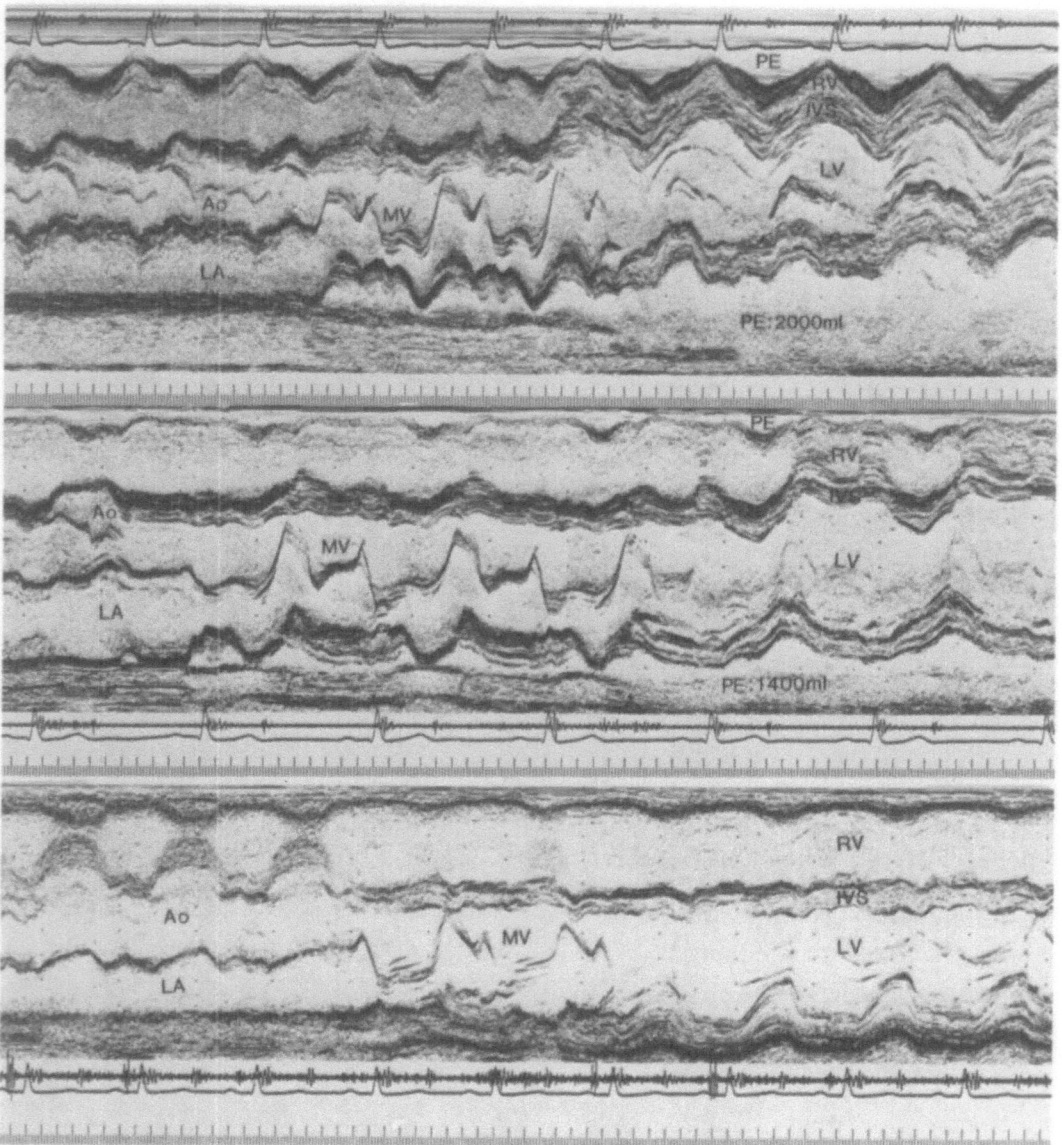

Figure 7.26. M-mode scan of a patient with large pericardial effusion before and after drainage. With large pericardial effusion (PE) (upper panel), an anterior and posterior echo-free space is evident. The anterior and posterior cardiac walls are moving in similar directions. After partial drainage of about 600 ml of the effusion (middle panel), the echo-free space is decreased and cardiac motion improves. With complete drainage of the pericardial effusion (lower panel), the echo-free space disappears and cardiac motion is normalized.

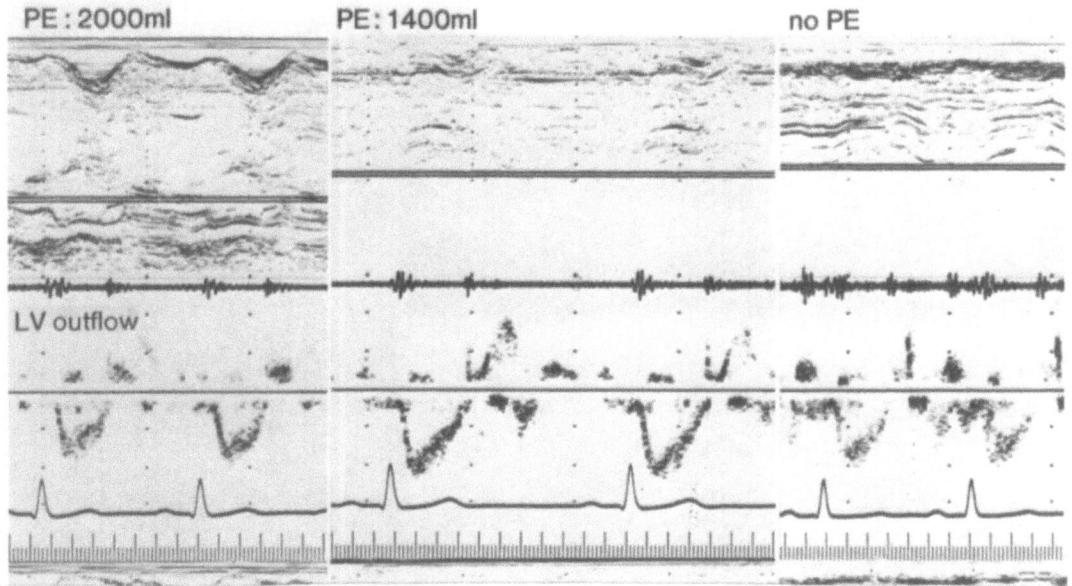

Figure 7.27. Pulsed Doppler echocardiogram of left ventricular outflow velocities from a patient with large pericardial effusion before and after drainage. With large pericardial effusion (left panel), the left ventricular outflow velocity shows decreased peak velocity due to the low output state. After partial drainage of the pericardial effusion (middle panel), the left ventricular outflow velocity illustrates the improvement of cardiac output that is manifested by an increment of peak velocity and ejection time. After complete drainage of the pericardial effusion (right panel), the left ventricular outflow velocity cannot reflect the improvement of cardiac output due to difficulty in obtaining the optimal Doppler angle in this condition.

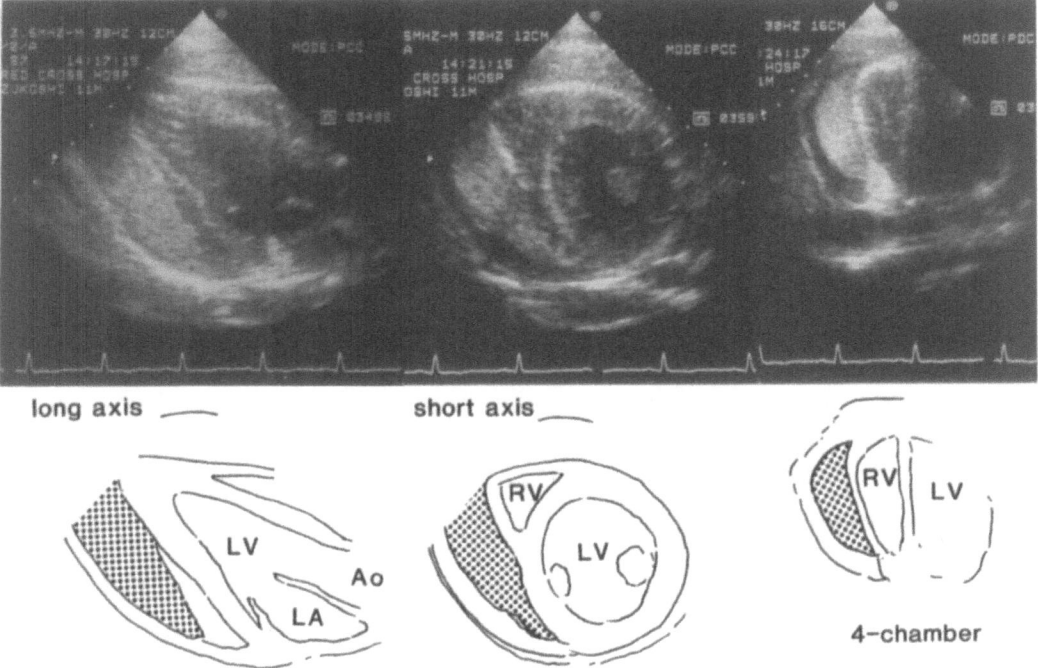

Figure 7.28. Long and short axis and four-chamger view of an 11 year-old boy with a pericardial hematoma. A hematoma attached to the right ventricular free wall is demonstrated as an echogenic mass (dotted area).

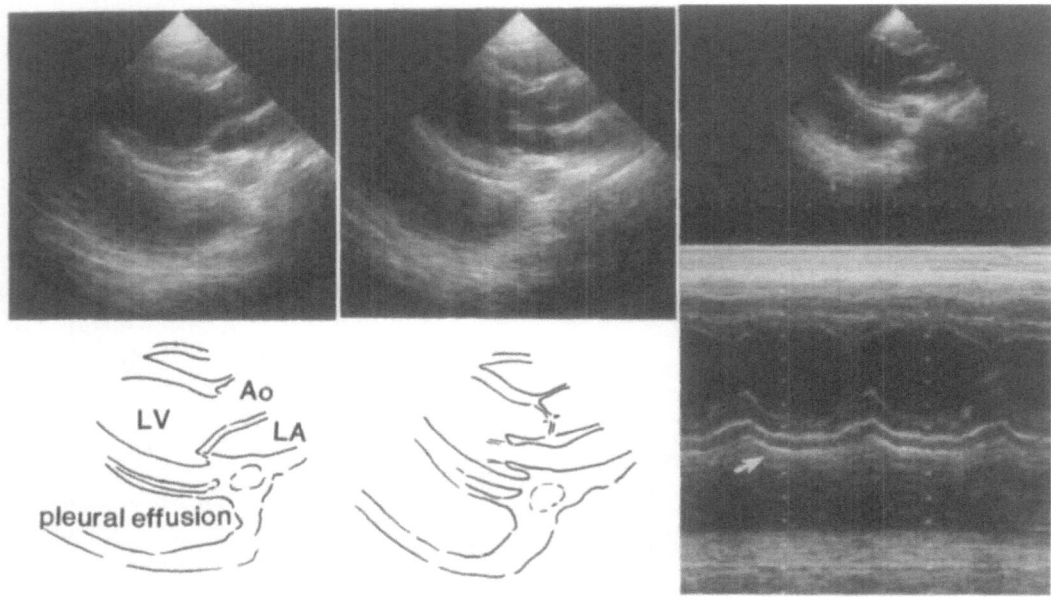

Figure 7.29.   Long axis and M-mode echocardiogram of a patient with large pleural effusion. The pericardial echo (arrow) is seen between the two echo-free spaces.

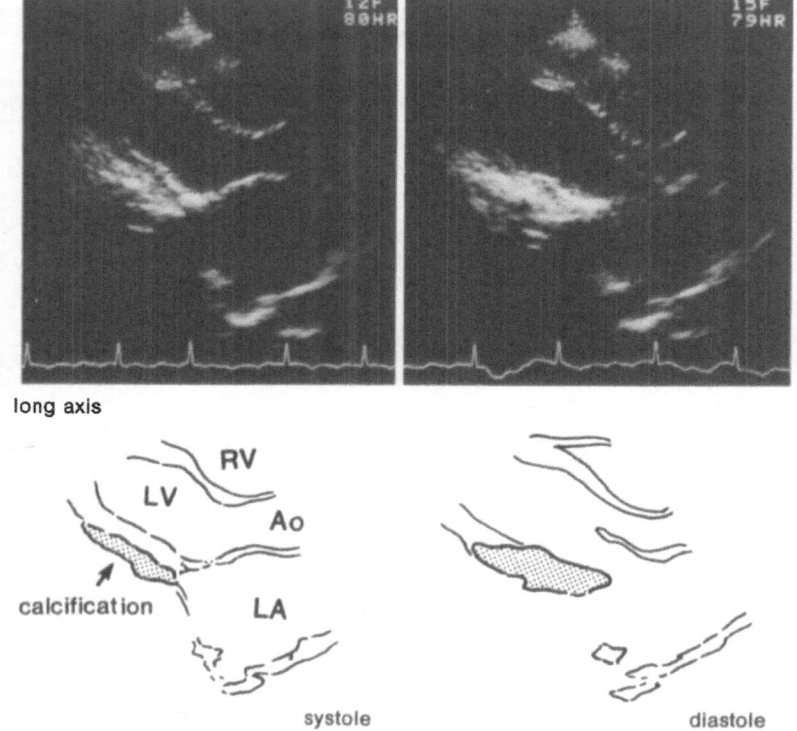

Figure 7.30.   Long axis view of a patient with constrictive pericarditis. The posterior pericardium has an increased echo intensity which might reflect calcification. Left atrial enlargement and reduced left ventricular cavity are also observed.

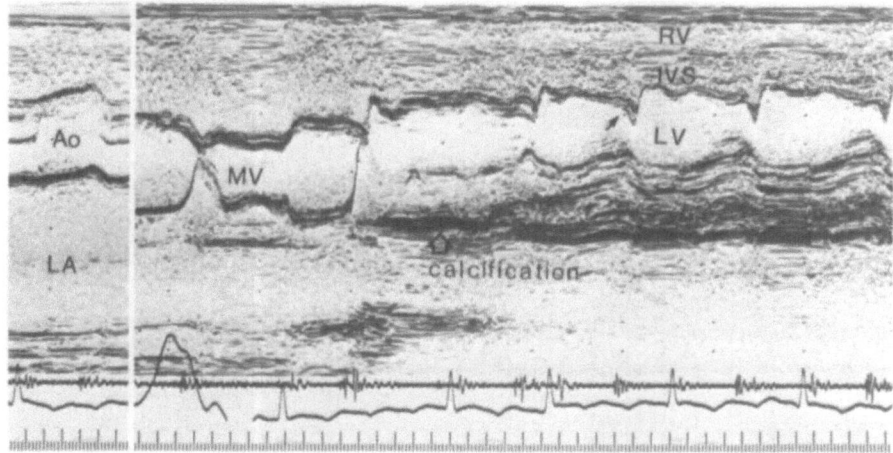

Figure 7.31. M-mode scan of a patient with constrictive pericarditis. Note the abnormal IVS motion (arrow), reduced left ventricular dimensions and enlargement of the left atrium. Posterior pericardial calcification is evident.

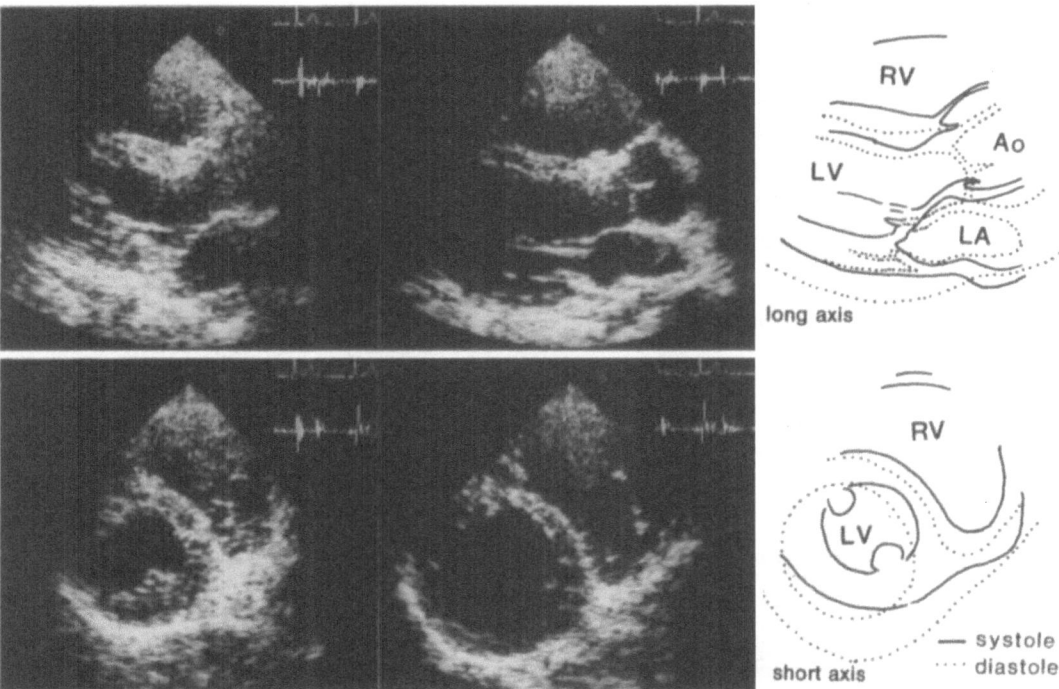

Figure 7.32. Parasternal long and short axis view of a patient with pericardial defect. The echocardiogram reveals the presence of right ventricular dilatation. The short axis view illustrates exaggerated displacement of the heart, with normal circular shape of left ventricle in diastole.

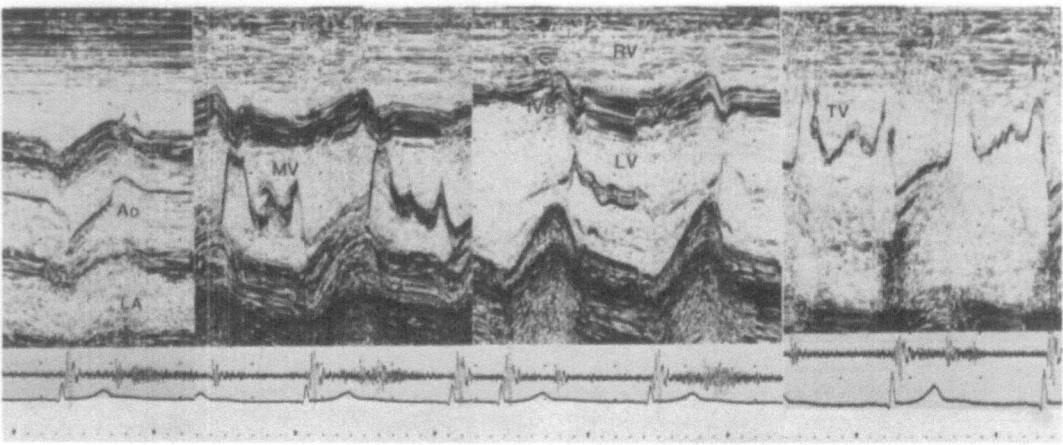

Figure 7.33. M-mode echocardiogram of a patient with a pericardial defect. Paradoxical IVS motion is present and the left ventricular posterior wall motion is exaggerated. In this patient, the tricuspid valve could easily be recorded.

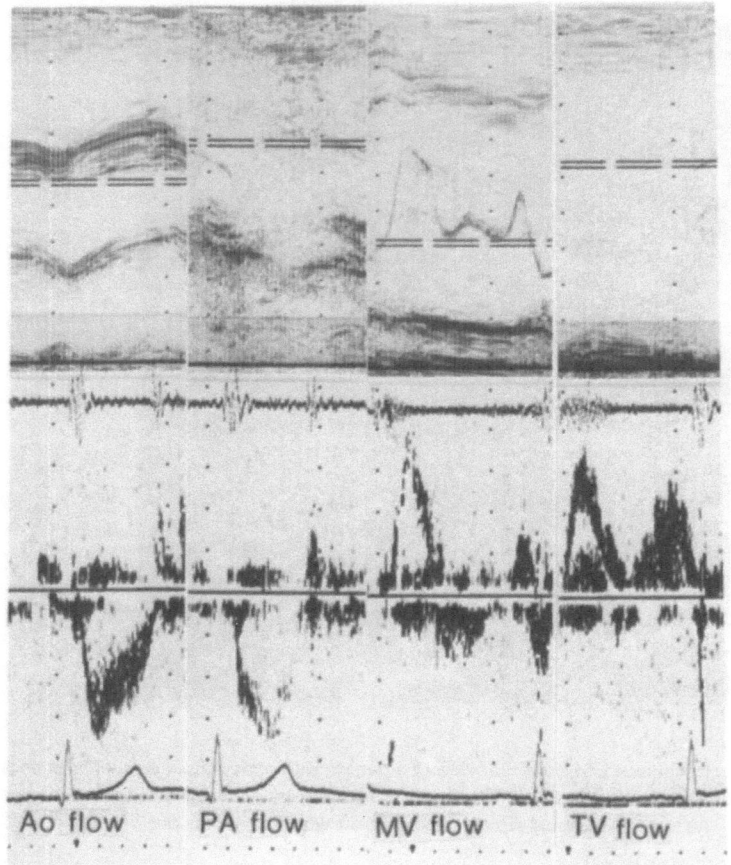

Figure 7.34. Pulsed Doppler echocardiogram of a patient with pericardial defect. Aortic and pulmonary flow velocity tracings are almost similar which suggests the absence of an intracardiac shunt. Transmitral and transtricuspid flows are also similar.

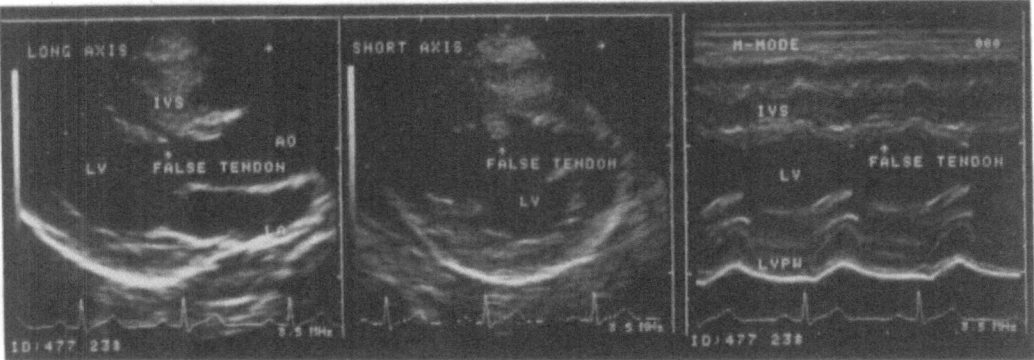

Figure 7.35. Parasternal long and short axis and M-mode echocardiogram of a patient with a false tendon. An abnormal dense echo band (arrow) is observed between the apical left ventricular posterior wall and basal interventricular septum.

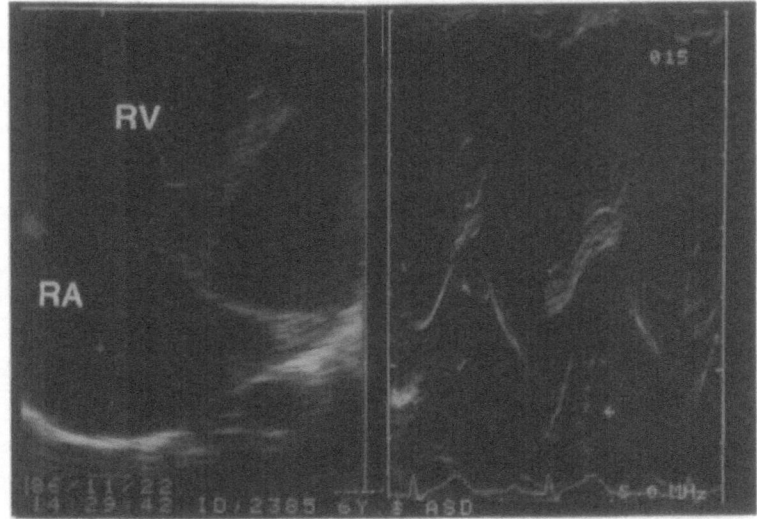

Figure 7.36. Two-dimensional and M-mode echocardiogram of a patient with Chiari network. Behind the tricuspid valve, the Chiari network is demonstrated as filamentous and mobile echoes.

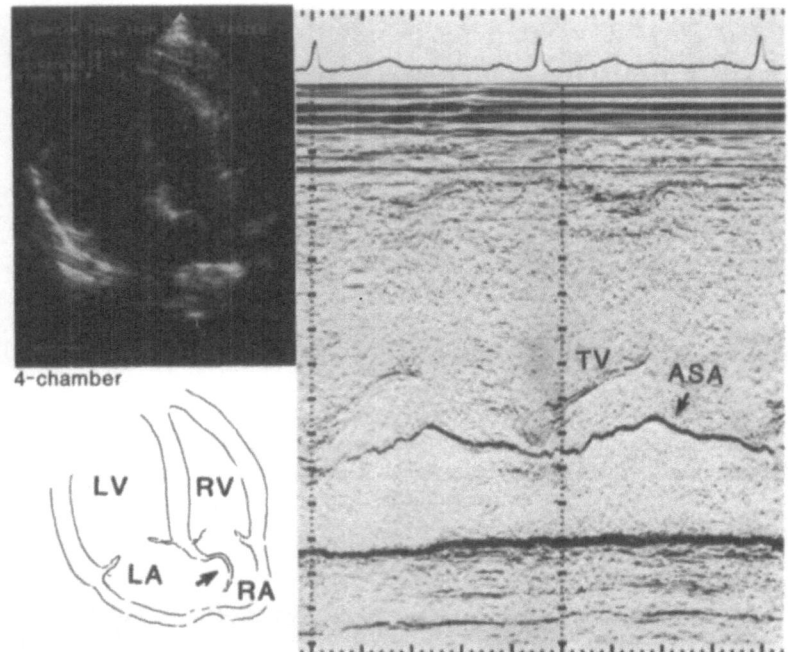

Figure 7.37.   Apical four-chamber view and M-mode scan of a patient with atrial septal aneurysm. This aneurysm protrudes into the right atrium. In M-mode one can see the wall motion of the atrial septal aneurysm (ASA).

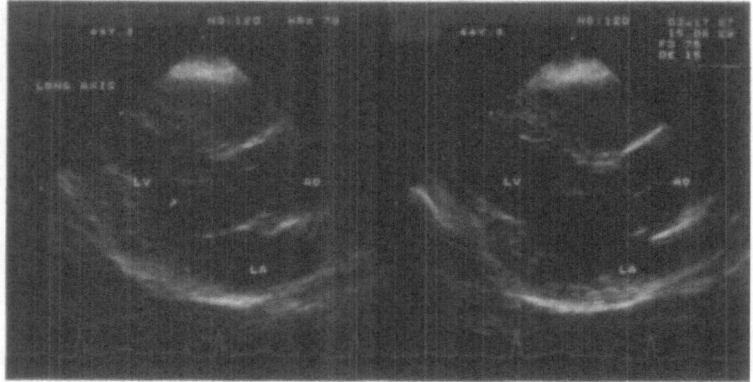

Figure 7.38.   Long axis view of an elderly patient with sigmoid septum. The basal potion of interventricular septum (arrow) impinges on the left ventricular outflow tract.

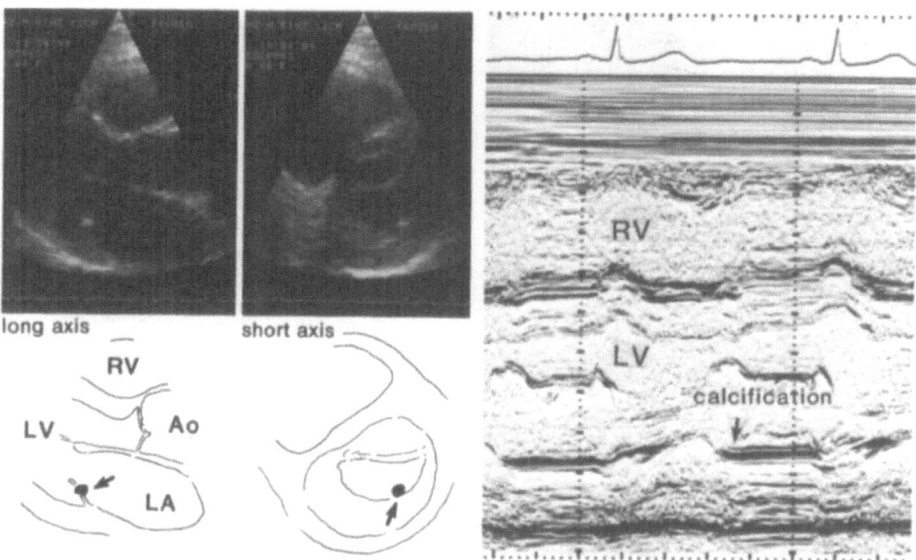

Figure 7.39. Two-dimensional and M-mode echocardiograms of a patient with mitral annular calcification. The calcified area (arrow) is located only in the posterior portion of the mitral annulus. In M-mode, dense echoes are observed behind the mitral valve.

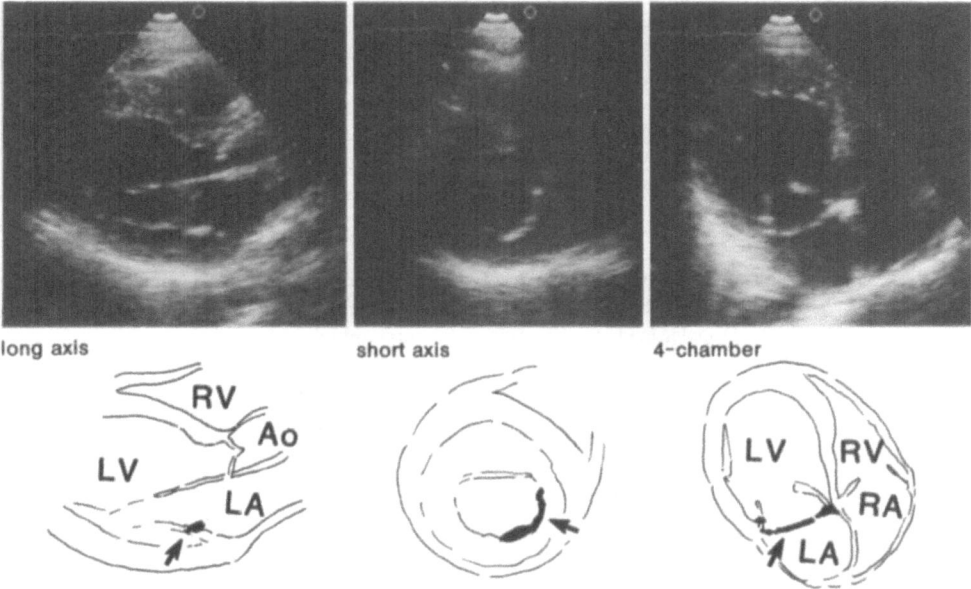

Figure 7.40. Long axis, short axis and four-chamber view of a patient with mitral annular calcification. In this patient, the calcification is located in the posterior and septal portion of the mitral annulus. In the four-chamber view, one notes the dense echo band behind the mitral valve due to relatively poor ultrasonic resolution.

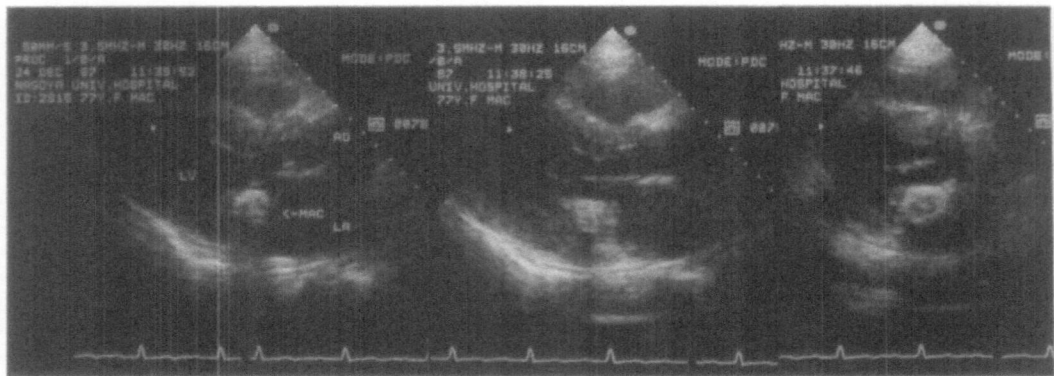

Figure 7.41.   Long and short axis view of a patient with large mitral annular calcification. The calcification is large enough to produce stenotic conditions in two-dimensional images.

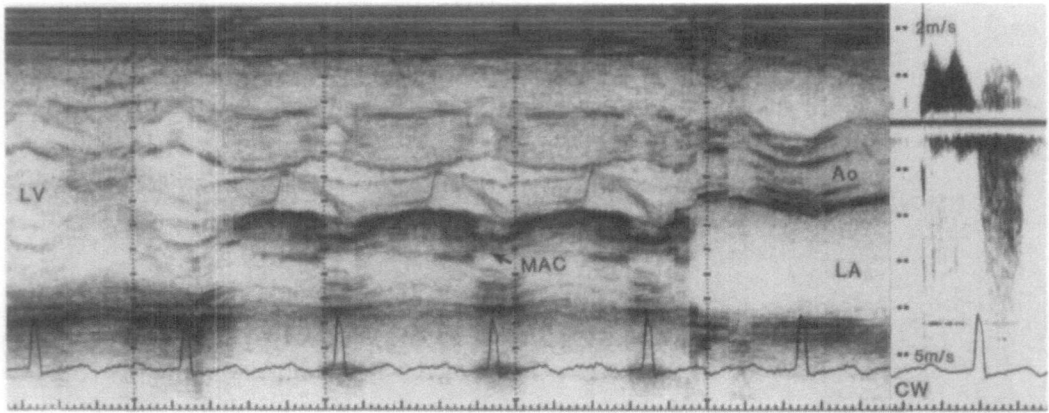

Figure 7.42.   M-mode scan and CW Doppler echocardiogram of a patient with large mitral annular calcification. In the M-mode scan, the dense echo band behind the mitral valve (MAC: mitral annular calcification) is observed. CW Doppler evidences stenotic and regurgitant mitral flow.

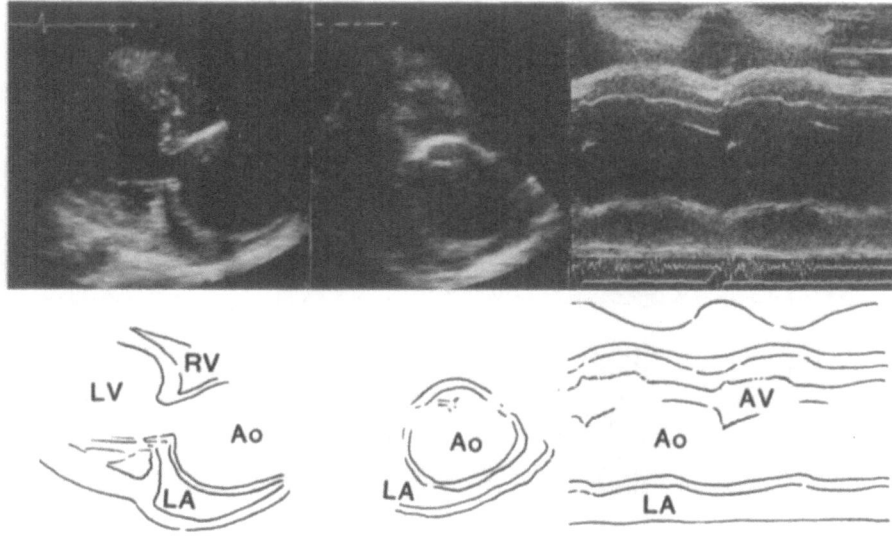

Figure 7.43. Two-dimensional and M-mode echocardiograms of a patient with an ascending aortic aneurysm. Severe dilatation of the ascending aorta with left atrial compression is observed.

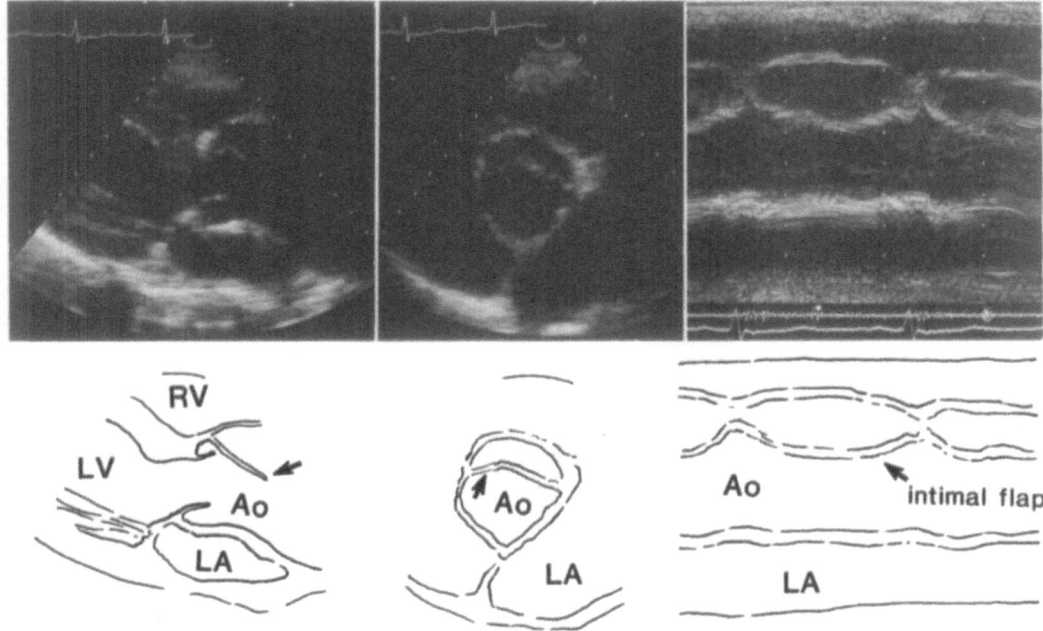

Figure 7.44. Two-dimensional and M-mode echocardiograms from a patient with a dissecting aortic aneurysm. The intimal flap is shown by the arrow.

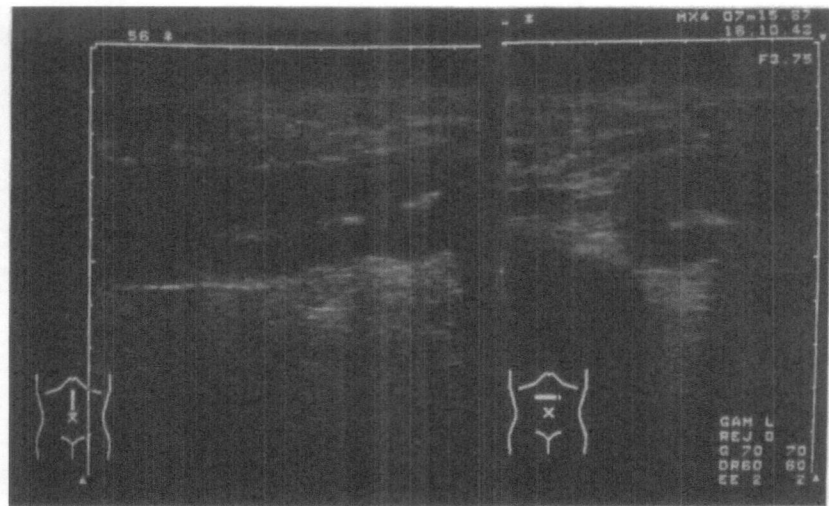

Figure 7.45. Two-dimensional image of a disecting abdominal aneurysm with intimal flap obtained by the linear scanner.

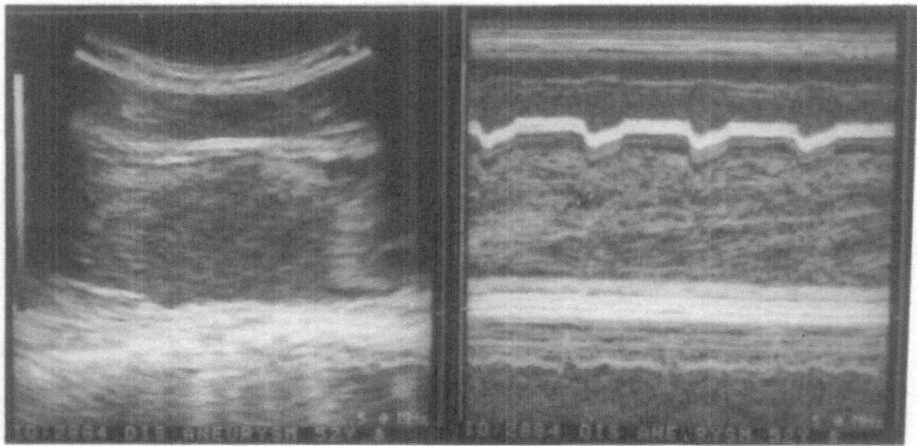

Figure 7.46. Transesophageal two-dimensional and M-mode echocardiograms from a patient with a dissecting thoracic aortic aneurysm. This echocardiogram is obtained using a flexible endoscope with axial convex scanner. The intimal flap and 'smoke-like' spontaneous echoes due to blood stasis in the false lumen can be clearly seen.

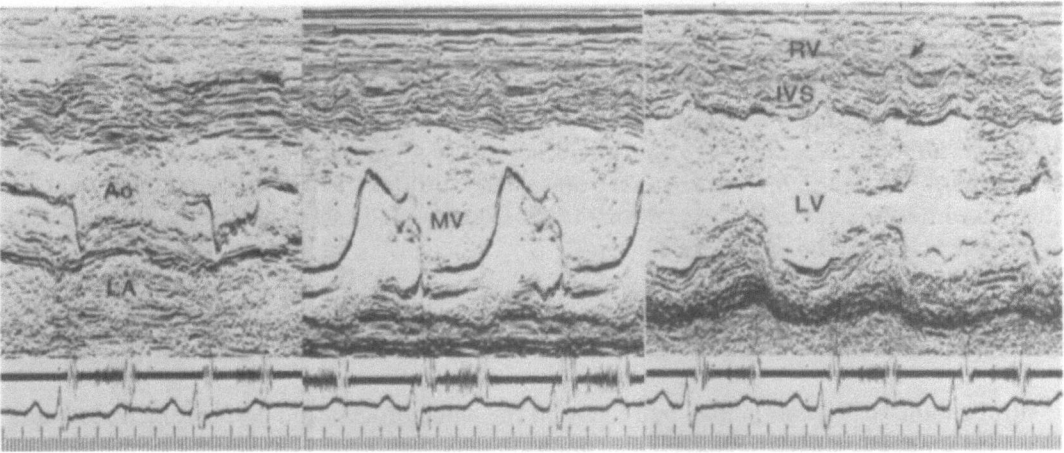

Figure 7.47. M-mode echocardiogram of a patient with primary pulmonary hypertension. The left panel shows hypertrophy of the right ventricular outflow tract. The right panel shows paradoxical motion of IVS without right ventricular dilatation (pressure overload).

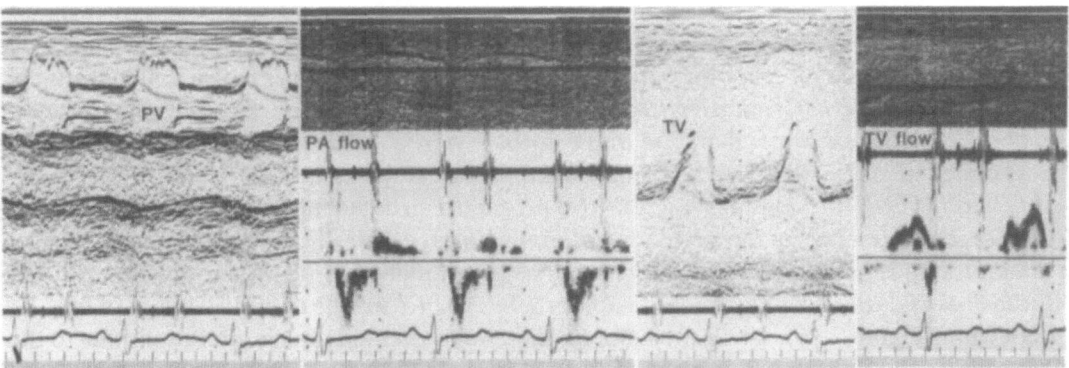

Figure 7.48. M-mode and pulsed Doppler echocardiogram of the same patient. The motion of the pulmonary valve (PV) cusps are clearly demonstrated. Pulmonary arterial (PA) flow shows a short acceleration time due to pulmonary hypertension. The right panel shows tricuspid valve (TV) flow with decreased rapid filling (R) and prominent atrial contribution (A) due to right ventricular pressure overload.

12. Chiari network

Chiari network is the residual tissue, which shows mobile and filamentous echoes within the right atrium (Figure 7.36) and is not pathological.

13. Atrial septal aneurysm

Atrial septal aneurysm is a congenital anomaly, which is located at the level of the foramen ovale (Figure 7.37). The clinical significance of this condition remains unclear.

14. Sigmoid septum

Elderly people sometimes have distortion of the basal portion of the interventricular septum so that it protrudes into the left ventricular outflow tract. This malformation is referred to as a 'sigmoid septum'. This entity is easily identified by two-dimensional echocardiography (Figure 7.38). The relatively narrow left ventricular outflow tract is often accompanied by increased outflow velocities. However, these patients usually show no symptoms related to this obstruction in clinical practice.

15. Mitral annular calcification

Mitral annular calcification may be related to the aging process and is sometimes accompanied by conduction disturbances. This condition mainly affects the posterior portion of the mitral annulus (Figure 7.39), but in rare cases the other portions can be involved (Figure 7.40). Sometimes this condition may be accompanied by mitral stenosis and/or regurgitation (Figures 7.41, 42).

16. Aneurysm of the aorta

Using two-dimensional echocardiography, one can evaluate the morphological changes of the aorta from parasternal, suprasternal and abdominal approach. In the case of an aneurysm, it is possible to demonstrate dilatation of the aorta (Figure 7.43). The presence of a dissecting aortic aneurysm is assessed by detecting the intimal flap (Figures 7.44, 45). Transthoracic and suprasternal echocardiography is a sensitive procedure in detecting ascending aorta and root disease, but often fails in the descending thoracic aorta, especially in patients with emphysema and adipositas. Because of the close anatomic connection of the esophagus with the thoracic aorta, transesophageal echocardiography can provide the definitive image of type III dissection (Figure 7.46). Using the Doppler method the hemodynamic alterations due to the dissection can be evaluated, in particular by using color Doppler flow mapping (see Figure 11.42).

17. Primary pulmonary hypertension

Primary pulmonary hypertension occurs in patients without evidence of other cardiac or pulmonary disease. Two-dimensional, M-mode and Doppler echocardiographically can provide qualitative and quantitative information about pulmonary hypertension (Figures 7.47, 48 and also Chapter 9).

Evaluation of left ventricular function

1. M-mode echocardiography

Until recently, the echocardiographic evaluation of left ventricular volume and systolic function has been performed by M-mode derived left ventricular end-diastolic and systolic dimension measurements. M-mode echocardiography more clearly identifies the endocardial surface of the left ventricle as compared with two-dimensional echocardiography. When recorded simultaneously with an electrocardiogram and a phonocardiogram, the timing of end-diastole and systole is easily recognized. Using this method of measurement, the left ventricular shape is assumed to be an ellipsoid and the ratio between the short and long axis dimension (D and L) is also assumed to be 1:2 through all cardiac cycles. This assumption has been justified by Pombo *et al.* and Popp *et al.* in the absence of left ventricular deformity or wall motion abnormalities. The assumption is that the left ventricular volume = $4/3 \times \pi \times L/2 \times (D/2)^2 = \pi/6 LD = \pi/6 \times 2D \times D^2 = \pi/3D^2 = D^3$ (Pombo's method). In cases with enlarged left ventricle, the shape of the left ventricle becomes more oval and the ratio of the long and short axis dimensions approaches 1. Therefore, the volume measurements by Pombo's method would be overestimated in this situation. To correct this error, Teichholz *et al.* reported that the left ventricular volume is $7.0/(2.4 + D) \times D^3$. Furthermore, to correct the changes in the ratio of long and short axis dimension between end-systole and diastole, Gibson *et al.* reported that the long axis dimension in end-systole is $4.18 + 1.14Ds$ and in end-diastole $5.90 + 0.98Dd$ on the basis of cinéangiographic measurements. However, these M-mode derived methods may sometimes be inadequate, since deformity of shape due to HOCM or segmental wall motion abnormalities in patients with ischemic heart disease can introduce significant errors in volume measurements. In recent advanced echocardiographic equipment, the dimensional and volume measurements are easily done on the CRT display using electronic calipers or a track ball (Figures 8.1, 2).

2. Two-dimensional echocardiography

Using area-length methods based on two-dimensional echocardiographic images, the left ventricular volume can be accurately measured, even in cases of left ventricular enlargement or in the presence of wall motion abnormalities. In this method, the left ventricular volume is calculated from the left ventricular area and long axis dimension on an apical long axis or two chamber view. On recent echocardiographic equipment, such measurements can easily be

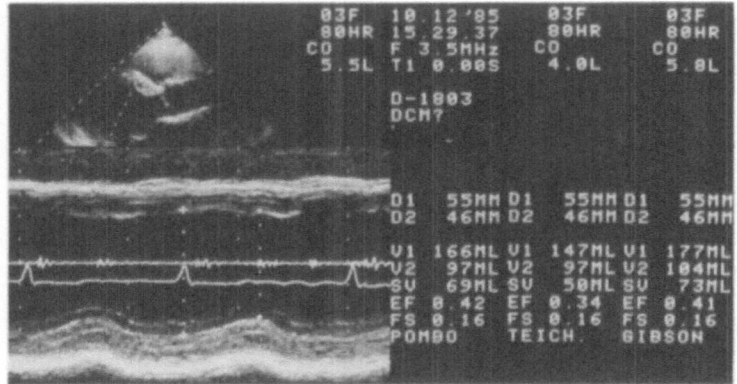

Figure 8.1. Parameters of left ventricular function in a normal subject, derived from M-mode echocardiogram. The evaluation of end-diastolic and systolic dimensions of the left ventricle are shown by dotted lines from the internal borders of IVS and left ventricular posterior wall. The calculated parameters that are obtained from Pombo's, Teichholz's and Gibson's methods are illustrated.

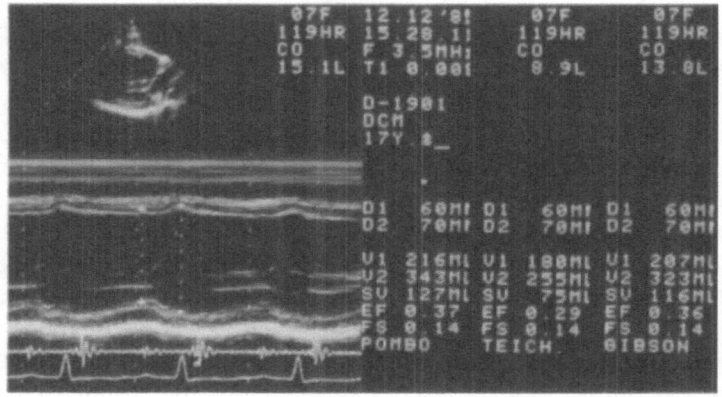

Figure 8.2. Parameters of left ventricular function derived from an M-mode echocardiogram in a patient with dilated cardiomyopathy. One can see a dilated and hypokinetic left ventricle. The over-estimated values obtained from three different methods (Pombo's, Teichholz's and Gibson's) are compared with those obtained by cardiac catheterization (EF = 25%).

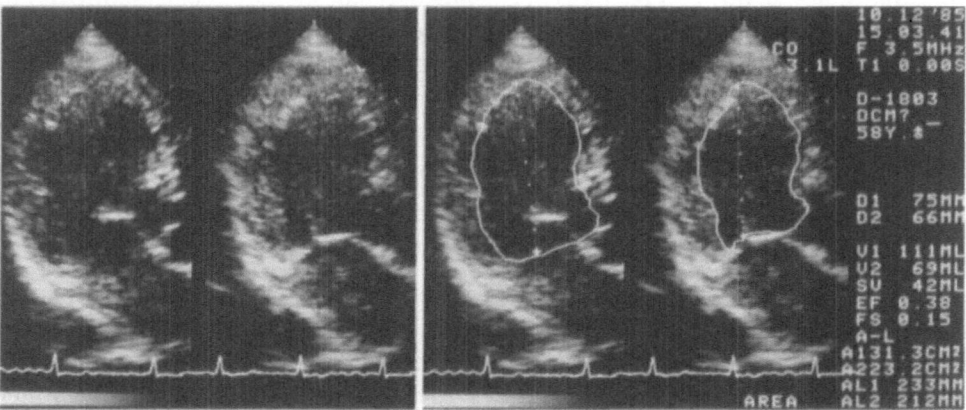

Figure 8.3. Evaluation of diastolic and systolic left ventricular volumes derived from two-dimensional images, using the apical long axis view. The left frame shows the endocardial surface of the left ventricle; the right frame illustrates its tracing and the area-length measurement.

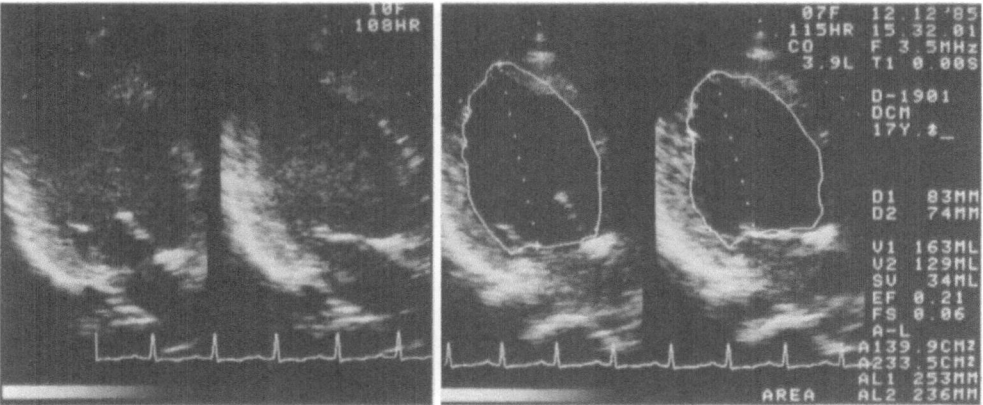

Figure 8.4. Apical long axis view demonstrating the evaluation of left ventricular diastolic and systolic volumes in a patient with dilated cardiomyopathy. In comparison with M-mode (Figure 8.2), the parameters derived from two-dimensional echocardiography are well correlated with those obtained by cardiac catheterization.

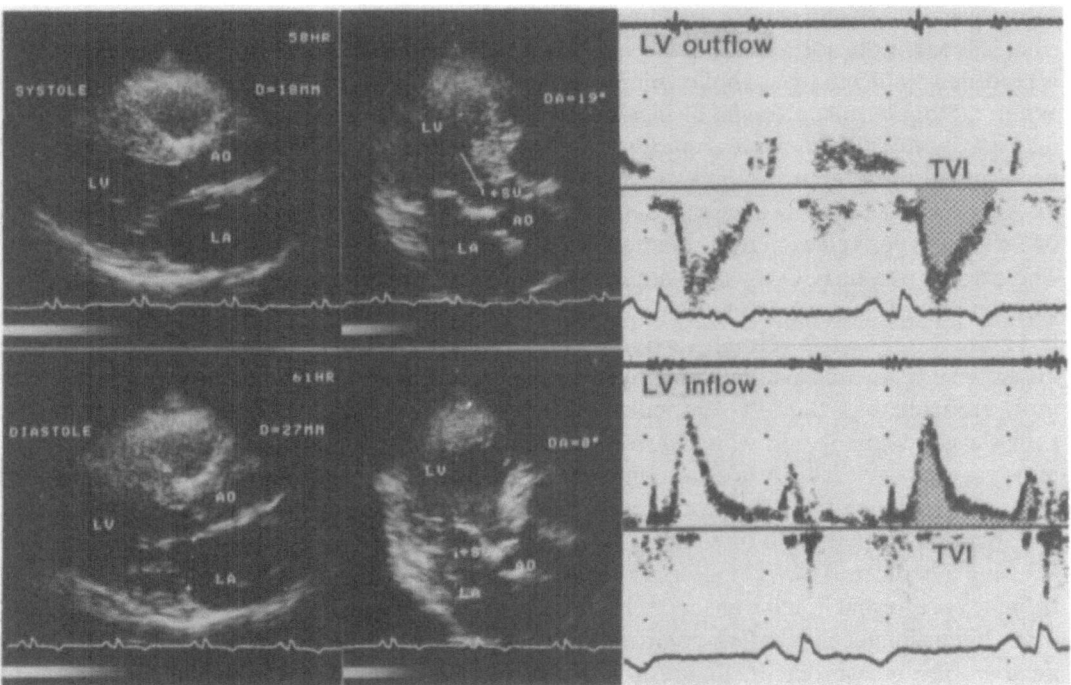

Figure 8.5. Evaluation of stroke volume and cardiac output derived by pulsed Doppler combined with two-dimensional echocardiography using left ventricular outflow and inflow tract. Upper shows the measurement of diameter (D) of the left ventricular outflow tract in the parasternal approach. The sample volume is placed in the left ventricular outflow tract. The right trace illustrates the left ventricular ejection flow with its flow velocity integral (FVI) shown by the dotted area. The lower panel shows the measurement of the mitral annular diameter. The sample volume is placed in the center of the mitral ring. The right panel illustrates the left ventricular inflow with its flow velocity integral (FVI) shown by the dotted area. Cross sectional area = $\pi(D/2)^2$. Stroke volume = Flow Velocity Integral (FVI) × Cross Sectional Area (CSA). Cardiac output = SV × Heart Rate.

made by tracing the left ventricular area in end-systole and diastole on the CRT display (Figures 8.3, 4). However, in clinical practice good quality two-dimensional images are sometimes difficult to obtain and it may be difficult to identify the entire endocardial surface. Therefore, the clinical application of two-dimensional method has some limitations.

3. Doppler method

A. Evaluation of systolic function

Instantaneous flow volume is calculated by flow velocity and cross-sectional area. In cardiac chambers and great arteries, the flow velocity profile is fairly flat at the level of the valve ring. For a flat velocity profile, the spatial mean velocity will be close to the spatial maximum velocity in the center of the lumen. The maximum velocity measured by the narrow Doppler beam, therefore, approximates the spatial mean velocity. The stroke volume (SV) is calculated by multiplying the pulsed Doppler derived flow velocity integral (FVI) by the cross-sectional area (CSA) of the valve being evaluated. The left ventricular stroke volume is obtained by the flow velocity integral of the left ventricular outflow or inflow tract and the cross-sectional area of the aortic or mitral ring, respectively. The left ventricular outflow velocity is recorded by placing the sample volume in the middle of the left ventricular outflow tract just below the aortic valve in the apical long axis view. The left ventricular inflow velocity is recorded by placing the sample volume in the center of the mitral ring using the same view. When a Doppler angle (angle of incidence between the Doppler ultrasound beam and the major axis of blood flow) is less than 20 degrees, the cosine of the angle is at least 0.94 and can be assumed to be approximately 1. The flow velocity integral is calculated by planimetric integration of the darkest envelope of the flow obtained (Figure 8.5). The cross-sectional area of each site is derived by annular diameters (D) from the parasternal long axis view as $\pi(D/2)^2$. The cardiac output (CO) is calculated by multiplying stroke volume by the heart rate. The correlation between thermodilution and Doppler measurements of cardiac output are shown in Figure 8.6. The left ventricular outflow method has a better correlation than the inflow method, since the mitral annular diameter may change during diastole and its measurement is more difficult than the left ventricular outflow tract. The Doppler derived peak velocity shows a good correlation with that obtained by a catheter tip manometer (Figure 8.7). A major source of variability in estimating stroke volume is the measurement of vessel diameter (D) or area. Since the area of a circular vessel is equal to $\pi(D/2)^2$, any error in the measurement of diameter will be squared in the final result.

Using a dedicated CW Doppler transducer, ascending aortic flow is more easily obtained from a suprasternal notch transducer position than the pulsed Doppler method (Figure 8.8). Two-dimensional echocardiographic measurement of aortic diameter is well correlated with angiographic measurement (Figures 8.9, 10). When the diameter of the ascending aorta just above the level of the aortic sinus from inner wall to inner wall is employed, the cardiac output calculated by the Doppler method has good correlation with thermodilution measurement (Figure 8.11). This technique is also applicable to treadmill exercise in normal subjects (Figures 8.12, 13) and in patients with coronary artery disease (Figures 8.14, 15) and artificial cardiac pacing (Figures 8.16, 17). Respiratory interference during exercise is not a major problem because the ultrasound beam traverses the mediastinum to reach the ascending aorta and does not come into contact with the lung. The CW Doppler method is more suitable than M-mode or two-dimensional echocardiography, where these difficulties are greatly en-

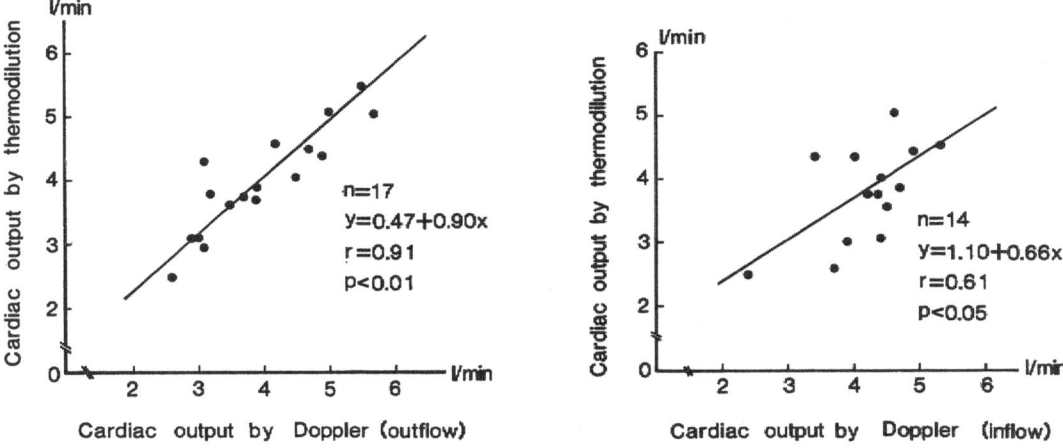

Figure 8.6. Correlationship of cardiac output between thermodilution and Doppler methods (LV outflow and inflow). The left graph shows the good correlation ($r = 0.91$) of the cardiac output (CO) obtained by pulsed Doppler of left ventricular outflow tract to those obtained by thermodilution method. The left ventricular inflow method has a relative good correlation ($r = 0.61$) with those obtained by the thermodilution method.

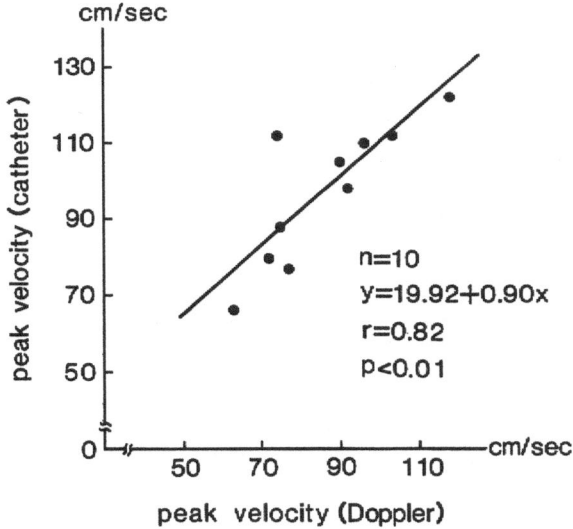

Figure 8.7. Correlation of peak velocity obtained by pulsed Doppler echocardiography and by catheter tip manometer ($r = 0.82$).

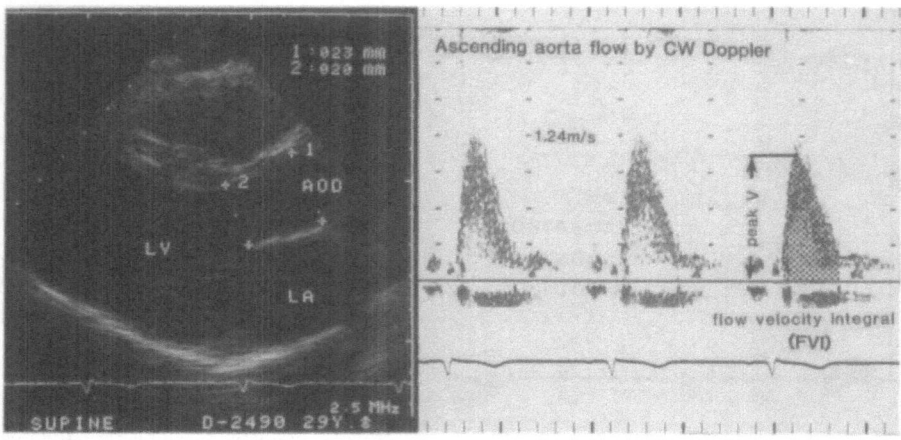

Figure 8.8. Measurements of aortic diameter and CW Doppler tracing of ascending aortic flow obtained from the suprasternal notch acoustic window. The cross-sectional area of the aorta was calculated from the internal diameter obtained at the level of the aortic annulus and the aortic root just above the sinus of valsalva during mid-systole. Peak flow velocity is measured from the maximal velocity of the envelope. The darkest envelope of the flow tracing is integrated to obtain flow velocity integral, which is shown by the dotted area.

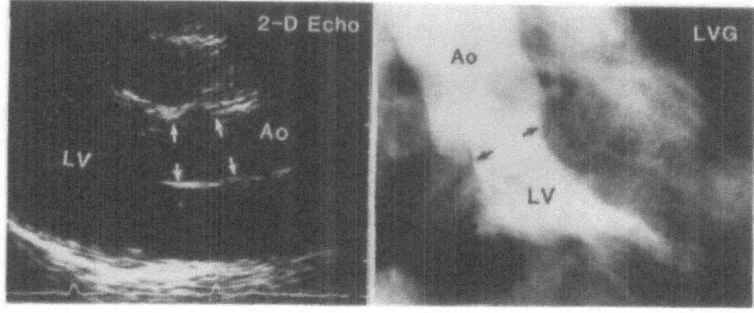

Figure 8.9. Left ventriculographic and two-dimensional echocardiographic measurement (inner to inner edge) of aortic annular diameter.

hanced, since only selected subjects with a suitable anatomic 'window' can be studied, often in a posture that makes exercise difficult or impossible. Since Doppler ultrasound has no dependency on left ventricular deformity or wall motion abnormalities, the Doppler derived stroke volume or cardiac output has potentially fewer theoretical problems in comparison with M-mode or two-dimensional measurements, and therefore is most suitable for clinical practice. The right ventricular stroke volume is also available using the pulsed Doppler method in right ventricular outflow tract or main pulmonary artery, therefore Qp/Qs can be calculated in patients with left-to-right shunt (see Figure 4.10).

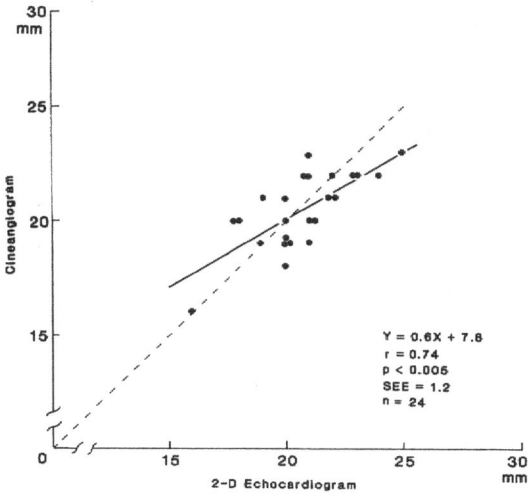

Figure 8.10. Regression analysis comparing aortic annular diameter measured by two-dimensional echocardiography (*x* axis) with angiographic measurement (*y* axis).

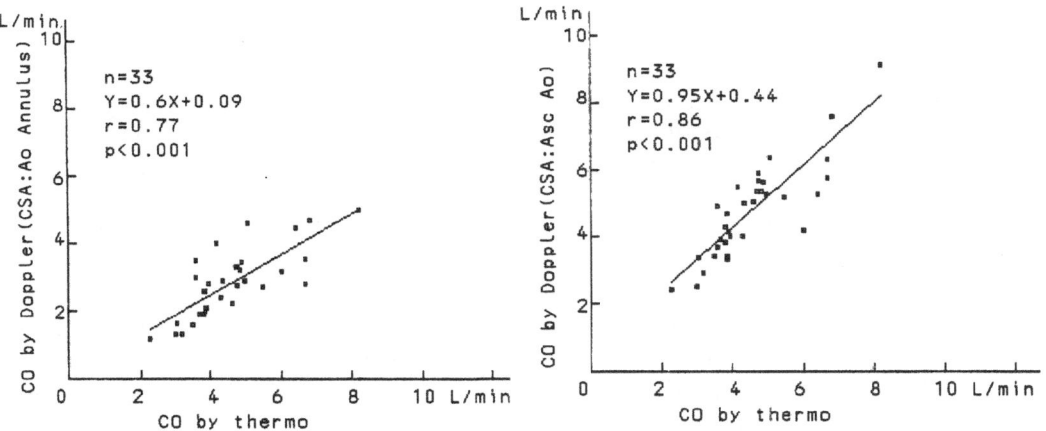

Figure 8.11. Correlation of cardiac output (CO) measurements between thermodilution and CW Doppler method using the cross-sectional area of aortic annulus in the left and the ascending aorta just above the aortic sinus in the right.

B. Evaluation of diastolic behavior

Until recently, left ventricular diastolic function has been evaluated from the pressure-volume relationship using cinéangiography and catheter tipped pressure manometers. However, this method is invasive, expensive and not possible in all patients. M-mode echocardiography has been used to examine left ventricular filling. Septal and posterior endocardial wall echoes can be digitized and, with computer assistance, continuous plots of left ventricular minor axis dimension vs. time and the rate of change of dimension vs. time can be generated. A reduction in the peak rate of dimension increase during rapid filling phase and/or an

Exercise Doppler ehchocardiography

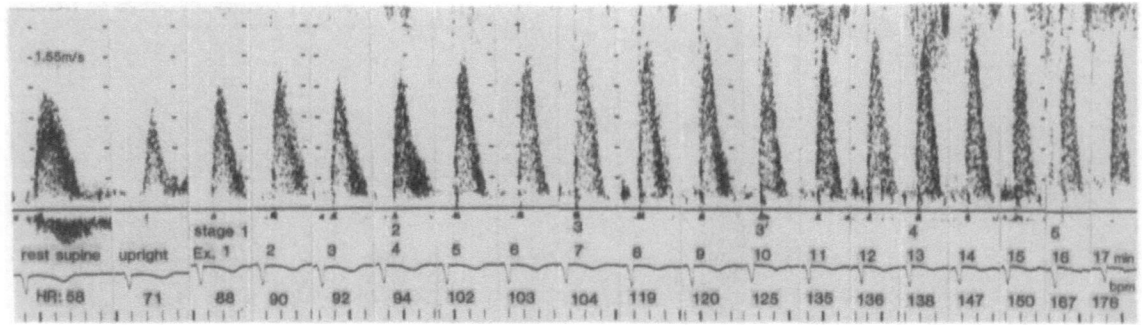

Figure 8.12.   CW Doppler tracing of the ascending aortic flow during treadmill exercise in a normal subject. During exercise, the ascending aortic flow gradually increases, but during the last three minutes it tends to decrease.

increase in the peak rate of dimension during the atrial contraction phase generally indicate impaired left ventricular diastolic function (Figures 8.18, 19). Because the left ventricular chamber is only viewed from one dimension in M-mode echocardiography, an irregularly shaped and/or asynchronously contracted left ventricle is difficult to evaluate.

In contrast, Doppler echocardiography is a noninvasive and an easily performed technique. The Doppler derived left ventricular inflow velocity may reflect the left ventricular volume changes in diastole (Figure 8.20). It provides good information about left ventricular diastolic behavior in patients with various heart diseases, irrespective of the presence of left ventricular deformity. Indices of left ventricular filling rate, calculated with this method, show good correlation with those obtained by contrast angiography (Figure 8.21) or radionuclide techniques. The transmitral flow velocity from the mitral ring to the apex is calculated from the shifted frequency using the Doppler equation. The pattern of transmitral flow velocity in diastole consists of two components. The first component corresponds to the rapid filling phase in early diastole, and the second one to the atrial contraction phase in late diastole. The peak velocity in the rapid filling phase (cm/sec), and in the atrial contraction phase (cm/sec), the ratio of peak velocity in the atrial contraction phase to that in the rapid filling phase and the deceleration half-time (msec), can be measured to analyze the left ventricular diastolic behavior (Figure 8.22).

Using quantitative analysis of cinéangiographic left ventricular volume curves, patients with chronic heart disease, regardless of lesions, have an abnormally decreased early diastolic filling rate of left ventricular volume and a larger increment in diastolic left ventricular volume due to atrial contraction. With the use of Doppler indices of left ventricular filling, many studies have shown that diastolic abnormalities often precede systolic dysfunction and can be detected in asymptomatic patients. The characteristics of abnormal left ventricular inflow velocity are decreased peak velocity in the rapid filling phase, prolonged deceleration half-time, and increased peak velocity in the atrial contraction phase (Figure 8.23). These findings suggest a grossly impaired left ventricular distensibility and a compensatory increase of atrial contribution to left ventricular filling. In contrast, in patients with increased chamber stiffness and with resultant 'restriction' of diastolic filling, rapid filling velocity may be increased, whereas atrial systole to the ventricular filling is normal or reduced. When end-diastolic pressure is significantly elevated, the flat portion of the ventricular function curve is approached and further increments in pressure would have less effect in augmenting left atrial

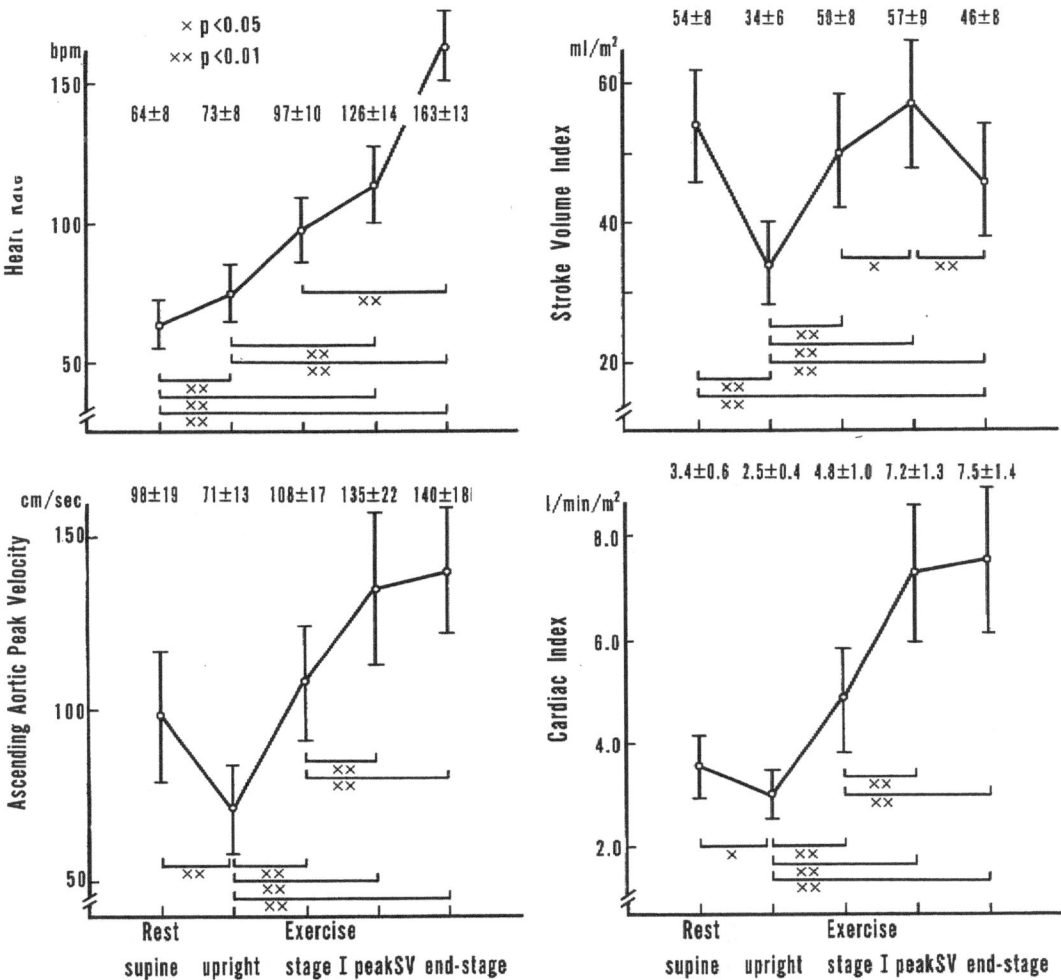

Figure 8.13. Changes in heart rate, ascending aortic peak velocity, stroke volume index and cardiac index during treadmill exercise in 21 normal subjects. The stroke volume index decreases from supine to upright position, reaches a peak value (peak stroke volume), and then decreases at the end-stage of exercise. However, the cardiac index progressively increases until the end-stage due to increased heart rate. The peak velocity progressively increases until the end stage of exercise.

contraction to filling volume (Figure 8.24). Thus, impaired relaxation and increased chamber stiffness result in sharply contrasting ventricular diastolic filling patterns that have been distinguished by a number of investigators. Figure 8.25 shows the relationship between the pulmonary wedge pressure (PWP) and Doppler derived A/R in patients with coronary artery disease. PWP over 20 mm Hg negatively correlates with A/R significantly, but not for PWP below 20 mm Hg. Therefore, it is important to appreciate that both types of diastolic dysfunction are often present to a variable degree in any types of heart disease.

This method is also applicable to exercise testing in patients with hypertrophic cardiomyopathy. Healthy subjects demonstrate a markedly increased rapid filling velocity of the left ventricle after mild dynamic exercise (Figure 8.26), while patients with hypertrophic cardio-

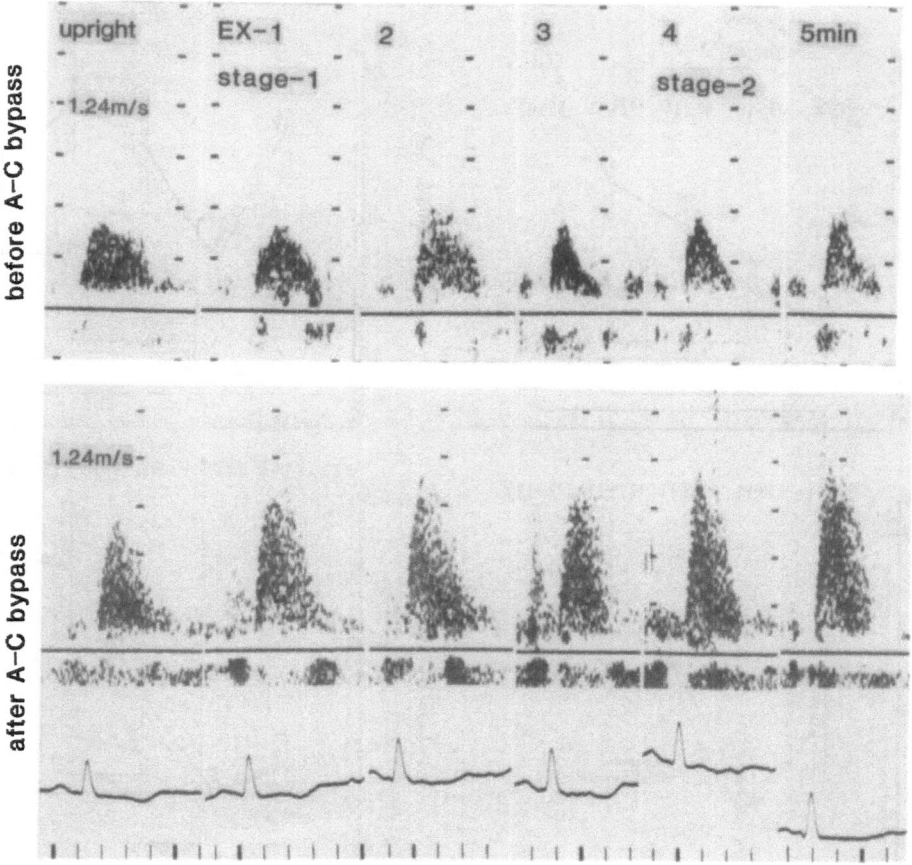

Figure 8.14. CW Doppler tracing of ascending aortic flow during treadmill exercise in a patient with angina pectoris before and after aorto-coronary (AC) bypass surgery. Before AC bypass, the increase of ascending aortic flow velocity is minimal during exercise possibly due to ischemia. After AC bypass, the ascending aortic flow velocity increases during exercise like normal subjects with improvements of coronary supply.

myopathy show only a minimal increment in this variable (Figure 8.27). The increase in flow velocity during the left atrial contraction phase during and after exercise is nearly parallel to the increase in rapid filling velocity of the left ventricle in healthy subjects, and much more marked in patients with hypertrophic cardiomyopathy. This augmented atrial contribution in dynamic exercise seems to be due to a compensatory mechanism for poor left ventricular distensibility in patients with hypertrophic cardiomyopathy. Usually after diltiazem administration in patients with hypertrophic cardiomyopathy, the left ventricular inflow velocity tends to increase more markedly in the rapid filling phase and, in contrast, less markedly in the atrial contraction phase at one minute post-exercise (Figures 8.28, 29, 30). The findings suggests that some kinds of drug can improve abnormal left ventricular diastolic behavior in patients with hypertrophic cardiomyopathy not only at rest but also after mild dynamic exercise. Exercise pulsed Doppler echocardiography can repeatedly and easily be used to estimate not only abnormal left ventricular distensibility in patients with hypertrophic cardiomyopathy but can also be used to evaluate the efficacy of drugs.

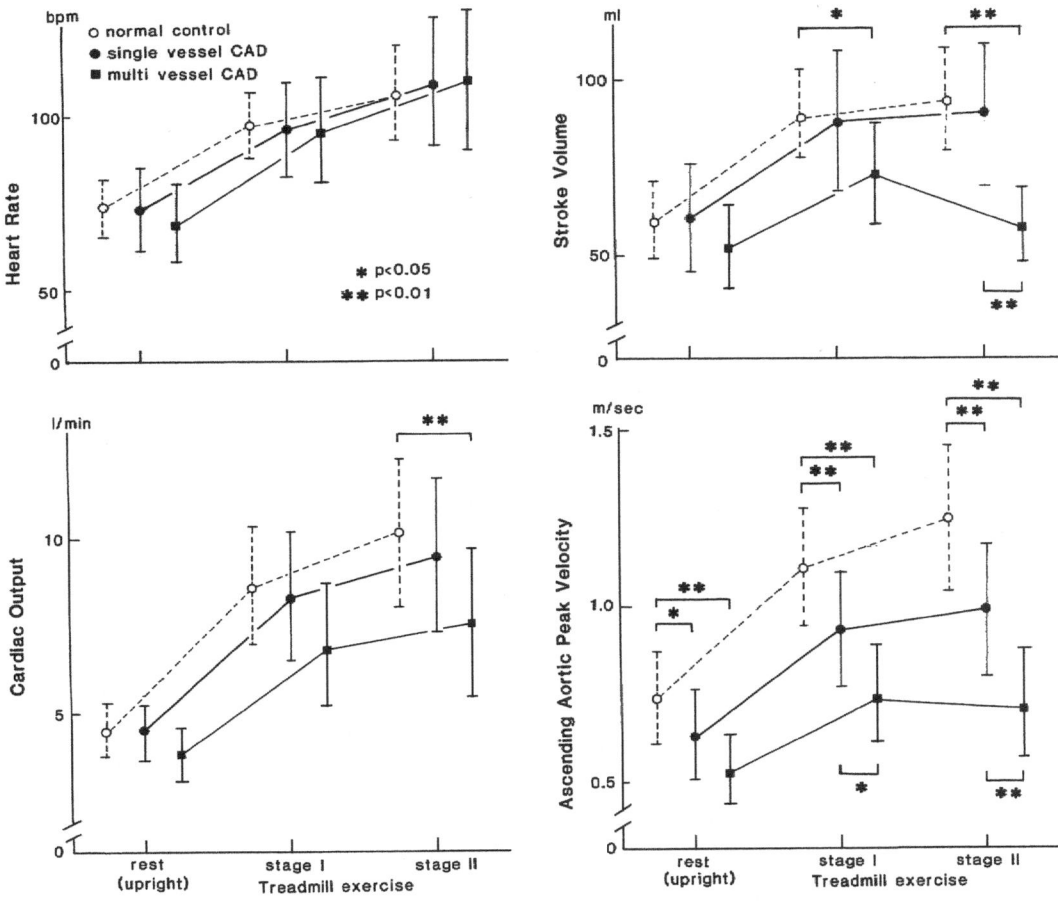

Figure 8.15. Changes in heart rate, stroke volume and cardiac output during treadmill exercise in patients with single vessel and multi vessel coronary artery disease (CAD) and healthy subjects.

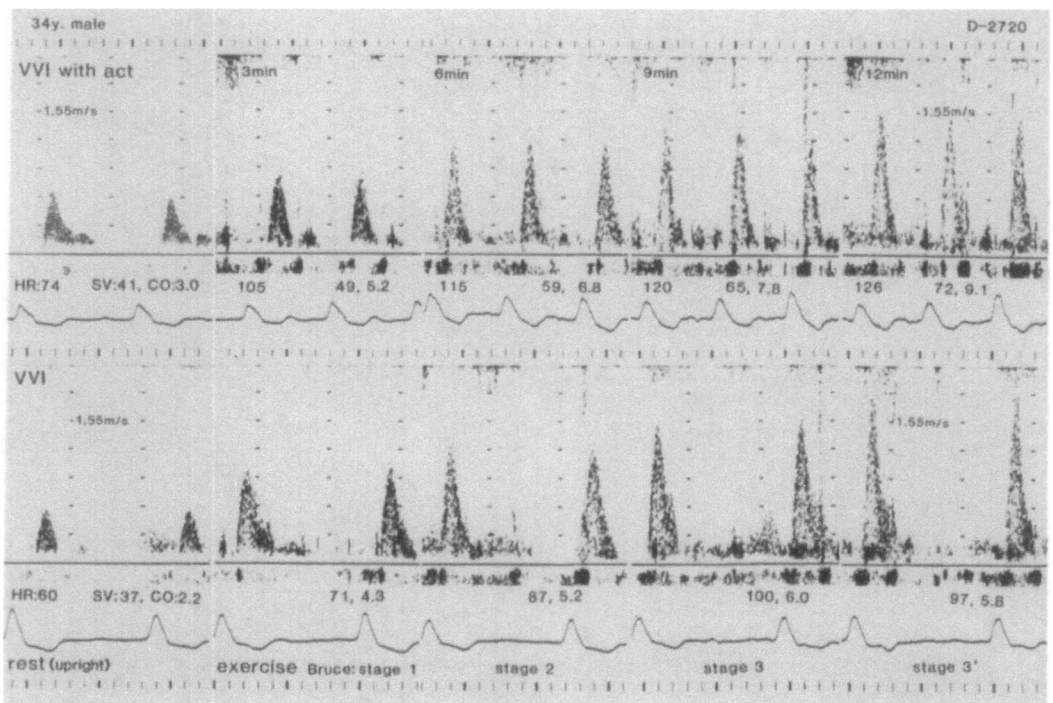

Figure 8.16.   CW Doppler tracing of the ascending aortic flow during treadmill exercise in a patient with and without an activity initiated rate responsive VVI pacemaker. With ventricular inhibited ventricular pacing (VVI) mode, the increase in ascending aortic flow velocity integral is larger than that with activity initiated mode (Act-VVI) during exercise.

→

Figure 8.18.   Serial recordings of M-mode and Doppler LV inflow velocity of a patient with hypertension administrating sublingual nifedipine. Before nifedipine administration, IVS and LV posterior motion in M-mode is reduced and LV inflow shows depressed rapid filling and increased atrial contribution to LV filling. After nifedipine administration, blood pressure (BP) decreases, IVS and LV posterior wall motion improve and LV inflow shows increases rapid filling velocity.

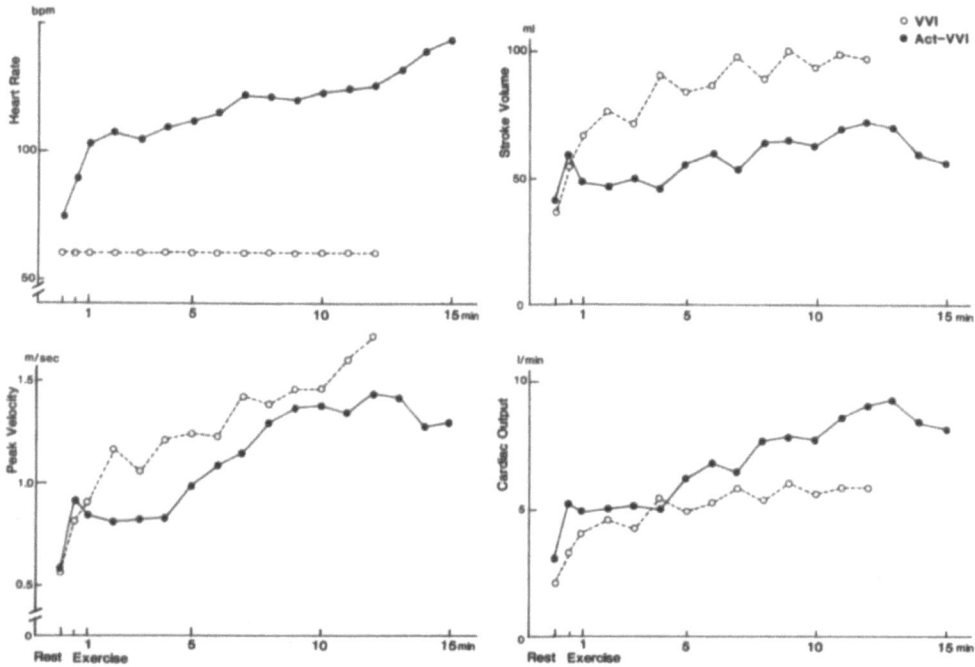

Figure 8.17. Series of changes in heart rate (HR), stroke volume (SV) and cardiac output (CO) during treadmill exercise in a patient with an activity initiated ventricular (Act-VVI) pacemaker. On exercise with the effect of circulating catecholamines, the increase in stroke volume is significantly greater in VVI pacing than VVI-act pacing, but the increase in cardiac output is less sufficient than VVI-act pacing in this patient. This finding suggests that the positive chronotropic response can provide the great contribution to increase in cardiac output during the exercise.

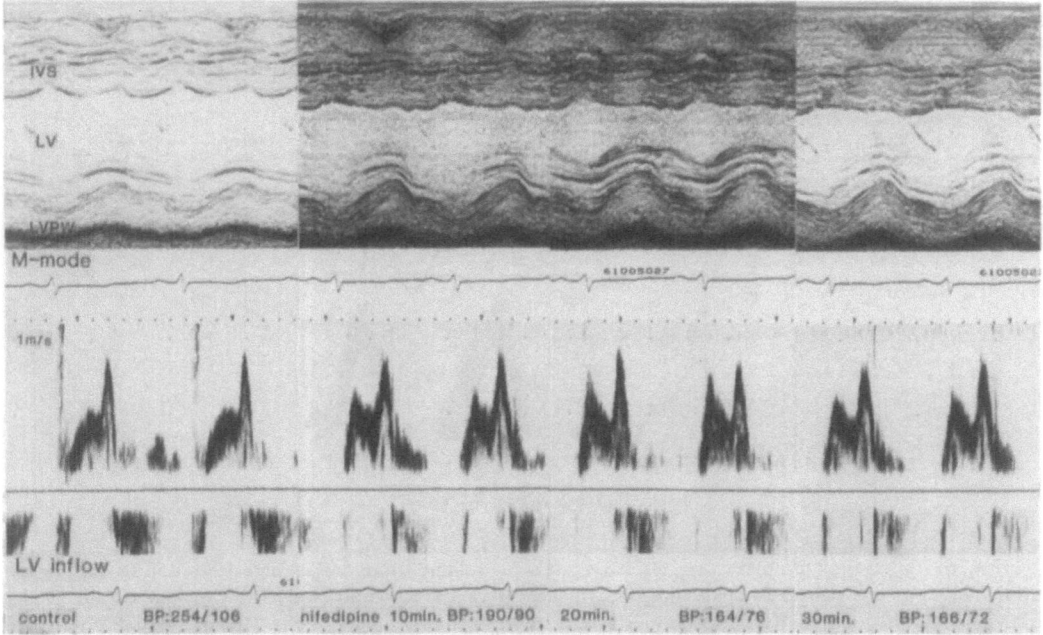

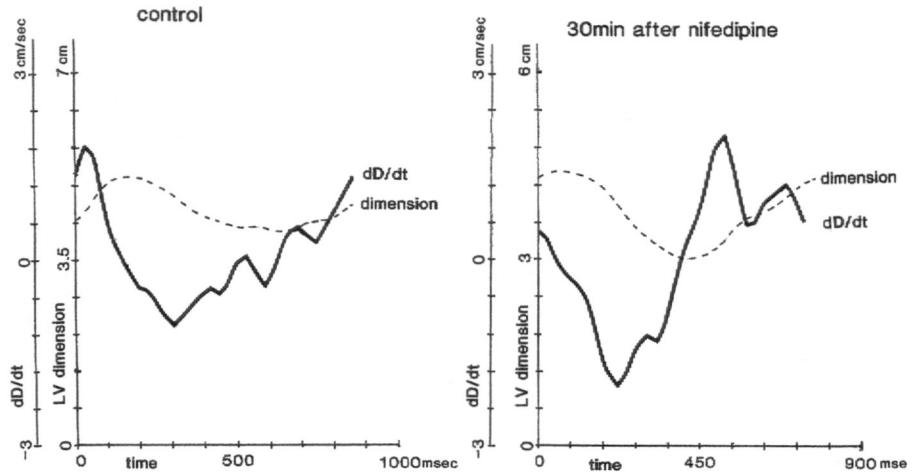

Figure 8.19. Computer-derived LV internal dimension and the rate of dimension change of a patient with hypertension (same patient as in Figure 8.18). Before nifedipine administration, negative (systolic) and positive (early diastolic) peak rate of dimension change is reduced. After nifedipine administration, these peak rates of dimensional changes improve. Positive peak rate of dimensional change is very similar to Doppler derived rapid filling velocity.

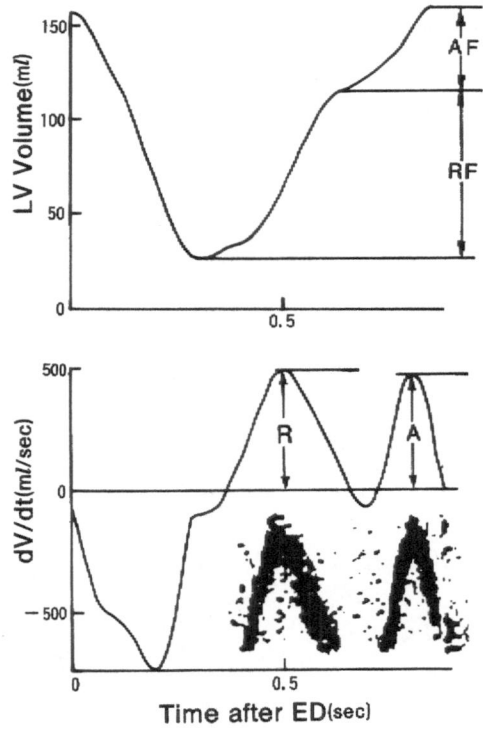

Figure 8.20. Interrelationship between the left ventricular volume curve and its first derivation (d*V*/d*t*) by left ventriculography and pulsed Doppler recording of the left ventricular inflow velocity. One can see the similar behavior of d*V*/d*t* and the left ventricular inflow velocity tracing in the same patient. RF and AF indicate the left ventricular volume during the rapid filling phase and the atrial contraction phase, respectively. R and A indicate the peak velocity in the rapid filling phase and the atrial contraction phase, respectively.

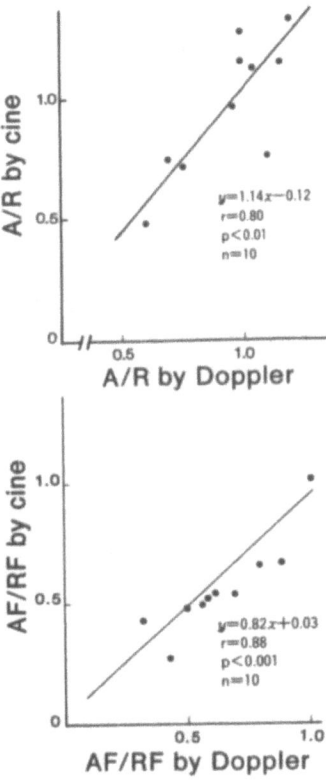

Figure 8.21. Correlation of AF/RF and A/R obtained by the pulsed Doppler method in comparison with those obtained by cineangiography (cine) (AF/RF *r* = 0.88 and A/R *r* = 0.80).

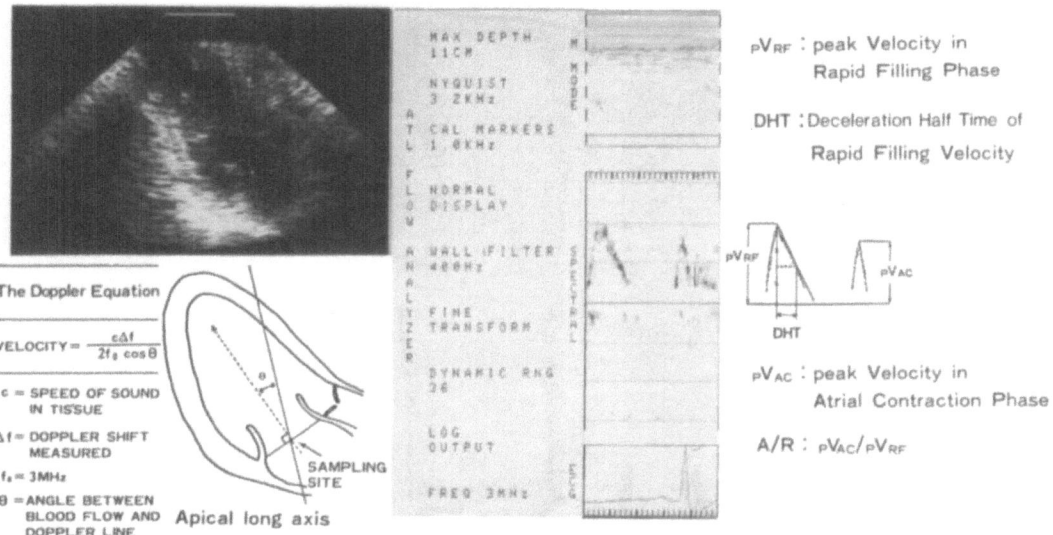

Figure 8.22. Transmitral flow velocity profile and the four variables derived from the transmitral flow velocity pattern. The measurements of transmitral flow velocity are the following: (1) the peak velocity in the rapid filling phase (P^V_{RF} cm/sec), (2) the peak velocity in the atrial contraction phase (P^V_{AC} cm/sec), (3) the ratio of peak velocity in the atrial contraction phase to that in the rapid filling phase (A/R) and (4) the deceleration half-time (DHT msec). The deceleration half-time is the time required for the maximal velocity curve of the rapid filling phase to fall its half velocity.

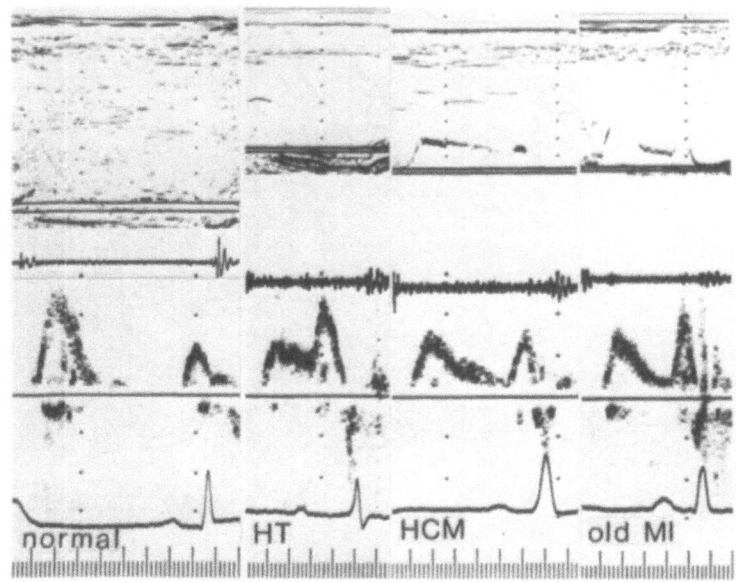

Figure 8.23. Transmitral flow velocity profile of a normal subject and patients with hypertension (HT), old myocardial infarction (MI) and hypertrophic cardiomyopathy (HCM). In comparison with a normal subject, transmitral flow of these patients shows decreased peak velocity in rapid filling phase and increased atrial contribution to left ventricular filling. The deceleration half-time also is prolonged.

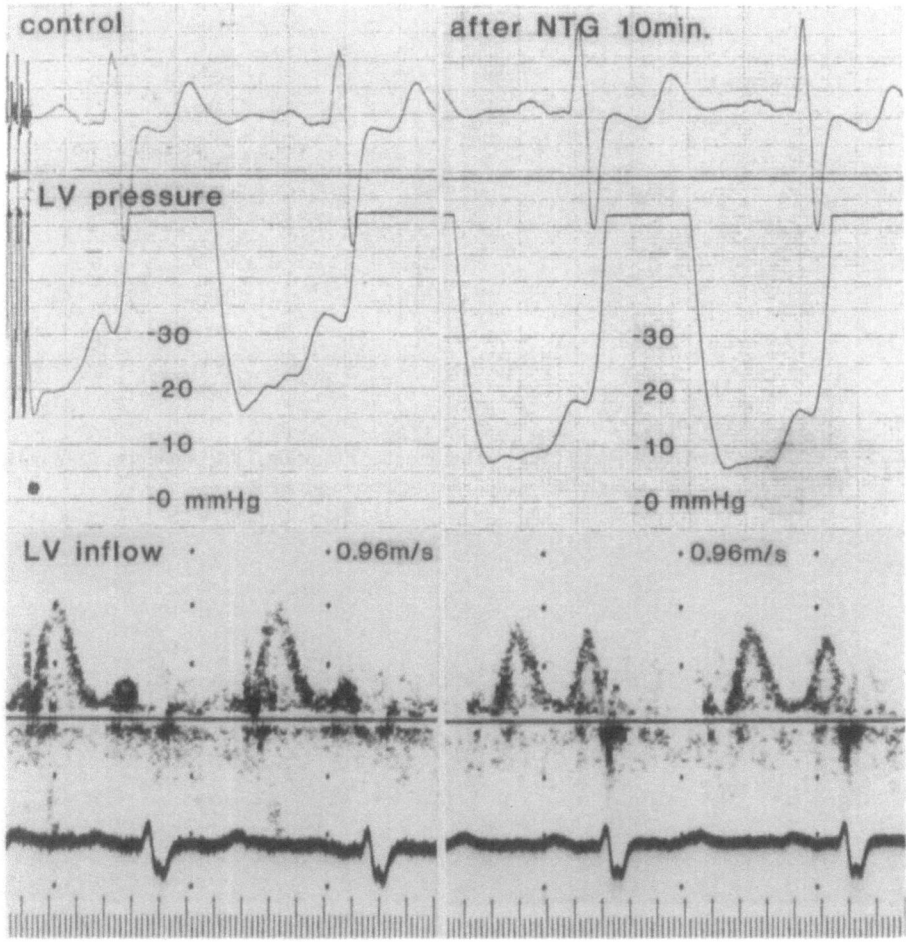

Figure 8.24. Changes in left ventricular (LV) pressure and inflow velocity tracing in a patient with dilated cardiomyopathy, before and after nitroglycerin (NTG) administration. In the control phase, the left ventricular inflow velocity tracing shows little atrial contribution to ventricular filling in the presence of a markedly increased left ventricular end-diastolic pressure. After 10 minutes of sublingual administration of nitroglycerin, end-diastolic pressure decreases markedly and left ventricular inflow velocity demonstrates the large atrial contribution to ventricular filling. The atrial contribution to ventricular filling tends to diminish when left ventricular filling pressure increases markedly.

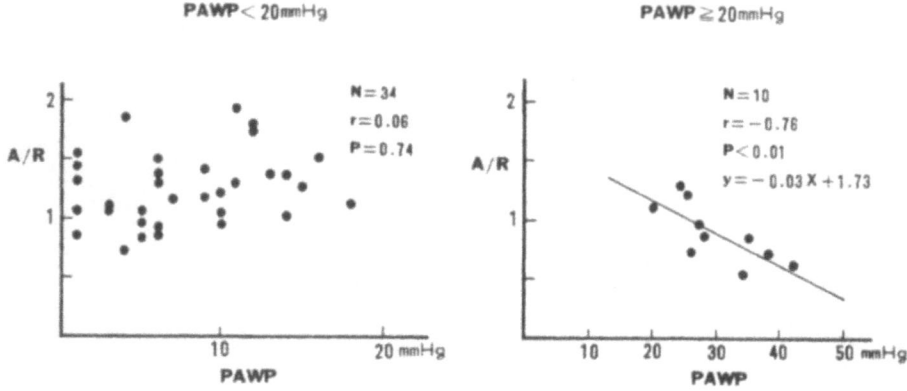

Figure 8.25.   Correlation between A/R and PWP greater or under 20 mm Hg. PWP greater than 20 mm Hg shows a
significantly negative correlation with A/R.

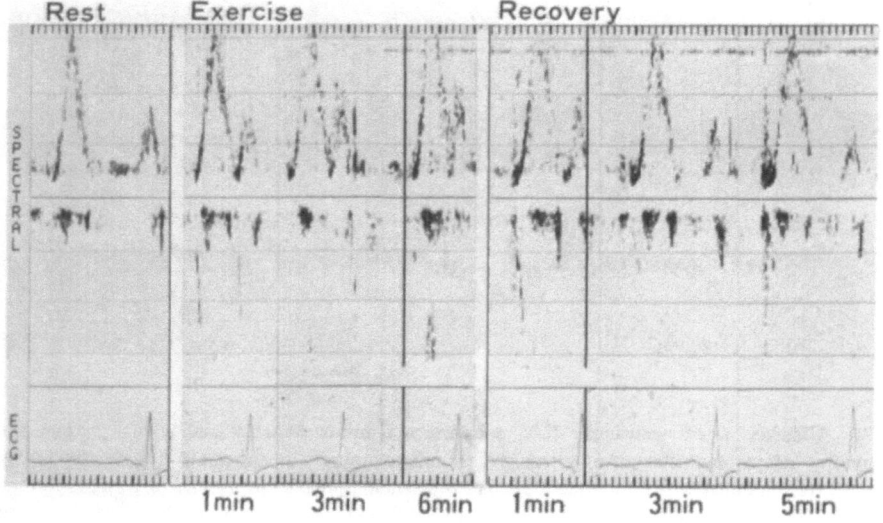

Figure 8.26.   Exercise pulsed Doppler echocardiogram in a 25 year-old healthy male. Peak velocity in the rapid
filling phase and that in the atrial contraction phase increase during exercise, but deceleration half-time shortens.
Rapid filling and the left atrial contraction flow tracings are not superimposed throughout the exercise testing.
During the recovery phase, these variables return gradually to rest levels except for the ratio of peak velocity in the
atrial contraction phase to that in the rapid filling phase. This variable does not change before, during, or after
exercise.

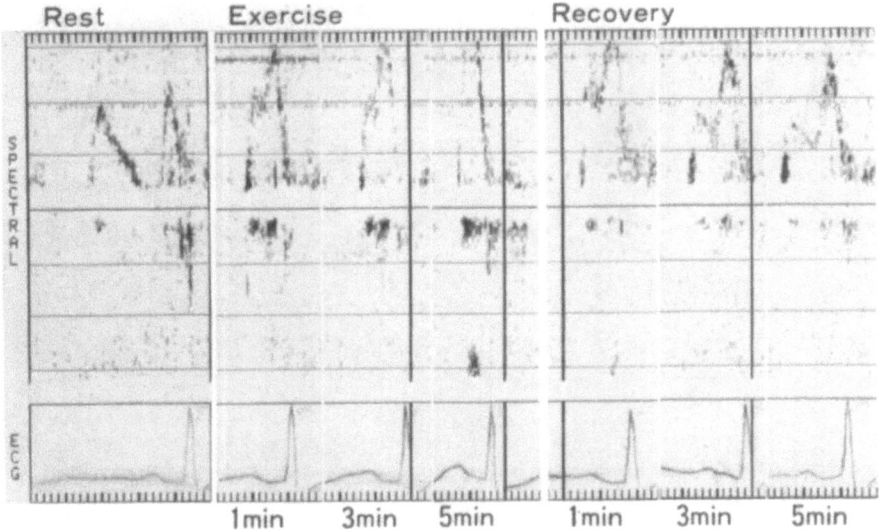

Figure 8.27. Exercise pulsed Doppler echocardiogram in a 51 year-old male with hypertrophic cardiomyopathy before diltiazem administration. At rest the transmitral flow velocity pattern shows decreased peak velocity in the rapid filling phase, prolonged deceleration half-time, and increased peak velocity in the atrial contraction phase and increased ratio of peak velocity in the atrial contraction phase to that in the rapid filling phase compared with findings in normal subjects. During exercise, peak velocity in the rapid filling phase increases very little, pressure half-time prolongs, and peak velocity in the atrial contraction phase and the ratio of peak velocity in the atrial contraction phase to that in the rapid filling phase increase markedly. During the fifth minute of exercise, at a heart rate of 86 beats/min, rapid filling and atrial contraction flow tracings overlap and could not be identified separately. After exercise, these two components separate again. Peak velocity in the rapid filling phase increases very little, pressure half-time prolongs while peak velocity in the atrial contraction phase and the ratio of peak velocity in the atrial contraction phase to that in the rapid filling phase increase markedly. These markedly increased Doppler variables represent the left atrial compensatory mechanism for the poor left ventricular distensibility during and after dynamic exercise.

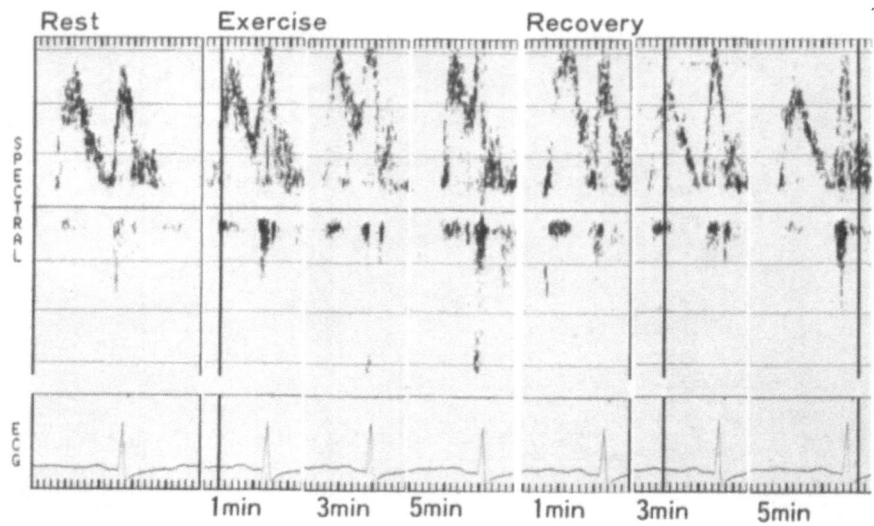

Figure 8.28. Exercise pulsed Doppler echocardiogram in the same case as Figure 8.27 after diltiazem administration (180 mg/day) for 1 week. The transmitral flow velocity pattern at rest shows increased peak velocity in the rapid filling phase, shortened deceleration half-time, increased peak velocity in the atrial contraction phase and unchanged ratio of peak velocity in the atrial contraction phase to that in the rapid filling phase. During exercise, peak velocity in the rapid filling phase increases, and deceleration half-time does not prolong as compared with the levels before diltiazem administration. During the fifth minute of exercise, at a heart rate of 82 beats/min, rapid filling and atrial contraction flow tracings do not fuse together. After 1 minute of exercise, peak velocity in the rapid filling phase and that in the atrial contraction phase increase, deceleration half-time shortens and the ratio of peak velocity in the atrial contraction phase to that in the rapid filling phase does not change. The increased peak velocity in the rapid filling phase and reduced deceleration half-time represent improved left ventricular distensibility as a result of diltiazem therapy, during and after dynamic exercise. The smaller in peak velocity in the atrial contraction phase and unchanged ratio of peak velocity in the atrial contraction phase to that in the rapid filling phase demonstrate that improvement of left ventricular distensibility by diltiazem does not necessitate the compensatory mechanism of the left atrial contraction.

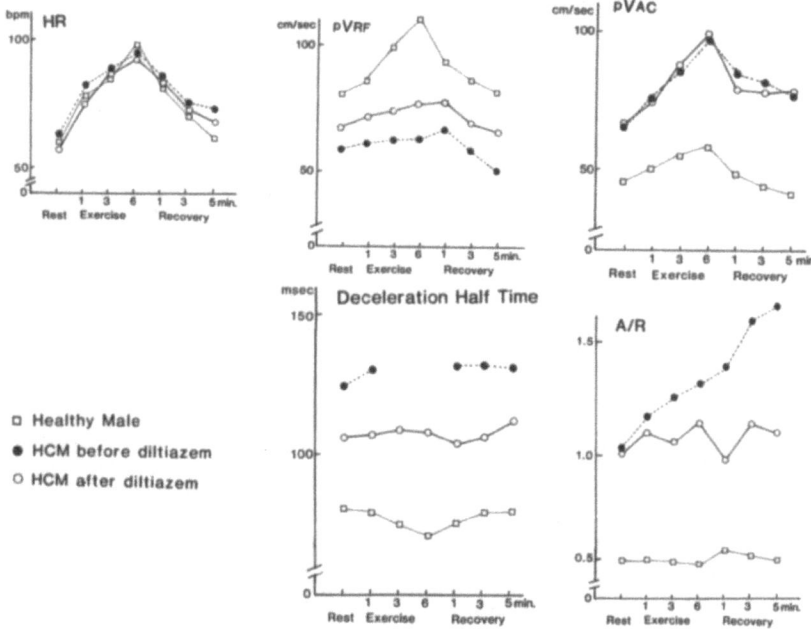

Figure 8.29. Serial changes in Doppler derived variables of a 25 year-old healthy male and a 51 year-old patient with hypertrophic cardiomyopathy with and without diltiazem in supine exercise.

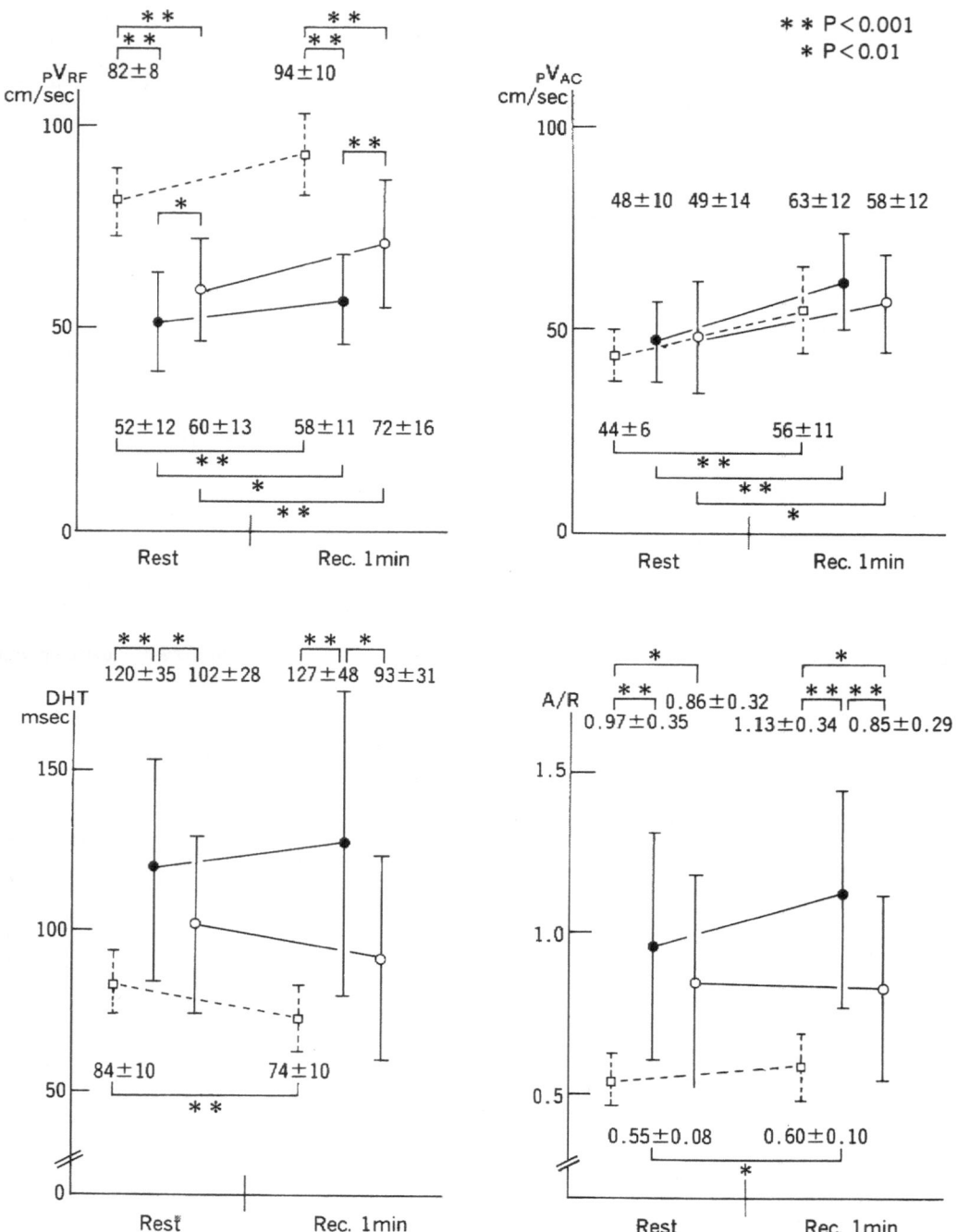

Figure 8.30. Changes in Doppler derived variables with exercise in 24 normal subjects (□) and 17 patients with hypertrophic cardiomyopathy with (○) and without (●) diltiazem.

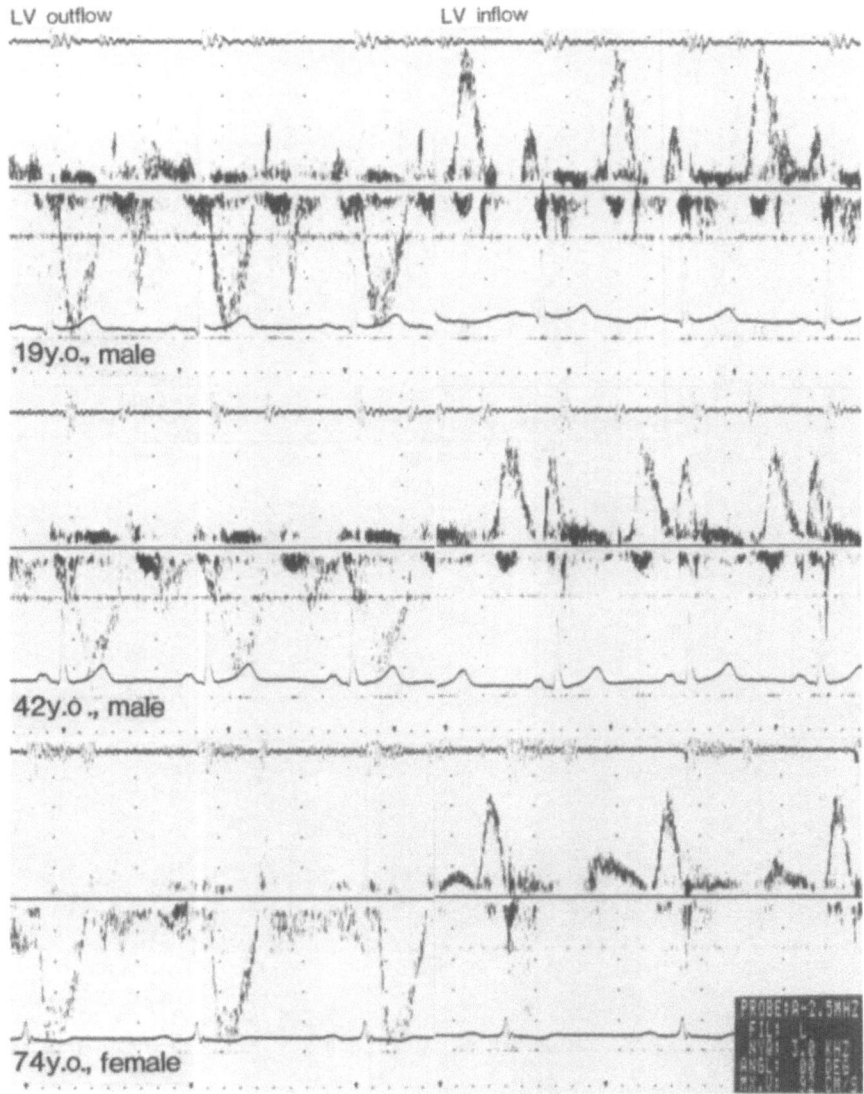

Figure 8.31. The left ventricular outflow and inflow velocity tracings in healthy young, middle-aged and elderly people. The peak velocity in left ventricular outflow is not altered with aging. In contrast, the peak velocity in rapid filling phase is decreased and deceleration half-time prolonged in elderly people.

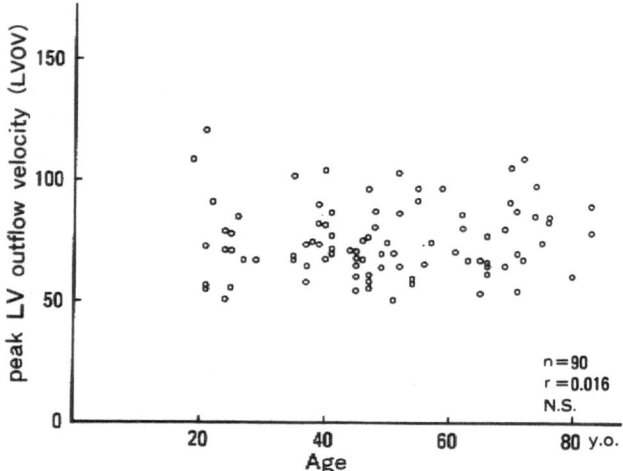

Figure 8.32.   Correlation between the peak velocity in left ventricular outflow tract and age.

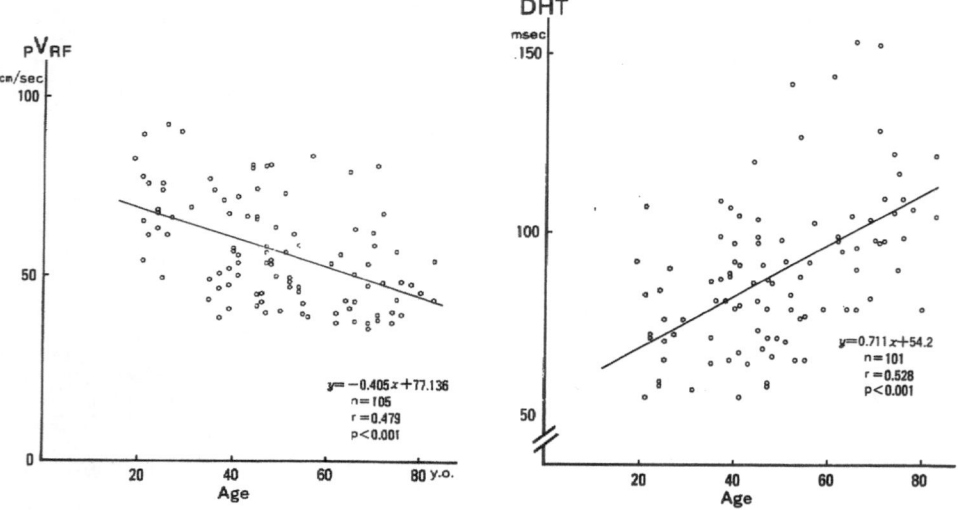

Figure 8.33.   Correlation between the peak velocity in left ventricular rapid filling phase or deceleration half-time
and age.

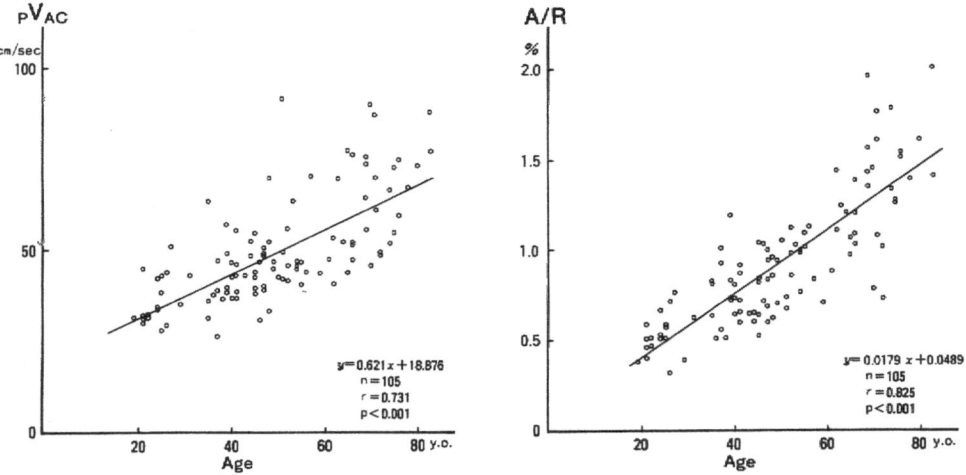

Figure 8.34. Correlation between the peak velocity in the atrial contraction phase or the ratio of peak velocity in the atrial contraction phase to that in the rapid filling phase (A/R) and age.

4. Age related changes in left ventricular function

It is generally accepted that the cardiovascular system is subject to the influence of aging. It is clinically important to consider age-related changes when evaluating left ventricular function, especially in elderly patients. Doppler derived left ventricular outflow and inflow velocity tracings in healthy young, middle-aged and elderly people are shown in Figure 8.31. The peak velocity of left ventricular outflow is not affected by aging (Figure 8.32). In contrast, the peak velocity in the rapid filling phase decreases and deceleration half-time increases in relation with age (Figure 8.33). The peak velocity in the atrial contraction phase and the ratio of peak velocity in the atrial contraction phase to that in the rapid filling phase (A/R) increases in relation with age (Figure 8.34).

CHAPTER 9

Pulmonary hypertension

Accurate assessment of pulmonary artery pressure has traditionally been obtainable only with invasive cardiac catheterization. However, recently M-mode and Doppler echocardiography has been helpful in identifying patients with normal and elevated pulmonary artery pressure.

1. M-mode echocardiographic evaluation

Pulmonary hypertension can produce characteristic pulmonary valve motions. We divided these findings into four types: (A) normal motion, (B) reduced E-F slope with diminished or absent *a*-dip, (C) systolic semiclosure, (D) gradual systolic closure (Figure 9.1). Our experience demonstrates that types C and D have a good correlation with cardiac catheterization (Figure 9.2).

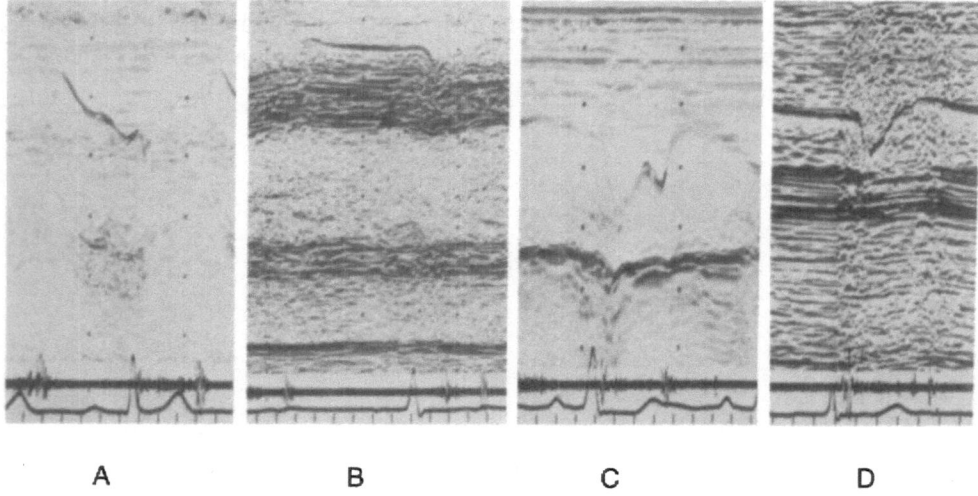

A   B   C   D

Figure 9.1. M-mode morphology of pulmonary valve motions. Type A: normal. Type B: reduced E-F slope without *a*-dip. Type C: systolic semiclosure with re-opening. Type D: systolic gradual closure.

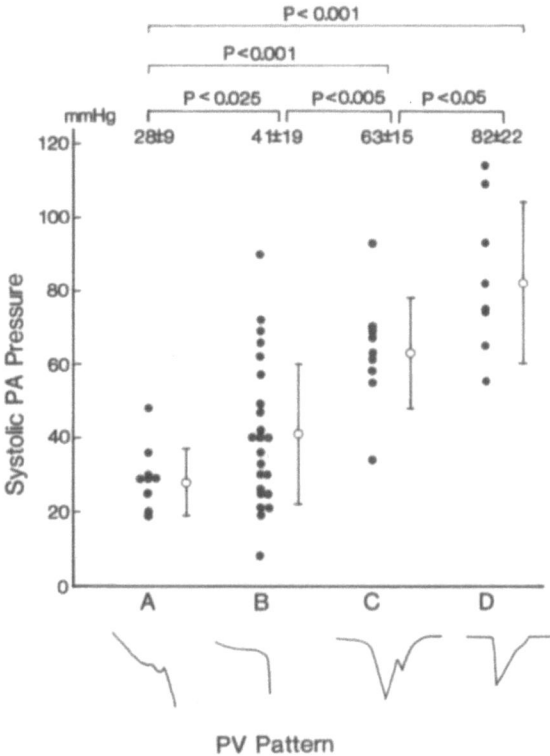

Figure 9.2.   Correlation between the types of pulmonary valve motion and systolic pulmonary artery pressure.

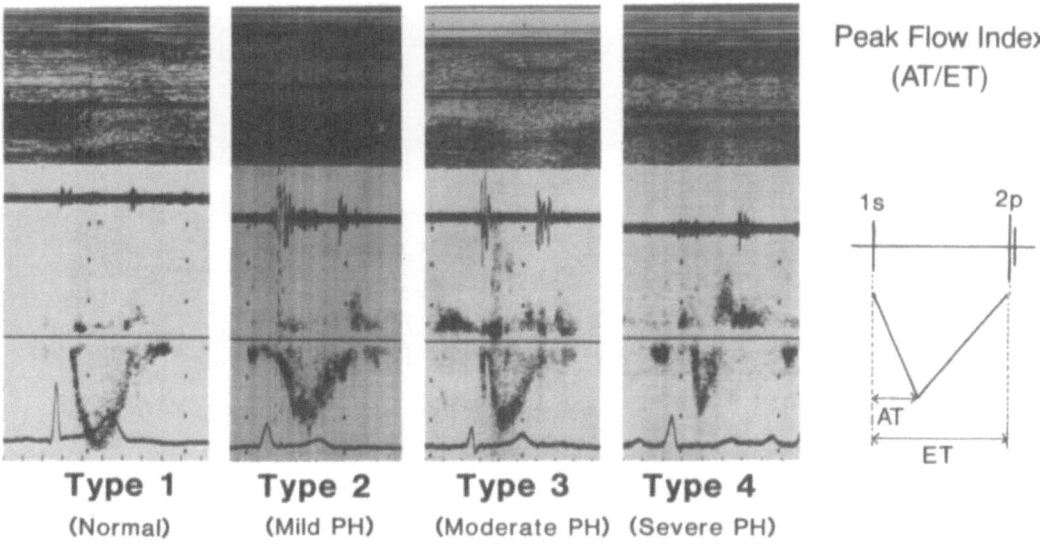

Figure 9.3.   Types of pulmonary flow patterns and the measurement of AT/ET. Type 1: pulmonary artery flow velocity accelerates slowly to a peak at midsystole, producing a 'dome-like' appearance. Type 2: triangular in shape. Type 3: pulmonary artery flow velocity accelerates rapidly to a peak in early systole, followed by rapid deceleration in midsystole. Type 4: pulmonary artery flow velocity accelerates rapidly to a peak in early systole, followed by rapid deceleration to a nadir in midsystole, and then exhibits a brief secondary increase in flow velocity in late systole. Acceleration time (AT) is measured from the onset of ejection to the time of peak flow velocity. Ejection time (ET) is measured from the onset to the end of systolic flow.

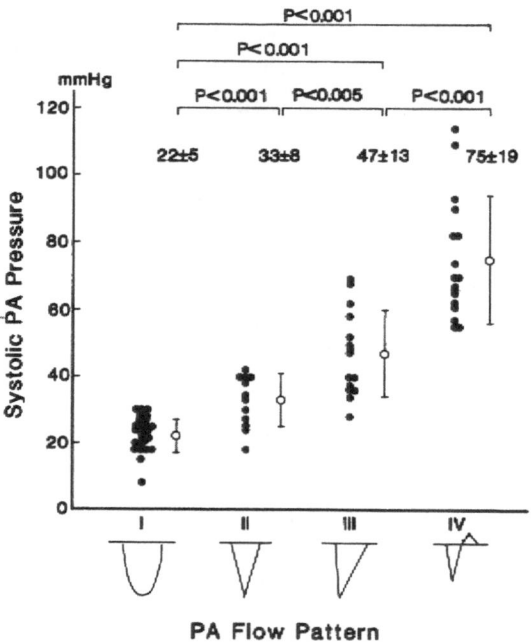

Figure 9.4. Correlation between the types of pulmonary flow patterns and systolic pulmonary artery pressure.

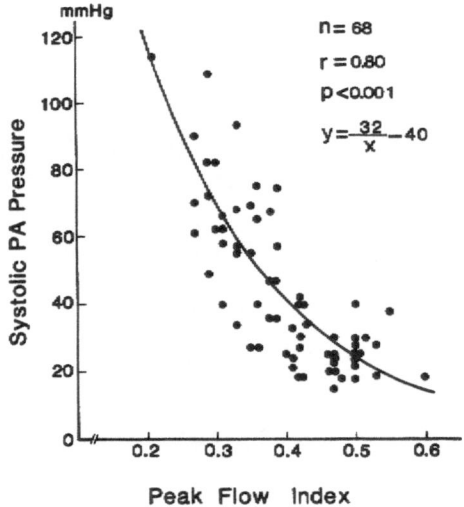

Figure 9.5. Correlation between the peak flow index and systolic pulmonary artery pressure.

2. Pulsed Doppler evaluation

Pulsed Doppler echocardiography is useful for the evaluation of pulmonary artery pressure. In normals, the pulmonary flow velocity accelerates smoothly, reaches peak flow velocity halfway through systole and then decelerates smoothly until ejection ends, producing a 'dome-like' appearance in the flow velocity curve. However, in the presence of pulmonary hypertension, this profile tends to be triangular and there is rapid acceleration to a peak velocity in early systole (decrease of acceleration time to ejection time; $AT/ET < 0.5$), followed by rapid deceleration in mid systole. In severe cases, a transient increase in flow velocity occurs in late systole, producing a 'spike and dome' appearance. In our laboratory, we have divided these flow patterns into four types according to the severity of pulmonary hypertension: Type 1: normal, Type 2: mild, Type 3: moderate and Type 4: severe (Figure 9.3). This classification has a good correlation with cardiac catheterization (Figure 9.4). The peak flow index (acceleration time over ejection time; AT/ET) also has a good hemodynamic correlation (Figure 9.5). However, these parameters yield equivocal results in certain situations. In idiopathic pulmonary dilatation, for example, the flow profile shows different patterns depending upon the site of sampling (see Figure 11.28). Also, normal subjects may show a shortened acceleration time or notching if the sample volume is positioned close to the posterior wall of the pulmonary artery. In the absence of pulmonary stenosis, continuous wave Doppler measurement of tricuspid regurgitation peak jet velocity using the simplified Bernoulli equation is also helpful and more quantitative in the estimation of right ventricular pressure (see Chapter 3, Section 11: Tricuspid Regurgitation). However, problems may be encountered in patients with a poorly recorded tricuspid regurgitant flow pattern or unusually high right atrial pressures. Therefore, in a given patient, either the pulmonary flow method or the tricuspid gradient method may be preferable, or the two methods may be used in combination.

CHAPTER 10

Echocardiographic evaluation of arrhythmia

M-mode echocardiography has been used to evaluate cardiac motion during altered electrical activity because of its rapid sampling rate and time correlation. However, M-mode echocardiographic studies are limited by an 'ice-pick' view of cardiac structures that becomes an impediment to quantitative segmental analysis during spontaneous alterations. In contrast, two-dimensional echocardiography is more comprehensive imaging technique, but has clinically many limitations due to its relative slow sampling rate. Recently, pulsed Doppler echocardiography has come to play an important role in explaining hemodynamic changes due to altered electrical activity, due to its ability to determine beat-to-beat changes in stroke volume and filling volume, irrespective of ventricular asynchrony. This method could also be used to evaluate the significance of atrial contribution to ventricular filling in the healthy or diseased subject.

1. Bundle branch block

The abnormal depolarization due to bundle branch block may affect left ventricular wall motion. Left bundle branch block (LBBB) produces a characteristic early systolic posterior displacement of the IVS (Figure 10.1). In patients with right ventricular endocardial pacing, this finding is also observed (Figure 10.2). In right bundle branch block (RBBB), no abnormal wall motion can be usually detected. Using pulsed Doppler echocardiography we can observe the marked delay of left ventricular ejection flow in patients with LBBB. On the contrary, in the case of RBBB the right ventricular ejection flow is delayed (Figure 10.3).

2. Wolf-Parkinson-White (WPW) syndrome

The altered sequences of ventricular activation due to the Wolf-Parkinson-White (WPW) syndrome should be accompanied by abnormal sequences of ventricular contraction, such as the early onset of anterior motion of the left ventricular posterior wall in patients with type A WPW (Figure 10.4). In the case of type B WPW, the IVS motion has an early posterior displacement and subsequently, paradoxical or hypokinetic motion during the ejection phase. With ajimalin-induced abolition of the delta wave, normalization of left ventricular posterior wall motion can also occur (Figure 10.5). These findings are quite similar to those in patients with LBBB. Right ventricular anterior wall motion can also be involved (Figure 10.6). Pulsed

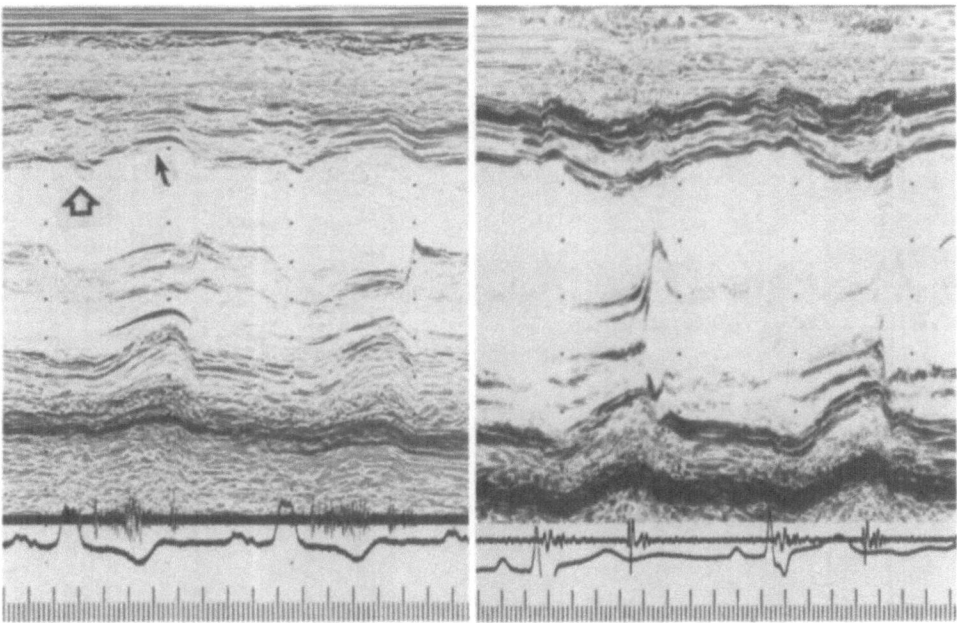

Figure 10.1. M-mode echocardiogram of a patient with a left bundle branch block (LBBB) and a right bundle branch block (RBBB) respectively. The left-hand side shows the early posterior motion of the IVS (large arrow) and paradoxical motion (small arrow) in the LBBB. The right-hand side shows a normal left ventricular wall motion in a patient with a RBBB.

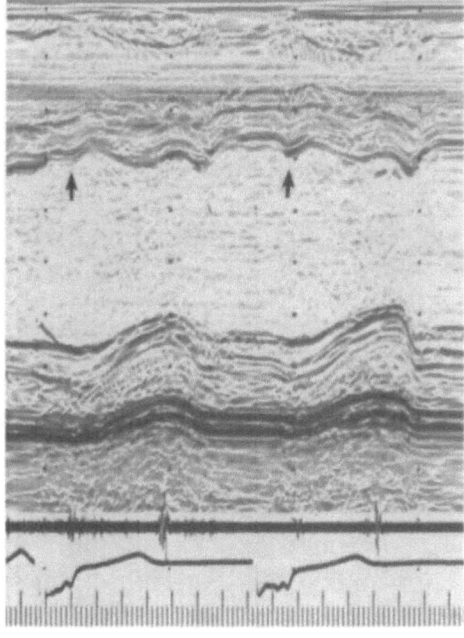

Figure 10.2. M-mode echocardiogram of a patient with right ventricular endocardial pacing. An early IVS posterior displacement is shown by the arrow.

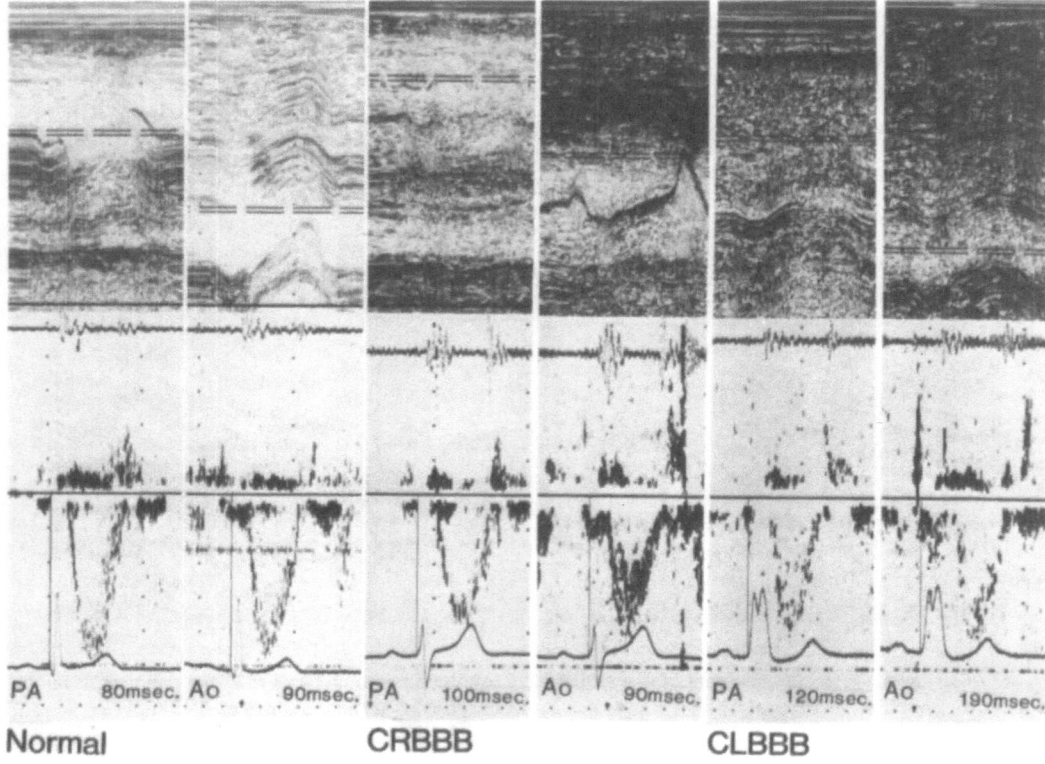

Figure 10.3. Pulsed Doppler echocardiogram of the pulmonary and aortic flow in a normal subject and a patient with a right bundle branch block (RBBB) and a left bundle branch block (LBBB). The left panel indicates the normal relationship of the beginning of pulmonary and aortic flow. RBBB illustrates the delayed beginning of pulmonary flow. The right panel demonstrates the delayed beginning of aortic flow in a patient with LBBB.

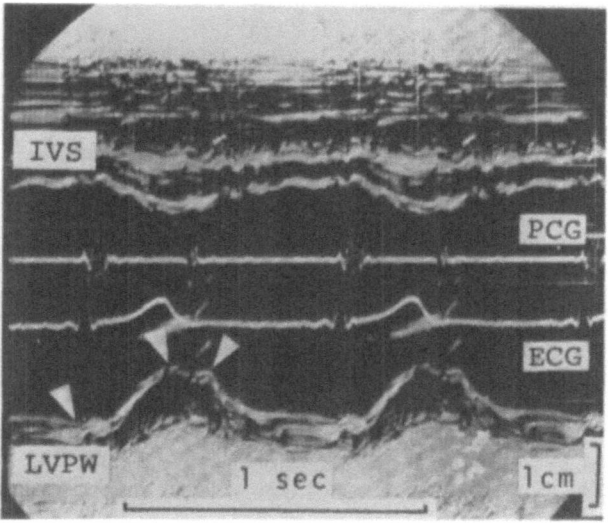

Figure 10.4. M-mode echocardiogram of a patient with type A WPW. The left arrow indicates the beginning of anterior motion of left ventricular posterior wall. The interventricular septal motion is almost normal.

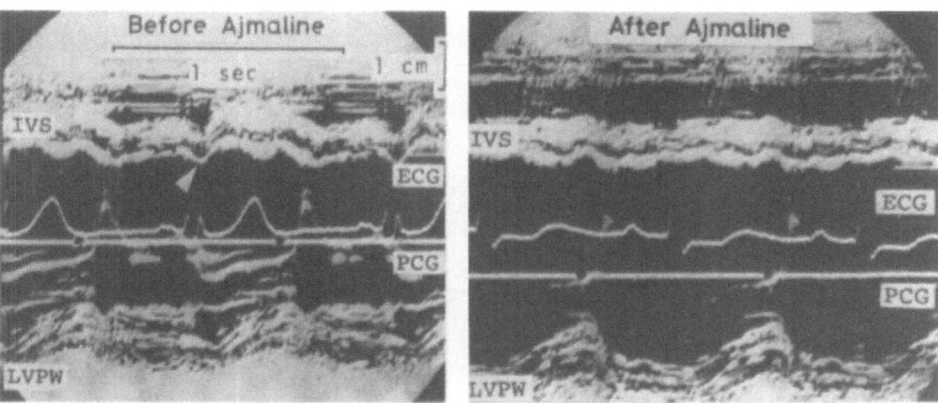

Figure 10.5.   M-mode echocardiogram demonstrating the normalization of atrioventricular conduction of a patient with type B WPW after intravenous ajimalin injection. The IVS paradoxical motion disappears and is replaced by a hypokinetic motion.

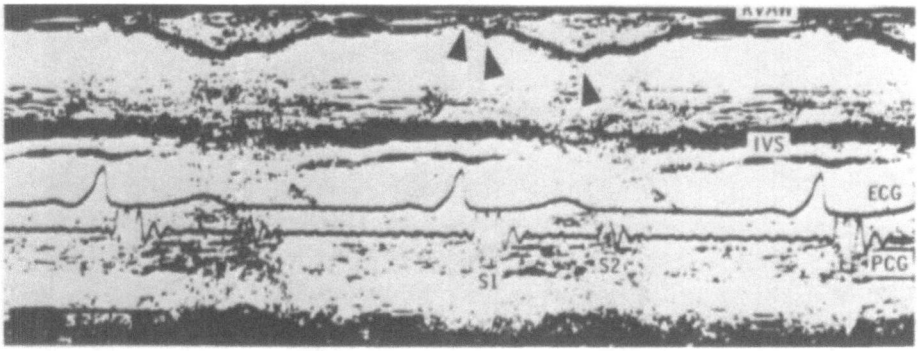

Figure 10.6.   M-mode echocardiogram illustrating the early posterior displacement of right ventricular anterior wall in a patient with type B WPW.

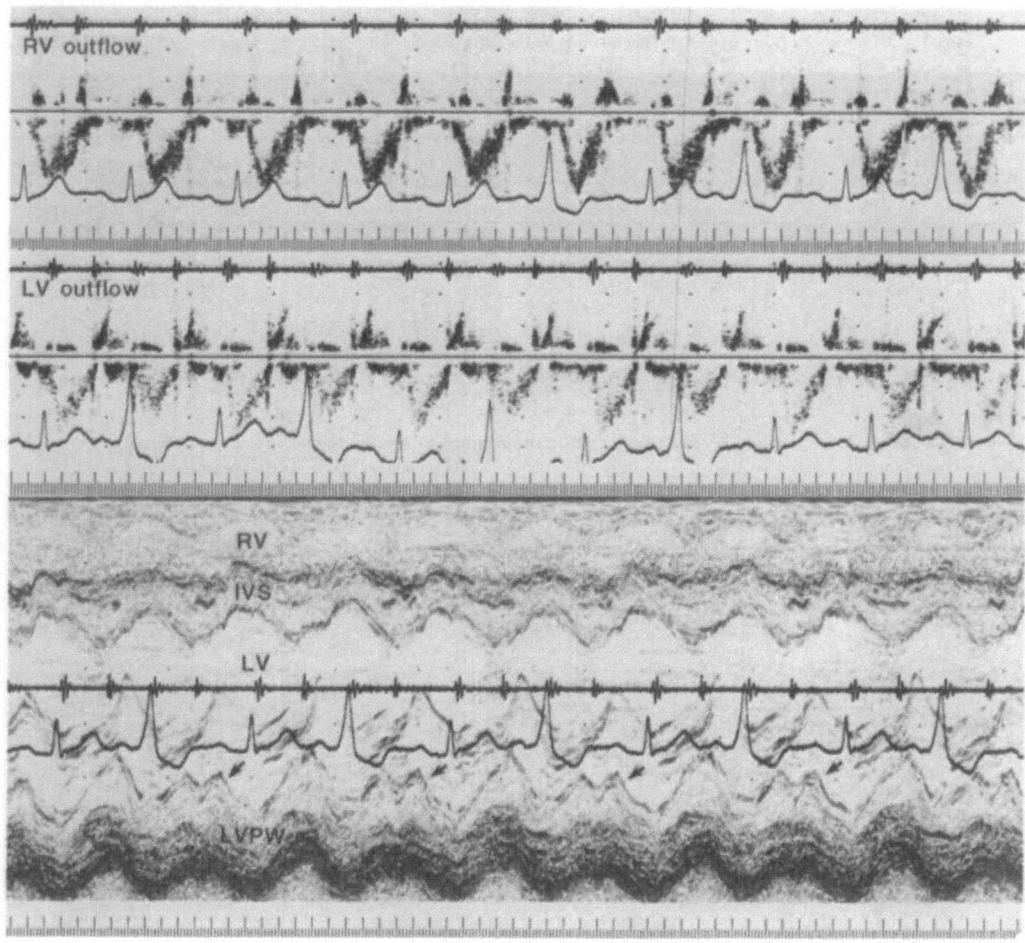

Figure 10.7.   Right ventricular and left ventricular outflow velocity and M-mode in a patient with type A WPW. Pulsed Doppler shows the relatively small left ventricular ejection flow during WPW beats. The right ventricular ejection flow shows no significant changes. M-mode shows the abnormal left ventricular posterior wall motion (arrow) during WPW beats.

Doppler echocardiography is a useful technique to evaluate the hemodynamic changes of both ventricles in patients with WPW syndrome. Usually, in type A WPW, the right ventricular outflow velocity is not affected. However, the left ventricular outflow velocity is relatively smaller than in the normal ventricular activation sequence (Figure 10.7). With type B WPW, the right ventricular outflow velocity is relatively smaller than in normal sinus beats, but the left ventricular outflow velocity shows no significant changes (Figure 10.8). These findings indicate the influence of early depolarization resulting in asynchronous contraction of the affected ventricle (type A in left ventricle and type B in right ventricle) to some degree.

3. Atrial fibrillation

During atrial fibrillation, the leaflets of mitral and tricuspid valves frequently show irregular oscillations in diastole after the E wave, in the M-mode echocardiogram (Figure 10.9). Sometimes, a well organized atrial contraction can produce left ventricular inflow and mitral valve re-opening which can be demonstrated by M-mode and pulsed Doppler echocardiography (Figure 10.10). In patients with atrial fibrillation, reduced diastolic cycle length and filling in the preceding cardiac cycle appear to be the underlying cause of the reduction in stroke volume, depending on Starling's law. Figure 10.11 shows left ventricular outflow and inflow in a 49 year-old female with atrial fibrillation. When the preceding R-R interval is so short as to interrupt the rapid filling of the preceding beat, left ventricular outflow velocity is not observed. When the pre-preceding R-R interval is significantly short, the left ventricular outflow velocity of the preceding beat disappears and the resultant diastolic phase of the preceding beat is relatively longer with a shorter preceding R-R interval. Therefore, the left ventricular outflow velocity of the beat with a shorter pre-preceding R-R interval is higher than the beat with a longer pre-preceding R-R interval (Figure 10.12). Figure 10.13 shows another patient with atrial fibrillation with a relatively slow ventricular rate. In this case, the preceding R-R interval is always long enough so as not to suppress the preceding rapid filling in each beat, and left ventricular inflow and outflow velocity is almost constant, irrespective of the preceding R-R interval. These findings suggest that the filling volume of the preceding beat is a major determinant of stroke volume in atrial fibrillation. In the case of atrial fibrillation due to mitral stenosis, the prolonged pressure half-time of transmitral flow reflects the longer R-R interval required to obtain a sufficient filling volume compared with idiopathic atrial fibrillation (Figure 10.14). After commissurotomy, a relatively short R-R interval can result in an adequate filling volume (Figure 10.15).

4. Atrial flutter

In atrial flutter, the electrical activation of the left atrium is constant and is sometimes detected as left atrial motion in the M-mode. During diastole the mitral valve re-opens with some degree of transmitral flow corresponding to consecutive atrial electrical activation (Figure 10.16).

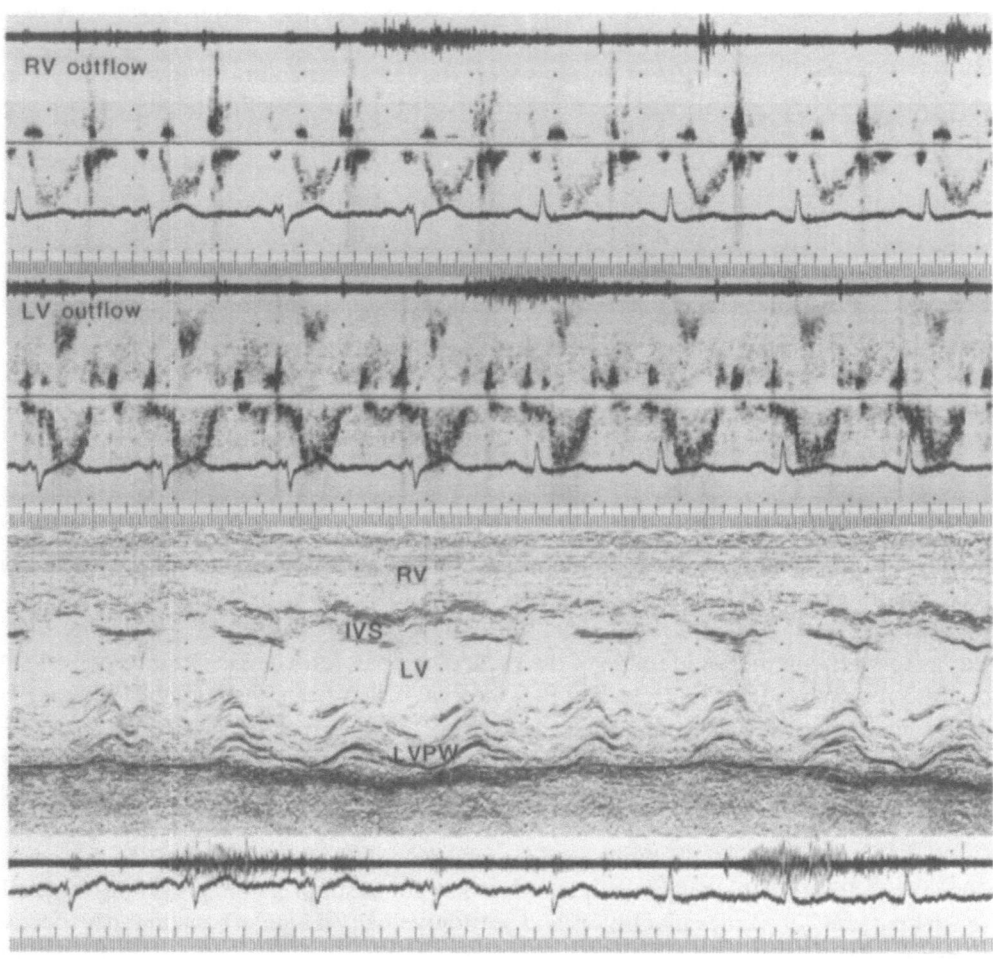

Figure 10.8.   Right ventricular and left ventricular outflow velocity and M-mode in a patient with type B WPW. The right ventricular outflow velocity is relatively smaller in WPW beat. Left ventricular outflow velocity shows no significant changes.

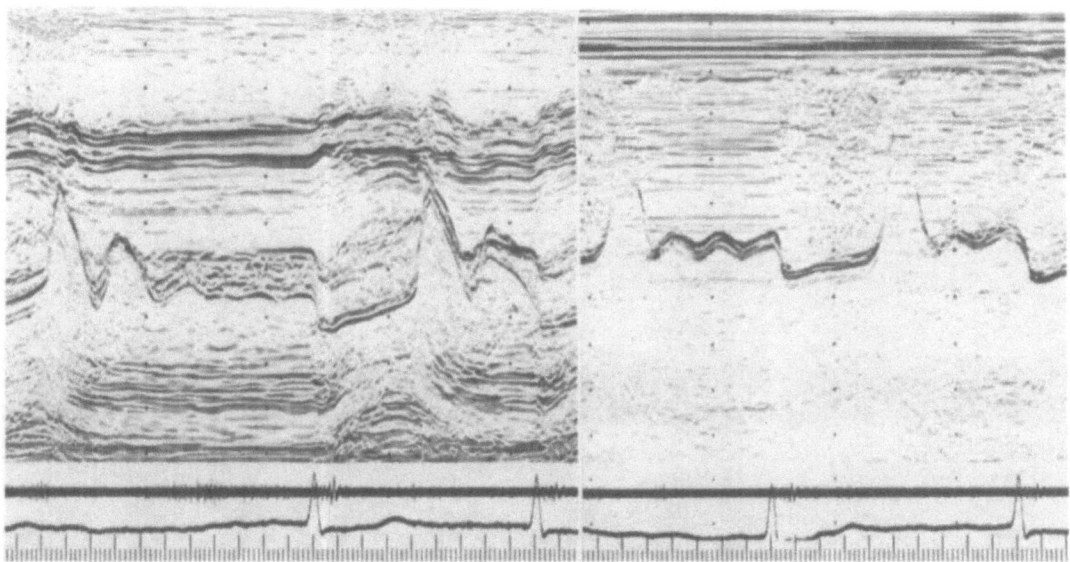

Figure 10.9. M-mode echocardiogram of mitral and tricuspid valve in a patient with atrial fibrillation. Diastolic oscillations of mitral and tricuspid leaflets are clearly seen.

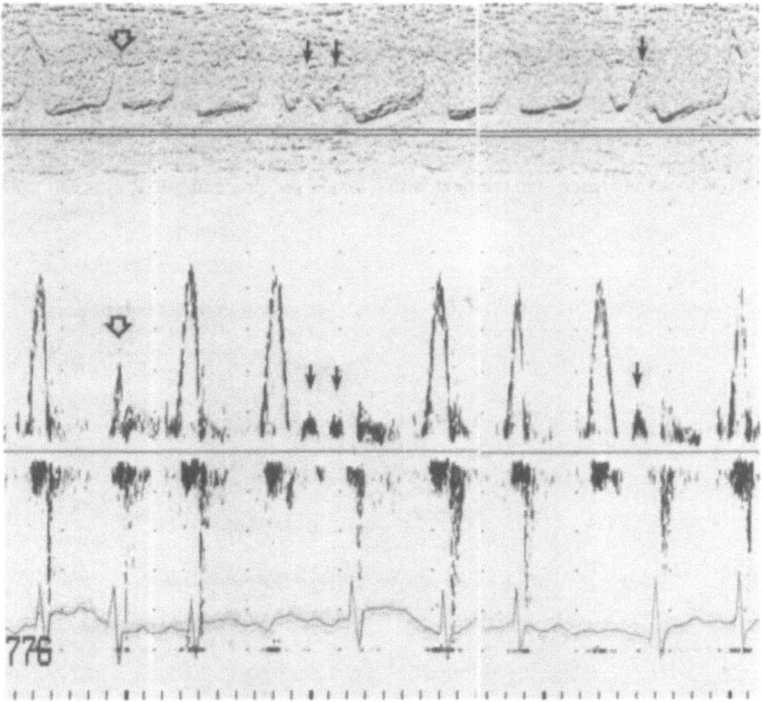

Figure 10.10. Pulsed Doppler echocardiography of left ventricular inflow in a patient with atrial fibrillation. After the rapid filling phase, reduced left ventricular inflow and mitral valve re-opening due to organized atrial contraction are shown by a small arrow.

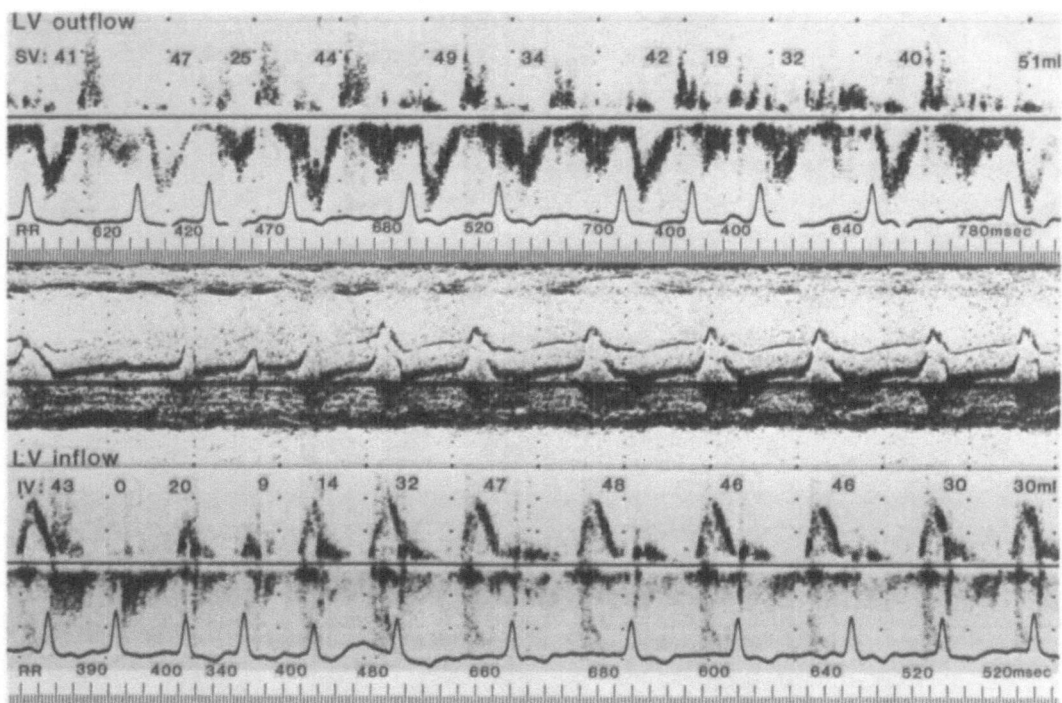

Figure 10.11. Pulsed Doppler echocardiography of left ventricular outflow and inflow in a patient with atrial fibrillation. When the preceding R-R interval is so short as to interrupt the rapid filling of the preceding beat, left ventricular outflow is not recorded. When the pre-preceding R-R interval is significantly short, the left ventricular outflow velocity of the preceding beat disappears and the resultant diastolic phase of the preceding beat is relatively longer with a shorter preceding R-R interval. Therefore, as shown by the large arrow, the left ventricular outflow velocity is higher than the beat with a longer pre-preceding R-R interval.

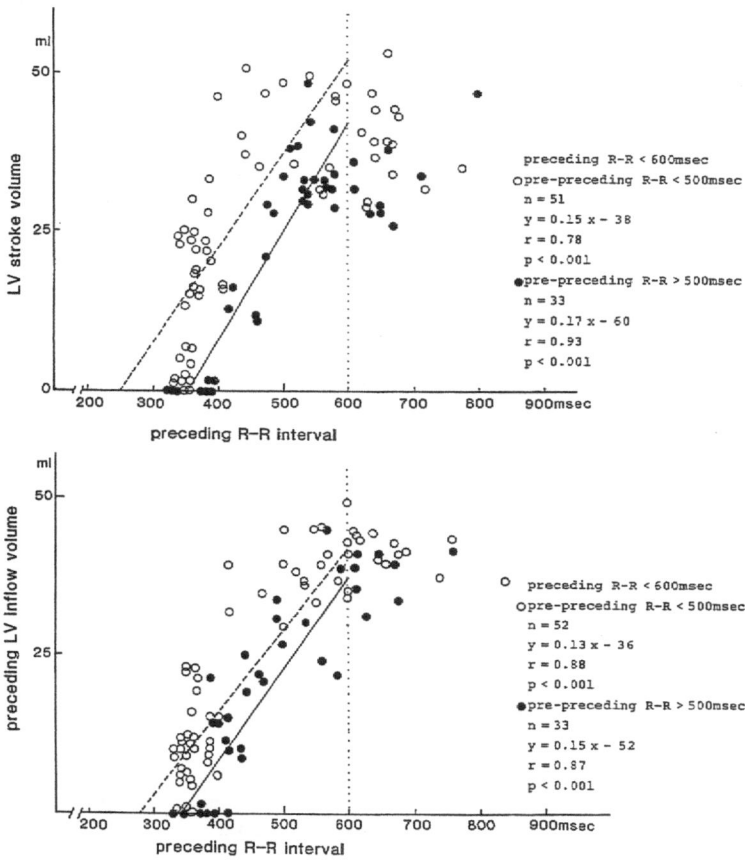

Figure 10.12. Relationship between the preceding R-R interval and left ventricular stroke volume and filling volume of the preceding beat. The pre-preceding R-R interval is divided into more and less than 500 msec. When the preceding R-R interval is under 600 msec, a significant positive correlation is observed between the preceding R-R interval and stroke volume or filling volume of the preceding beat. Stroke volume and filling volume of the preceding beat are constant, independent of the preceding R-R interval when the R-R interval is longer than 600 msec. With a similar preceding R-R interval, a larger stroke volume is found in a shorter pre-preceding R-R interval.

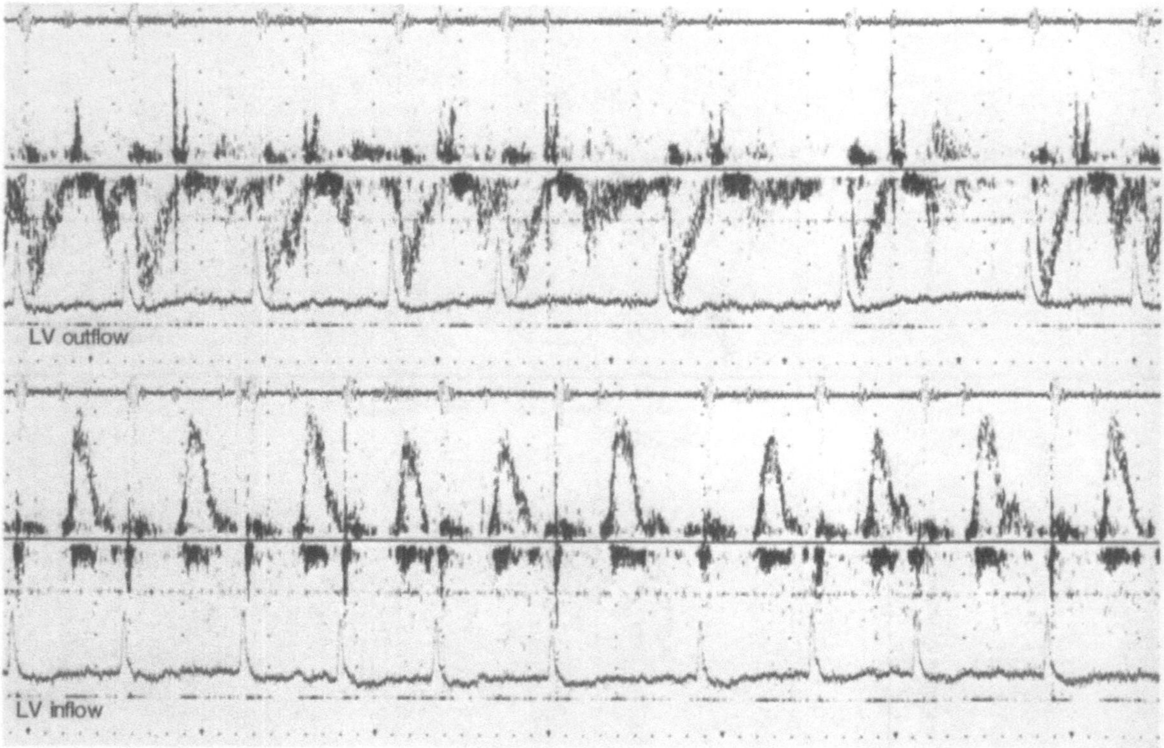

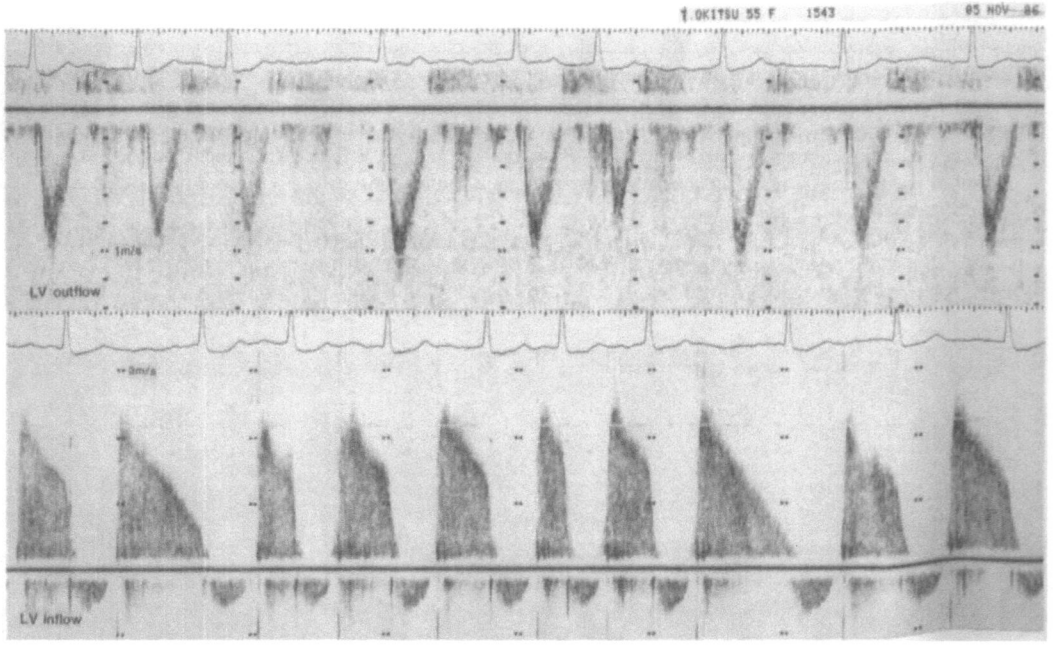

Figure 10.13. Pulsed Doppler echocardiography of left ventricular outflow and inflow in a patient with atrial fibrillation of long R-R interval.

Figure 10.14. Pulsed Doppler echocardiography of left ventricular outflow and inflow in a patient with mitral stenosis and atrial fibrillation. The pressure half-time of transmitral flow is significantly prolonged and the left ventricular ejection flow is reduced in a relatively long coupling interval.

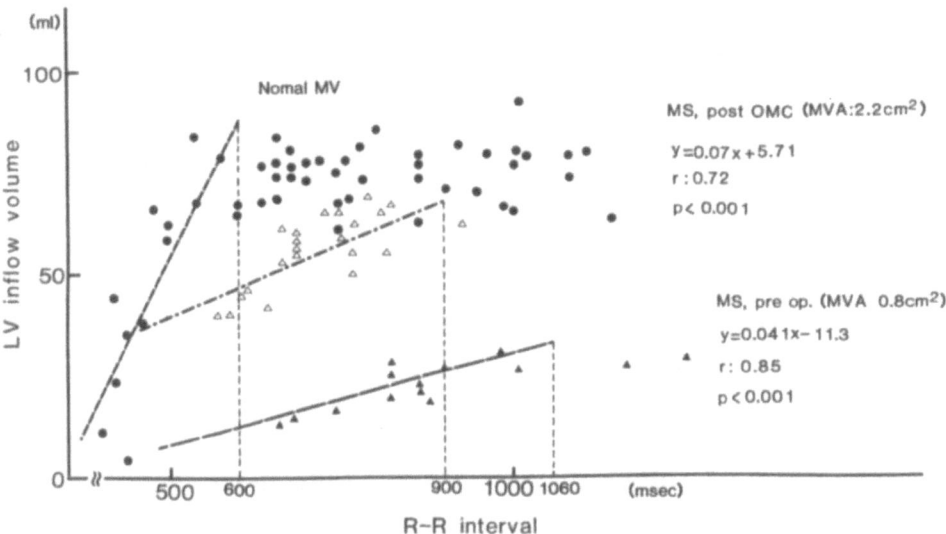

Figure 10.15. Relationship between the preceding R-R interval and left ventricular stroke volume and filling volume of the preceding beat in patients with normal mitral valve, mitral stenosis and post-commissurotomy. The regression line between the preceding R-R interval and left ventricular filling volume of the preceding beat shifts markedly to the right and downward in a patient with mitral stenosis (white triangle) compared with that of a subject with lone atrial fibrillation (black circle). However, this regression line shifts to the left and upward after commissurotomy of the mitral valve.

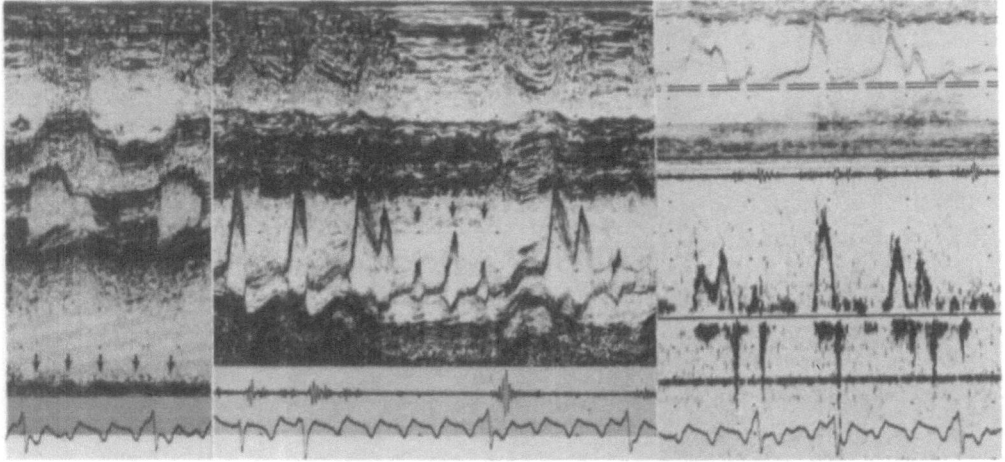

Figure 10.16. M-mode and pulsed Doppler echocardiography of a patient with atrial flutter. The left figure illustrates the anterior motion of the posterior LA wall by an arrow. The re-opening of mitral valve during diastole is shown in the center. The right-hand illustration demonstrates some degree of transmitral flow according to electrical activation.

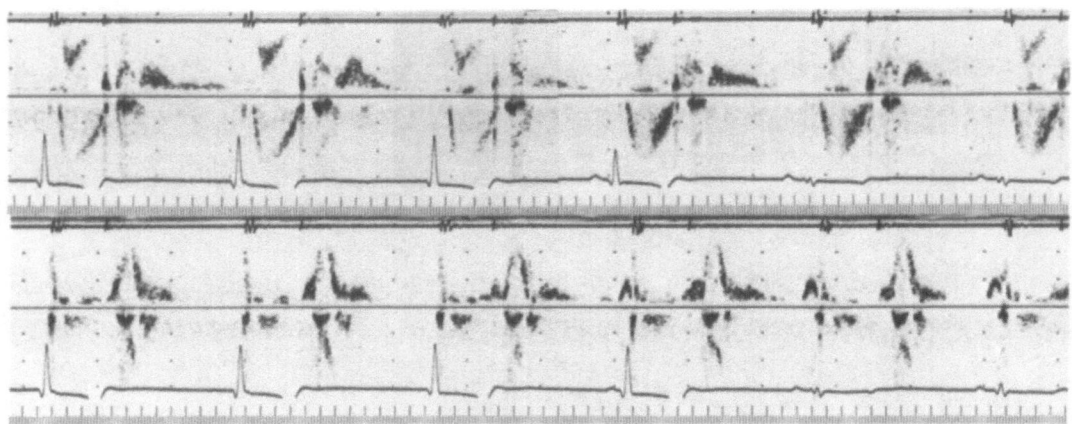

Figure 10.17. Pulsed Doppler echocardiography in a patient with ectopic atrial rhythm. It is possible to appreciate three different kind of rhythms with and without a P wave in ECG. In the presence of a P wave, the left ventricular inflow due to atrial contraction is evident. However, the left ventricular ejection flow is almost constant in the presence or absence of a P wave, due to the small atrial contribution to ventricular filling in this young patient (16 years old).

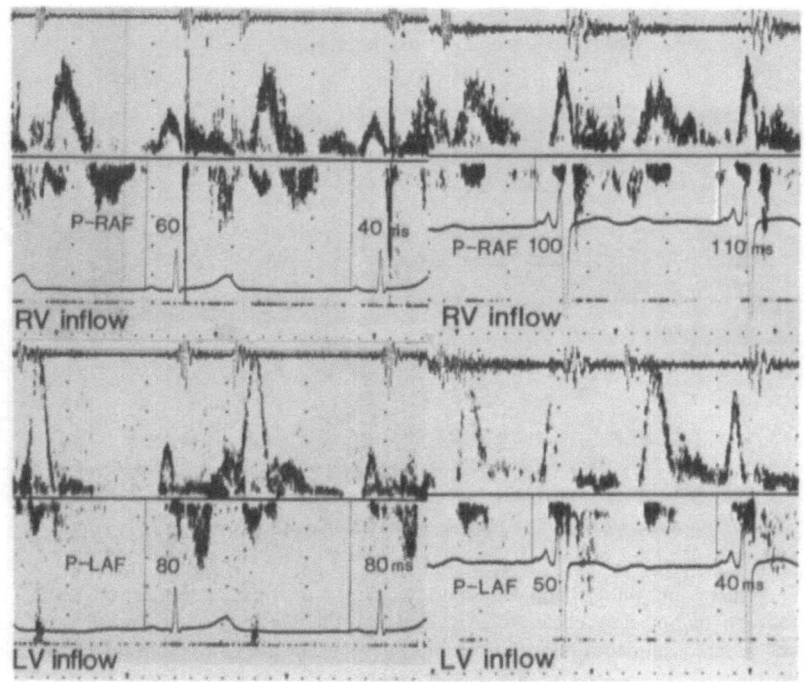

Figure 10.18. Right and left ventricular inflow velocity recording in a 25 year-old man with normal sinus rhythm and a patient with LA rhythm. In the normal subject (left), right atrial ejection flow began at 40 to 60 msec after the onset of the P wave and left atrial ejection flow began at 80 msec after the onset of the P wave. Note that the onset of the right ventricular inflow due to atrial ejection preceded the left ventricular one by 20 to 40 msec. In a patient with LA rhythm (right), right atrial ejection flow began at 90 to 100 msec after the onset of the P wave, and left atrial ejection flow began at 40 to 50 msec after the onset of the P wave. It is noteworthy that the beginning of the left ventricular inflow, due to atrial ejection, preceded the right ventricular one by 40 to 60 msec.

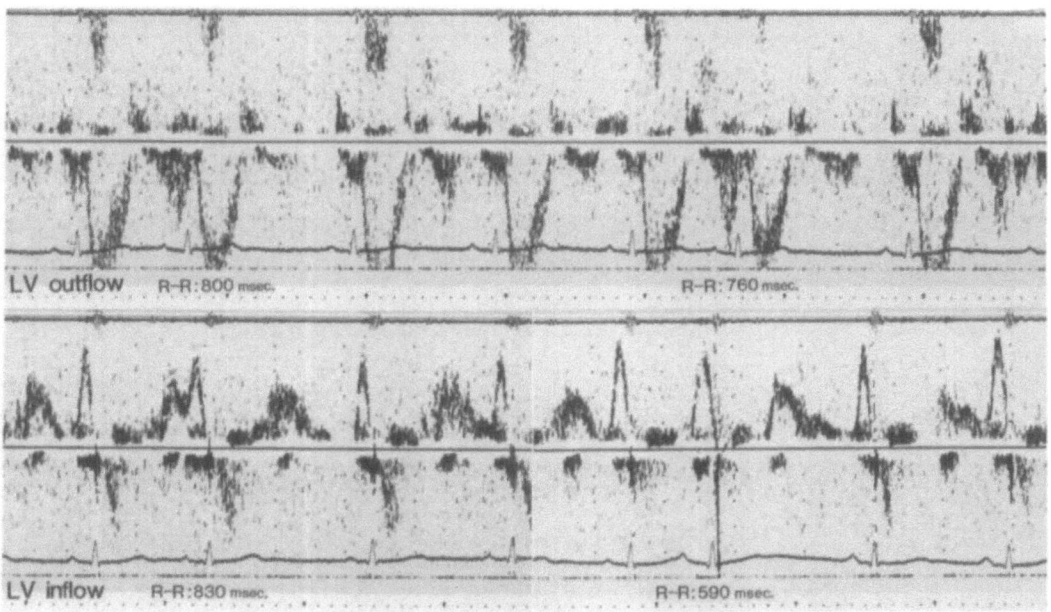

Figure 10.19. Pulsed Doppler echocardiogram of left ventricular outflow and inflow in a patient with SVPCs. Left ventricular inflow illustrating the atrial contribution superimposed on rapid filling velocity.

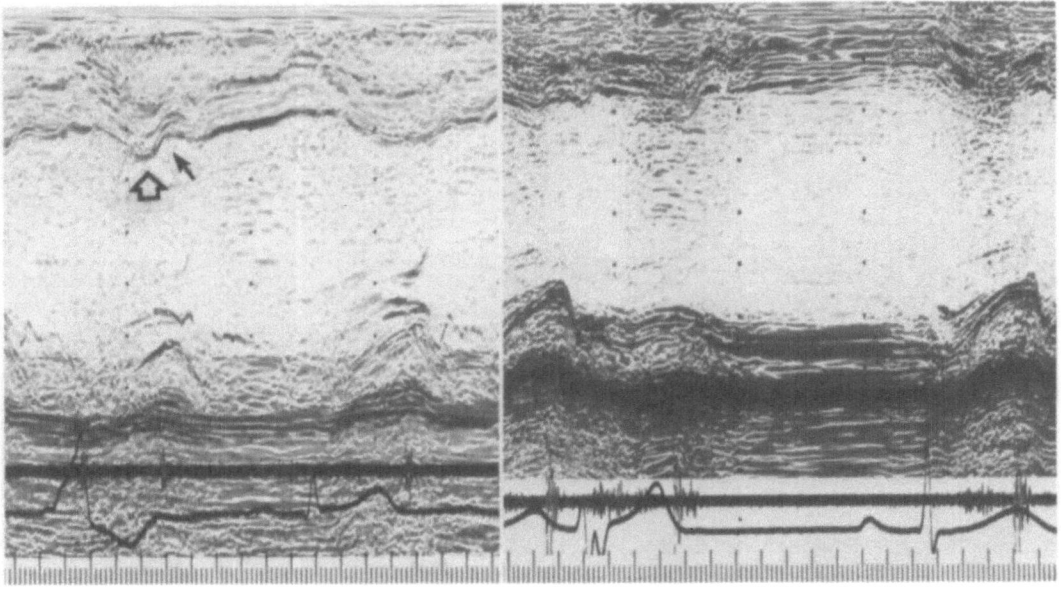

Figure 10.20. M-mode echocardiogram in two different patients with VPCs of left bundle branch block (LBBB) and right bundle branch block (RBBB) configuration. On the left is shown the early posterior motion of IVS with subsequent paradoxical motion during the VPC of LBBB configuration. The right-hand side illustrates the reduced systolic motion of left ventricular posterior wall in a patient with VPC of RBBB configuration.

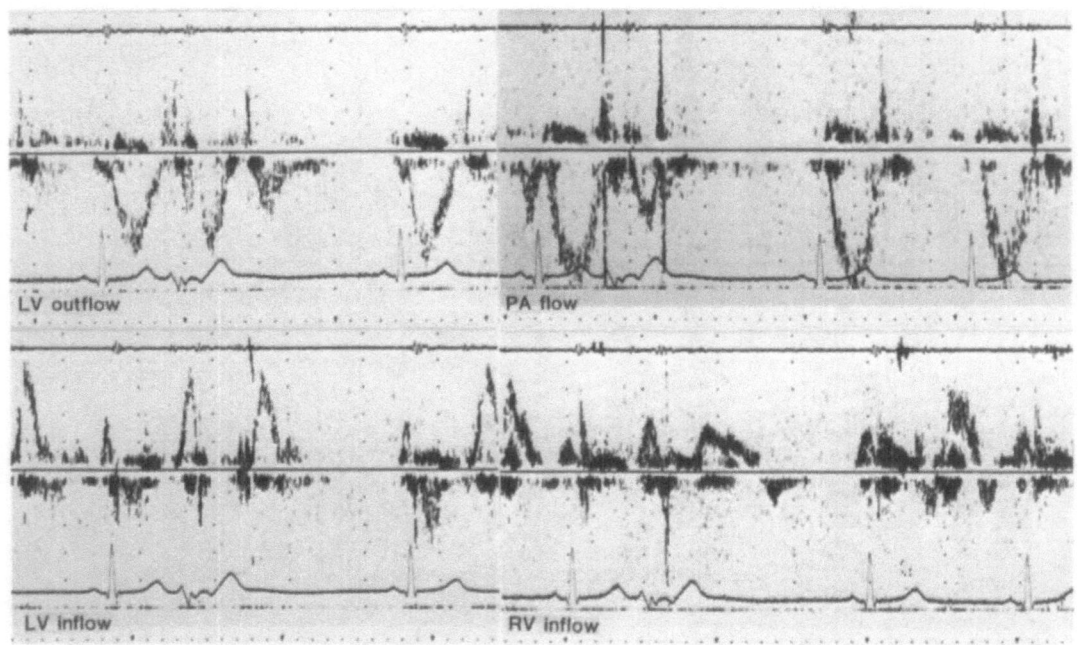

Figure 10.21. Left and right ventricular outflow and inflow velocity tracings of extrasystole of LBBB configuration (right ventricular origin). Right ventricular inflow is more profoundly depressed than the left side due to earlier right ventricular depolarization. As a result, right ventricular outflow peak velocity is lower than the left.

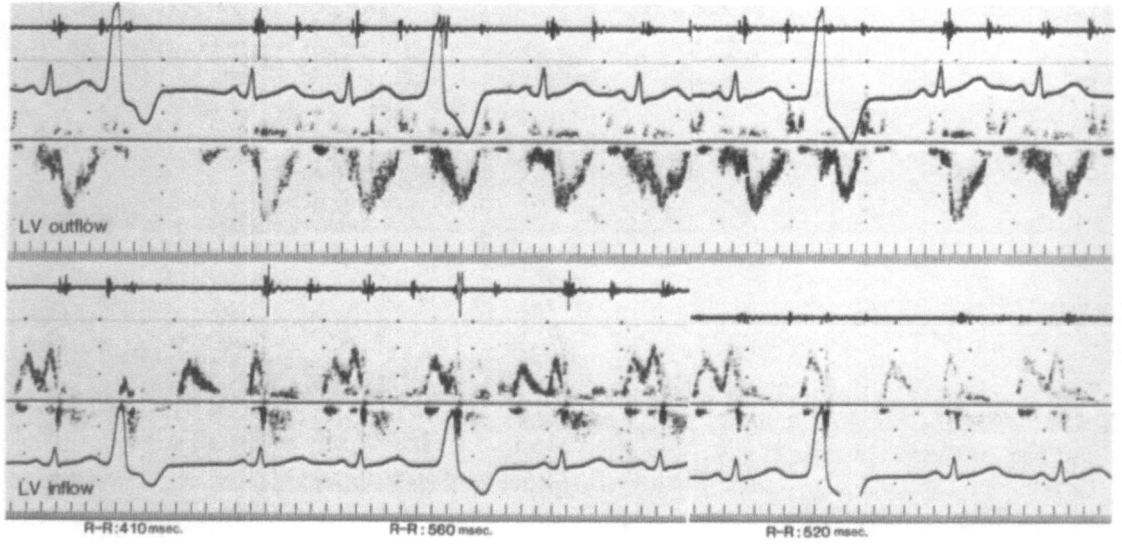

Figure 10.22. Left ventricular (LV) outflow and inflow velocity tracings in a 42 year-old female with extrasystole of three different coupling intervals. The extrasystole of shorter coupling interval (R-R interval of 410 msec) interrupts preceding rapid filling almost completely and produces no LV outflow velocity. The LV outflow velocity of subsequent postextrasystolic beat shows increased peak velocity and flow velocity integral compared with these of basic sinus beat. The extrasystole of longer coupling interval (R-R interval of 560 msec) makes no interruption of the preceding rapid filling and results in almost the same LV outflow velocity tracing as a basic sinus beat. The LV outflow velocity of postextrasystolic beat shows almost no change. The extrasystole of moderate coupling interval (R-R interval of 520 msec) makes an incomplete interruption of preceding rapid filling and moderately decreased LV outflow peak velocity and flow velocity integral are resulted.

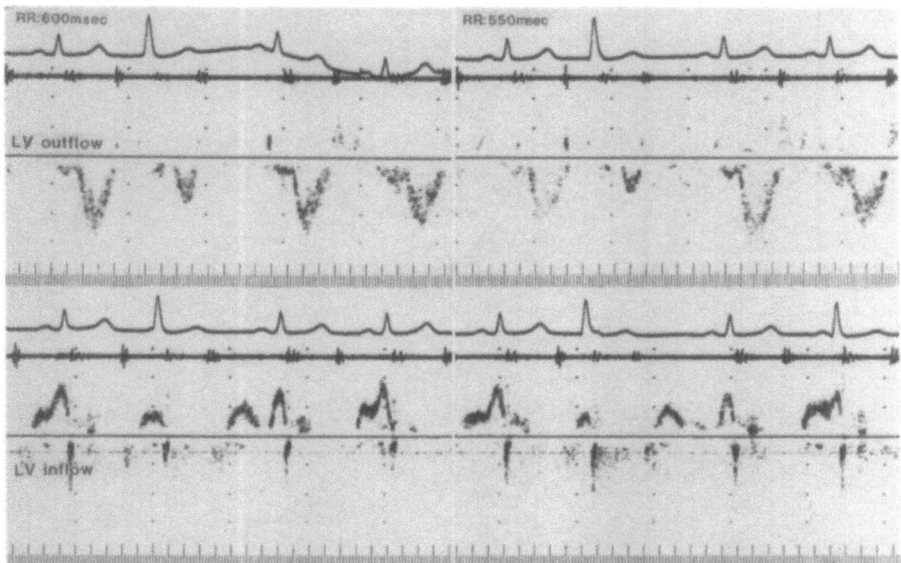

Figure 10.23. Left ventricular (LV) outflow and inflow velocity tracings in a 58 year-old male with old myocardial infarction and extrasystole of two different coupling intervals. In this patient, LV inflow velocity tracing in basic sinus beat shows depressed rapid filling and increased left atrial contribution to ventricular filling. The extrasystoles of two different coupling intervals result in different interruptions of preceding rapid filling. However, there are little LV outflow velocity tracings in both two extrasystoles. In this patient, the LV outflow velocity of extrasystole has no definitive dependency on preceding filling volume.

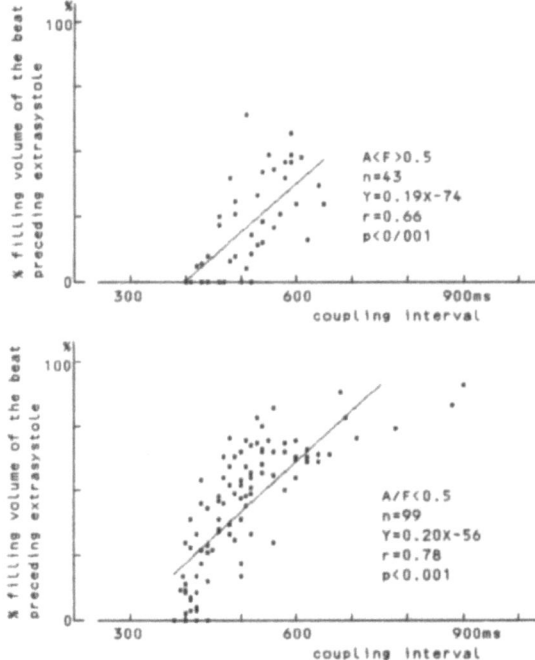

Figure 10.24. Correlation between coupling intervals and percentage filling volume of the beats preceding VPC in patients with A/F over and under 0.5. A significant correlation between coupling intervals and percentage filling volume of the beats preceding VPC in patients with A/F over and onder 0.5 were observed. The regression line in patients with A/F over 0.5 shifted downward significantly compared with that in patients with A/F under 0.5 (*p* < 0.001). A/F = the relative contribution of left atrial contraction to ventricular filling, VPC = ventricular premature contraction.

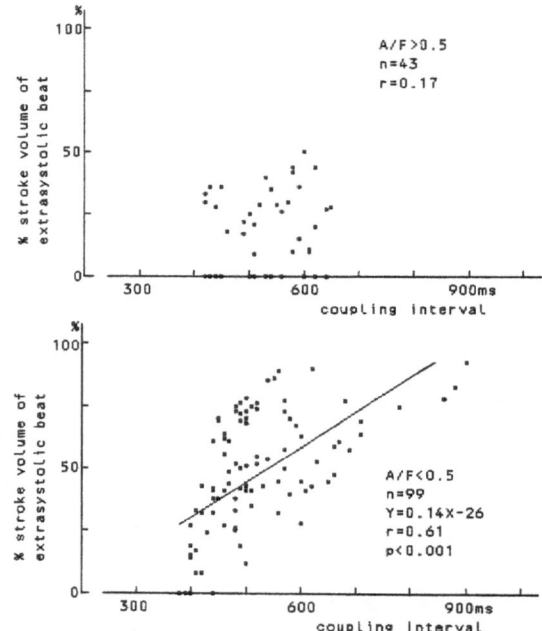

Figure 10.25. Correlation between coupling intervals and percentage stroke volume of VPCs in patients with A/F over and under 0.5. In patients with A/F under 0.5, a significant positive correlation between percentage stroke volume of 99 VPCs and coupling intervals was present. In contrast, patients with A/F over 0.5 had no significant correlation between percentage stroke volume of 43 VPCs and coupling intervals. Abbreviations as in Figure 10.24.

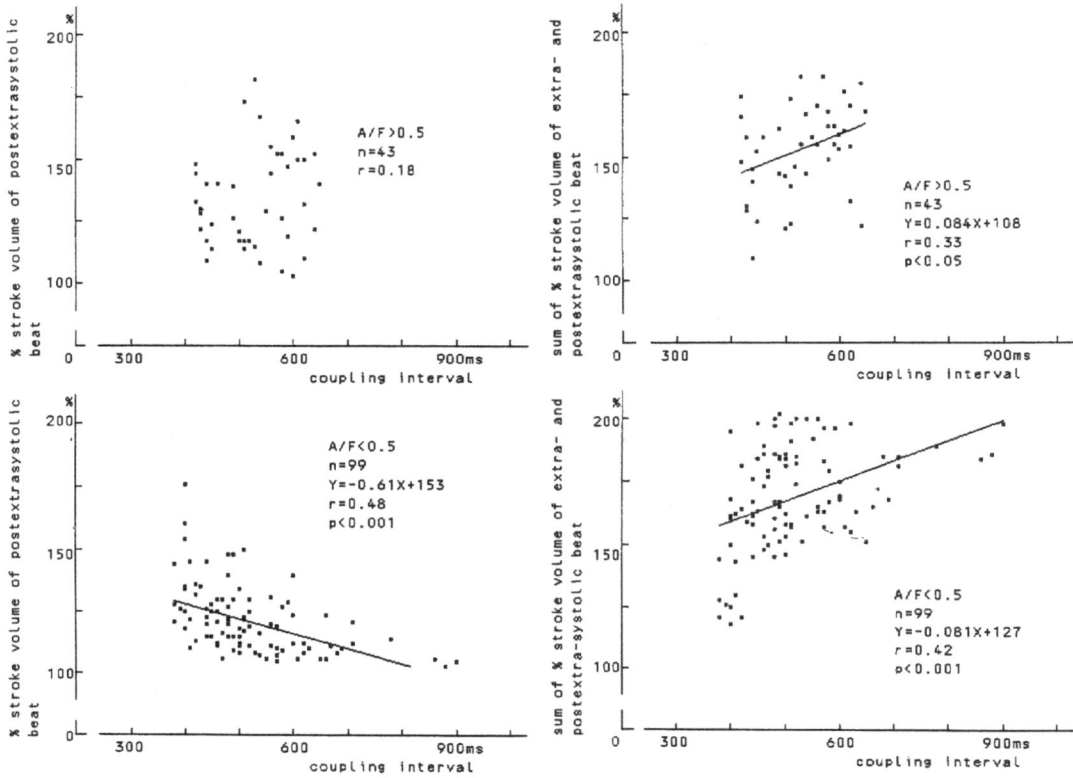

Figure 10.26. Correlation between coupling intervals and percentage stroke volume of postextrasystolic beats in patients with A/F over and under 0.5. A significantly negative correlation was observed between percentage stroke volume of 99 postextrasystolic beats and coupling intervals in patients with A/F under 0.5, but not in patients with A/F over 0.5. A/F = the relative contribution of left atrial contraction to ventricular filling.

Figure 10.27. Correlation between coupling intervals and the sum of percentage stroke volume of VPCs and postextrasystolic beats in patients with A/F over and under 0.5. Significant correlations between coupling interval and the sum of percentage stroke volume of VPCs and postextrasystolic beats in patients with A/F over and under 0.5 were observed. The regression line in patients with A/F over 0.5 shifted downward significantly compared with that in patients with A/F under 0.5 ($p < 0.001$). Abbreviations as in Figure 10.26.

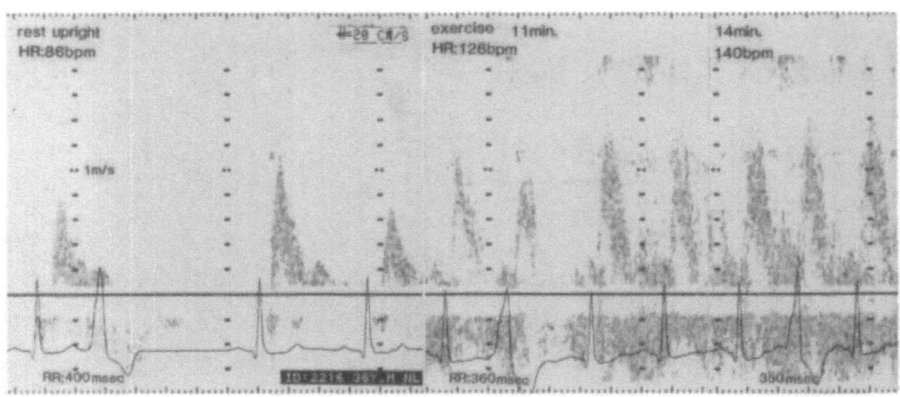

Figure 10.28. Exercise Doppler echocardiogram of a 38 year-old sportsman with VPCs. At rest, the VPC shows no ejection flow in the coupling interval of 400 msec. During exercise, the VPCs become more frequent with relatively short coupling interval but all the VPCs are accompanied by adequate ejection flow.

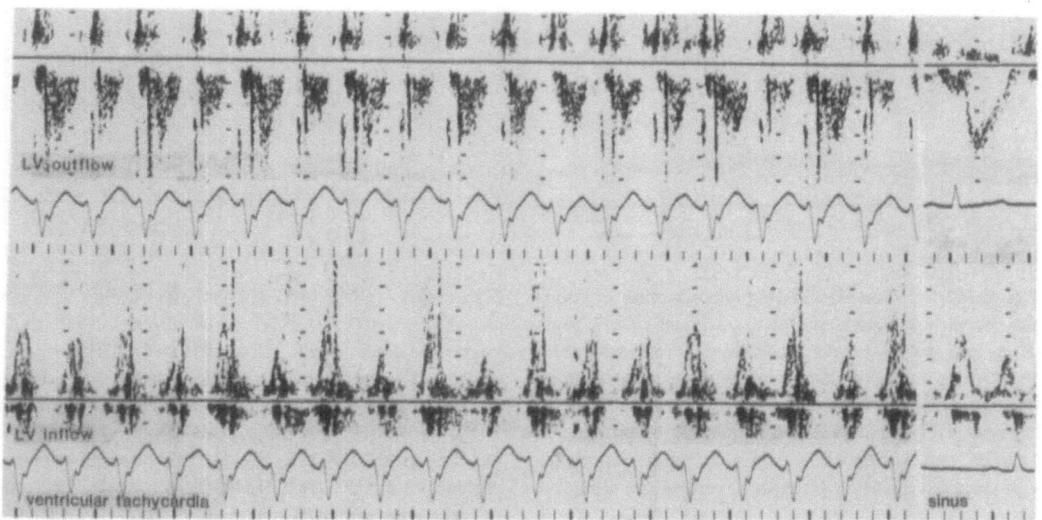

Figure 10.29. Left ventricular (LV) outflow and inflow velocity tracings in a 37 year-old man with ventricular tachycardia. LV inflow velocity is interrupted by the premature onset of the next systole and an impairment of stroke volume results.

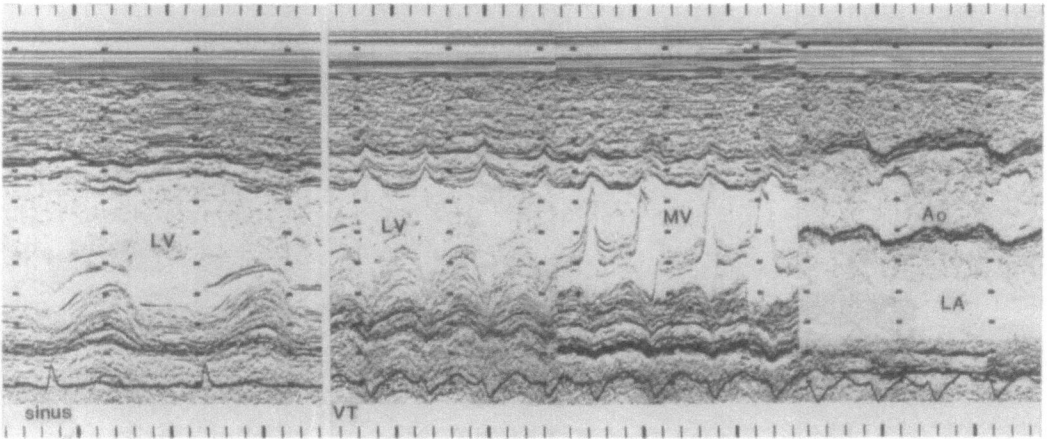

Figure 10.30. M-mode echocardiogram of ventricular tachycardia in a 37 year-old man. Compared with normal sinus rhythm (left), the left ventricular (LV) dimension is reduced. Mitral valve opening is limited by early onset of the next systole. Aortic valve opening is observed only once in every two beat.

5. Ectopic atrial rhythm

In case of ectopic atrial rhythm, the mechanical activation of the heart can be involved. However, a significant hemodynamic derangement does not usually constitute a common finding using pulsed Doppler echocardiography (Figure 10.17). In patients with LA rhythm, the electrical and mechanical activation of the LA is earlier than RA, therefore this diagnosis can be done by demonstrating the early beginning of the left ventricular inflow due to atrial contraction preceding the right ventricular one (Figure 10.18).

6. Supraventricular premature contraction

In supraventricular premature contractions (SVPC), the rapid filling velocity is superimposed by the atrial contribution (Figure 10.19). Therefore, the left ventricular ejection flow is relatively unchanged when compared with VPC of the same coupling interval.

7. Ventricular premature contraction

Ventricular premature contractions (VPCs) alter the motion of the IVS and/or the left ventricular posterior wall due to abnormal depolarization (Figure 10.20). Much work concerning non-invasive evaluation of hemodynamic changes due to VPCs has been reported using M-mode and two-dimensional echocardiography. However, these methods have some limitation since asynchrony of ventricular contraction may result in errors in volume measurements. The use of Doppler-determined cardiac flow parameters enables us to evaluate some instantaneous characteristics of intracardiac blood flow and hemodynamic derangement due to VPCs, irrespective of ventricular asynchrony. The hemodynamic effects of VPCs depend on several factors including the site of origin, the degree of prematurity and the

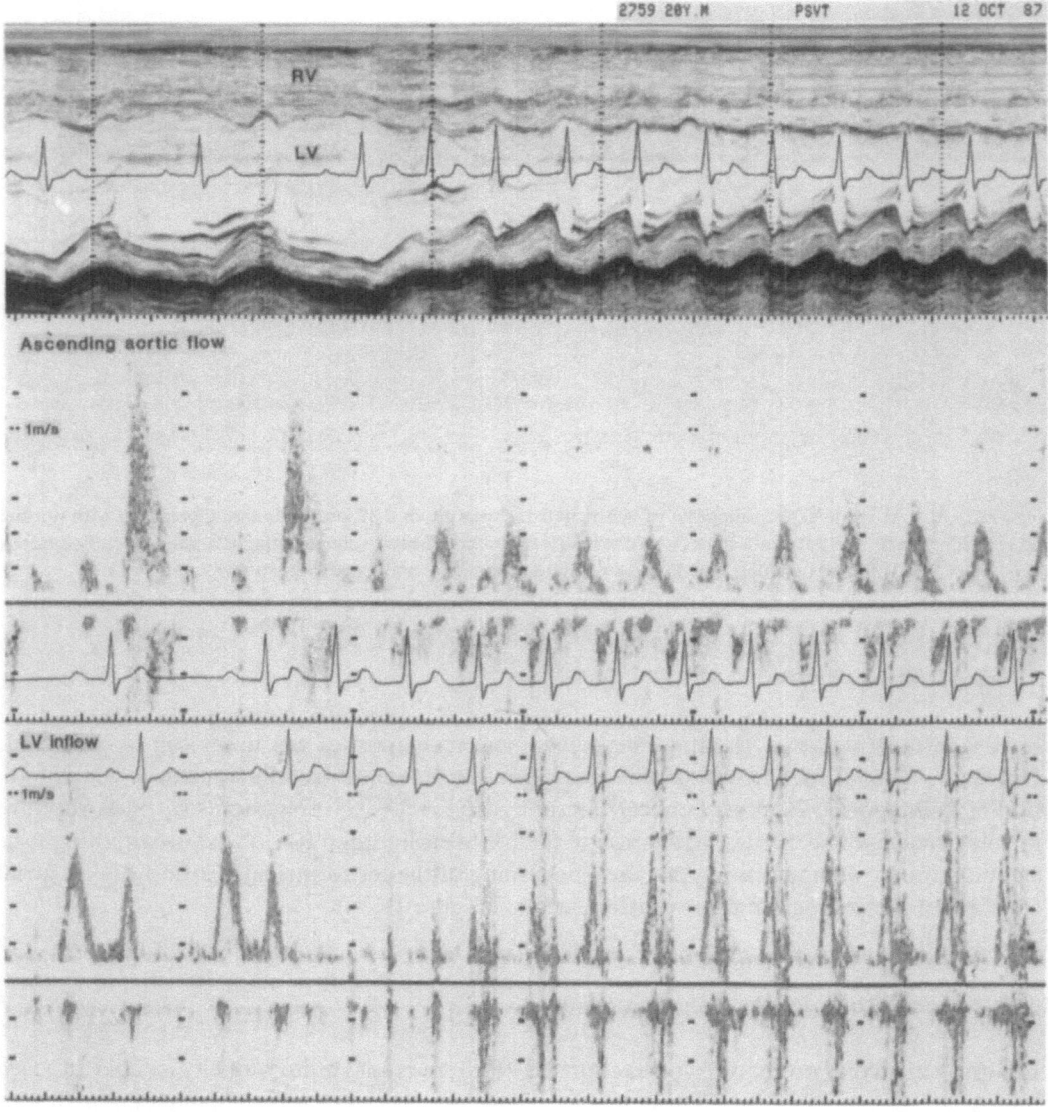

Figure 10.31. M-mode and left ventricular (LV) outflow and inflow velocity tracings in a 20 year-old man with supraventricular tachycardia. Compared with normal sinus rhythm (left), the left ventricular (LV) dimension is reduced. LV inflow velocity is interrupted by the premature onset of the next systole and the impairment of stroke volume results, especially in the beginning of tachycardia.

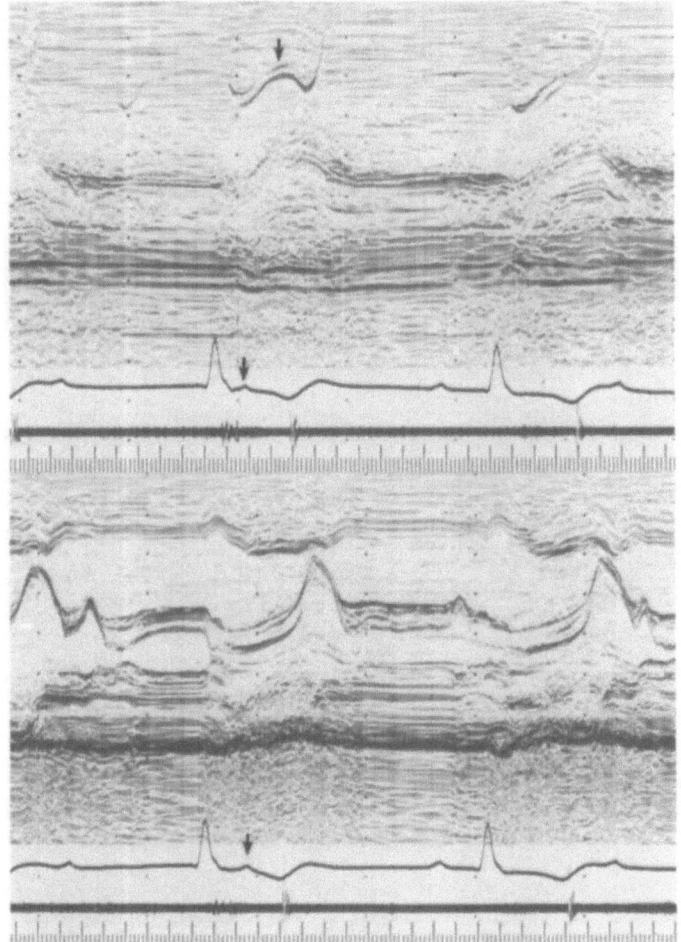

Figure 10.32. M-mode echocardiogram of the tricuspid and mitral valves in a patient with complete AV block. During systole, the tricuspid valve shows an anterior displacement (arrow) immediately after P wave. In contrast, the mitral valve is closed during the same phase.

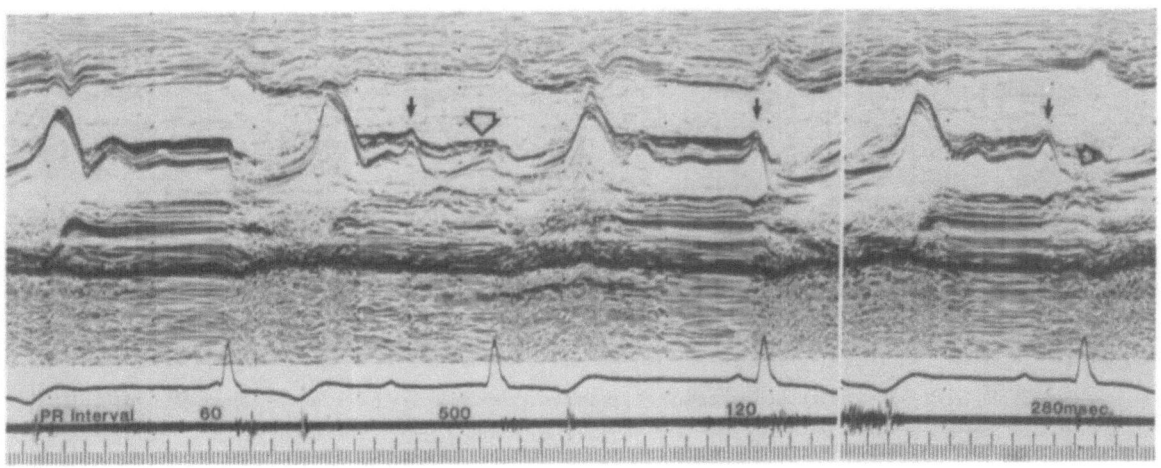

Figure 10.33. M-mode echocardiogram illustrating the 'shoulder' formation (large arrow) of the mitral valve after the A wave (small arrow) during a long PR interval in a 23 year-old patient with congenital AV block.

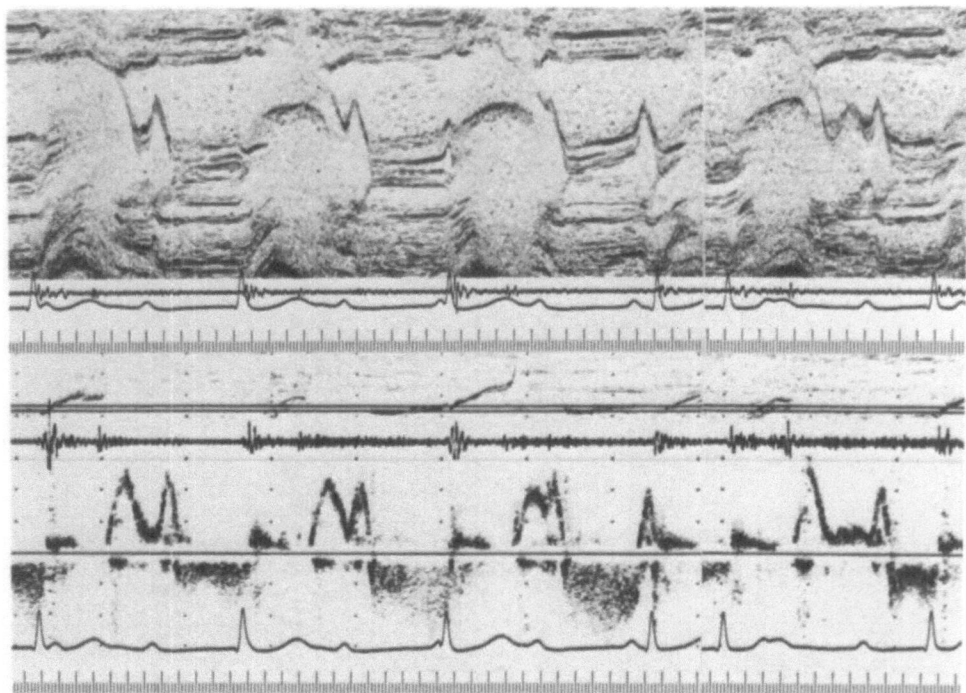

Figure 10.34. M-mode and pulsed Doppler echocardiogram of a patient with complete AV block. In a long PR interval, the mitral valve shows an incomplete closure in M-mode and mild diastolic mitral regurgitation is evidenced in this phase by pulsed Doppler echocardiography.

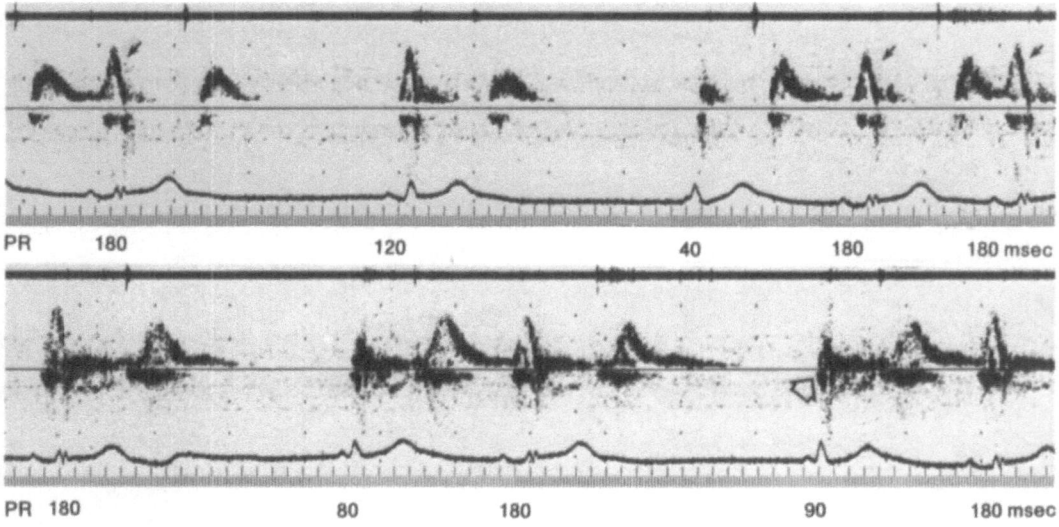

Figure 10.35. Pulsed Doppler echocardiogram of a patient with complete AV block. We can appreciate that the left ventricular inflow due to atrial contraction almost disappears in PR intervals less than 100 msec (40, 80, and 90 msec).

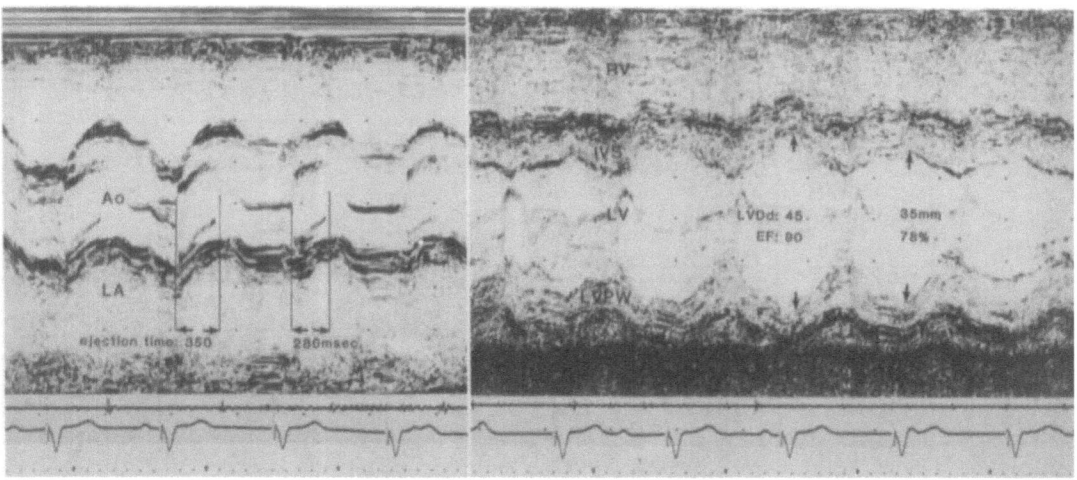

Figure 10.36. M-mode echocardiogram of a patient with VVI pacing. During the pacing beat with a preceded P wave, the longer ejection time and larger left ventricular end-diastolic dimension and ejection fraction (EF) compared to those without are clearly noted.

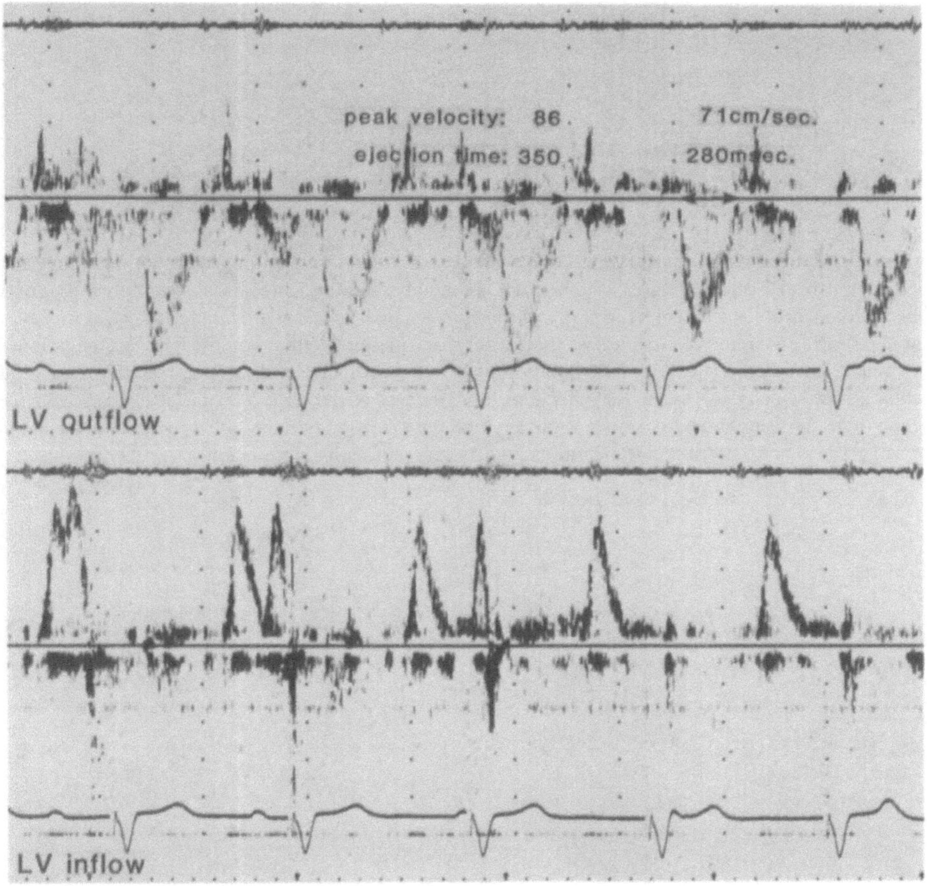

Figure 10.37. Pulsed Doppler echocardiogram directly illustrating atrial contribution to left ventricular filling and increased left ventricular ejection flow during the pacing beat with preceded P wave in a patient with VVI pacing.

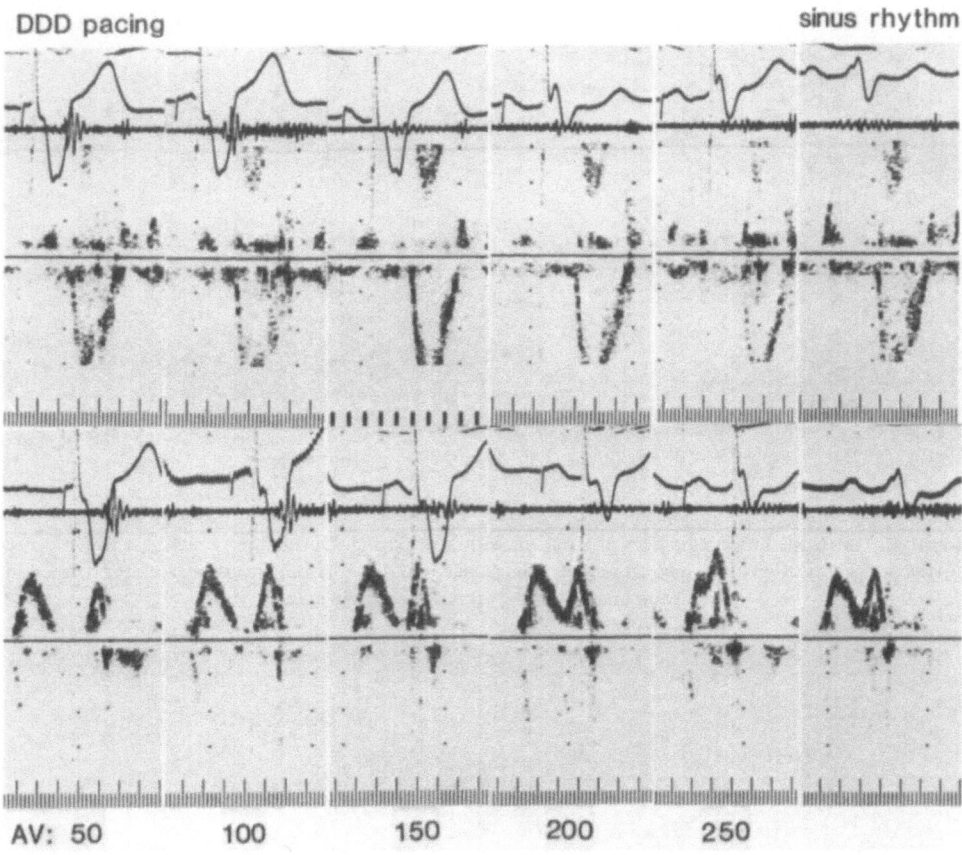

Figure 10.38. Left ventricular outflow and inflow velocity during AV sequential pacing with various AV intervals and sinus rhythm in a 67 year-old man in whom a DDD pacemaker was implanted because Mobitz II type of AV block continued after an acute episode of inferior myocardial infarction. The left ventricular outflow velocity curve in AV sequential pacing at AV interval of 50 msec is smaller than that in sinus rhythm because left ventricular inflow due to LA ejection is interrupted prematurely by the onset of left ventricular contraction, resulting in a reduced left ventricular inflow velocity. AV sequential pacing with AV interval of 100, 150, 200 and 250 msec shows a similar left ventricular outflow velocity curve as the sinus rhythm since left ventricular inflow due to LA ejection is not prematurely interrupted by left ventricular contraction.

VVI pacing   sinus rhythm

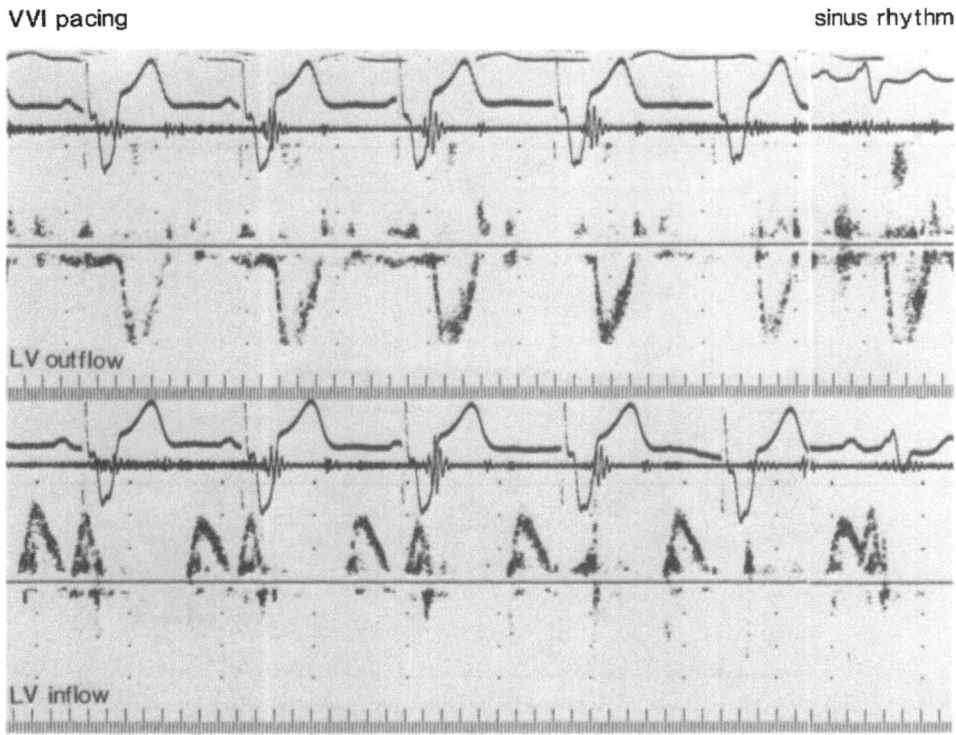

LV outflow

LV inflow

Figure 10.39. Left ventricular outflow and inflow velocity during VVI pacing in a 67 year-old man implanted with a DDD pacemaker. When a P wave precedes the ventricular pacing spike, left ventricular inflow due to LA contraction is clearly recognized in left ventricular inflow velocity recordings. The left ventricular outflow velocity curve is larger in beats with a preceding P wave than in those without.

frequency of VPCs, and the underlying heart disease. If both left and right ventricular outflow and inflow velocity can be recorded, the different hemodynamic derangement between left and right ventricle can be evaluated (Figure 10.21). The degree of prematurity also affects hemodynamic derangement in VPCs. Earlier premature occurrence of a VPC is generally preceded by an incomplete degree of ventricular filling and is thereby initiated by a lower than usual end-diastolic volume, the resultant stroke volume then being concomitantly diminished as well (Figure 10.22). This indicates that the hemodynamic performance in extrasystole would be mainly affected by the filling volume at the onset of ventricular contraction with the resultant Starling's law. In cases of decreased left ventricular rapid filling or, in other words, increased left atrial contribution to left ventricular filling, the significance of coupling intervals in VPCs in left ventricular performance is less important, possibly due to depressed left ventricular diastolic behavior and loss of synchronized atrial contraction (Figures 10.23, 24, 25). The augmentation of left ventricular stroke volume by postextrasystolic beats is more prominent in VPCs of shorter coupling intervals in patients with smaller atrial contribution to ventricular filling, but the compensation by this increase is less sufficient in VPCs of shorter coupling intervals (Figure 10.26, 27). Therefore, VPCs may reduce cardiac output to a substantial degree, depending on their frequency of occurrence and degree of prematurity. In patients with larger atrial contribution to ventricular filling, the augmentation of postextrasystolic beats has no definitive relation to prematurity. This suggests a significant contribution of the left ventricular diastolic behavior to left ventricular performance during VPCs. In exercise

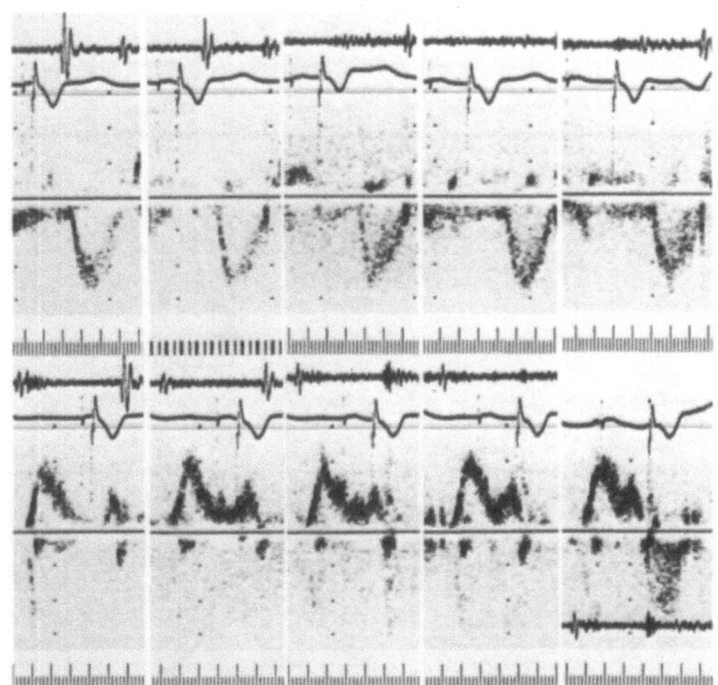

Figure 10.40.   Left ventricular outflow and inflow velocity during AV sequential pacing with various AV intervals in a 29 year-old woman in whom a previously implanted VVI pacemaker was exchanged for a DDD pacemaker because of battery failure. A smaller left ventricular inflow velocity curve during LA ejection phase in AV sequential pacing is seen when compared to Figure 10.39. Therefore, the left ventricular outflow velocity tracing shows no significant changes with alternation in AV intervals. At an AV interval of 250 msec, atriogenic diastolic reflux by LA relaxation is shown in late diastole.

VVI pacing   29yrs. female

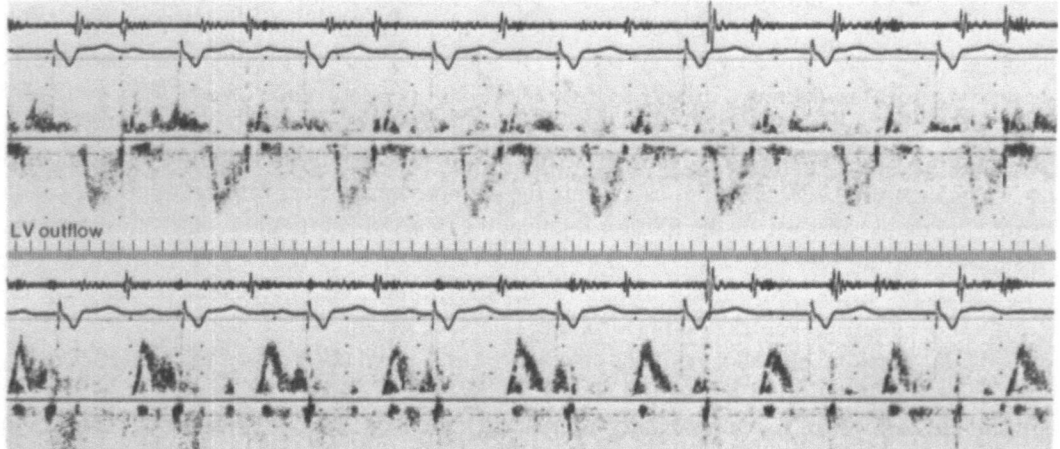

Figure 10.41.   Left ventricular outflow and inflow velocity during VVI pacing in a 29 year-old woman. Left ventricular inflow due to LA contraction is observed immediately after a P wave appearing in diastole, but the left ventricular outflow velocity curve remains almost unchanged, irrespective, of the presence of a preceding P wave, because of the smaller LA contribution to left ventricular filling. Atriogenic diastolic reflux is also seen in long PR interval (first and second beats).

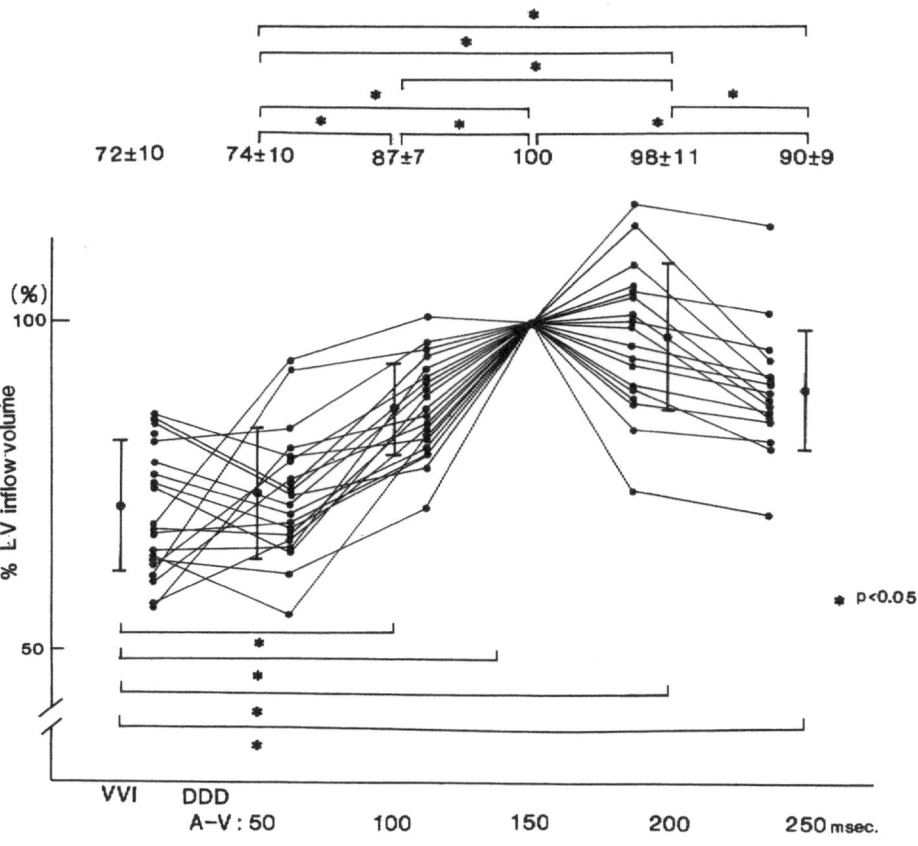

Figure 10.42. Percent changes in left ventricular inflow volume with conversion of the pacing mode and alternations in AV intervals. The percent left ventricular inflow volume is significantly smaller at AV intervals of 50, 100 and 250 msec than at an AV interval of 150 msec. It is also significantly smaller in VVI pacing than in AV sequential pacing with AV interval of 100, 150, 200 and 250 msec.

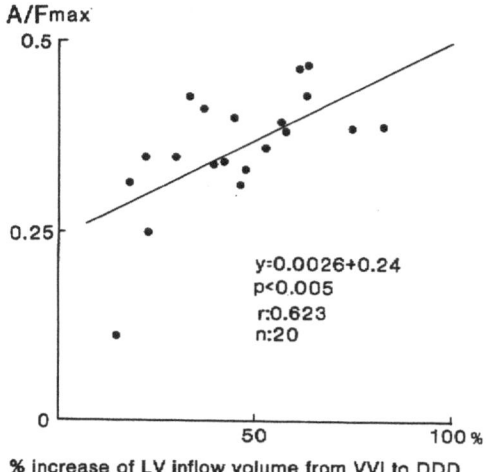

Figure 10.43. Relationship between the percentage increase of left ventricular inflow volume from VVI to DDD and the ratio of atrial contribution to ventricular filling (A/F_{max}).

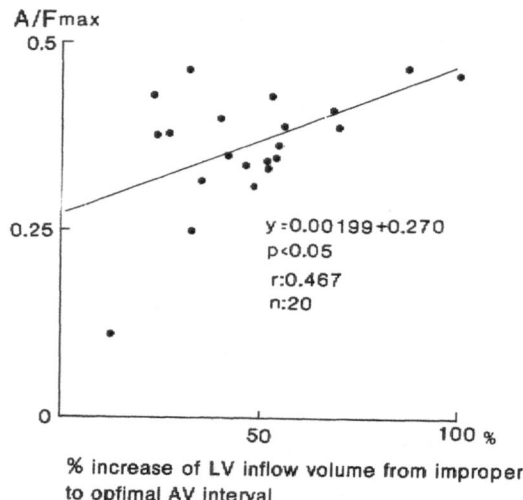

Figure 10.44. Relationship between the percentage increase of left ventricular inflow volume from improper to optimal AV interval and the ratio of atrial contribution to ventricular filling (A/F_{max}) in patients with DDD pacing.

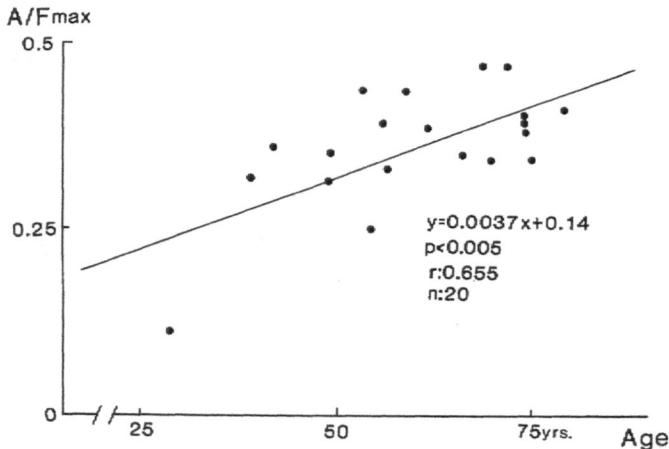

Figure 10.45. Relationship between aging and the ratio of atrial contribution to ventricular filling (A/F_{max}) in patients with DDD pacing.

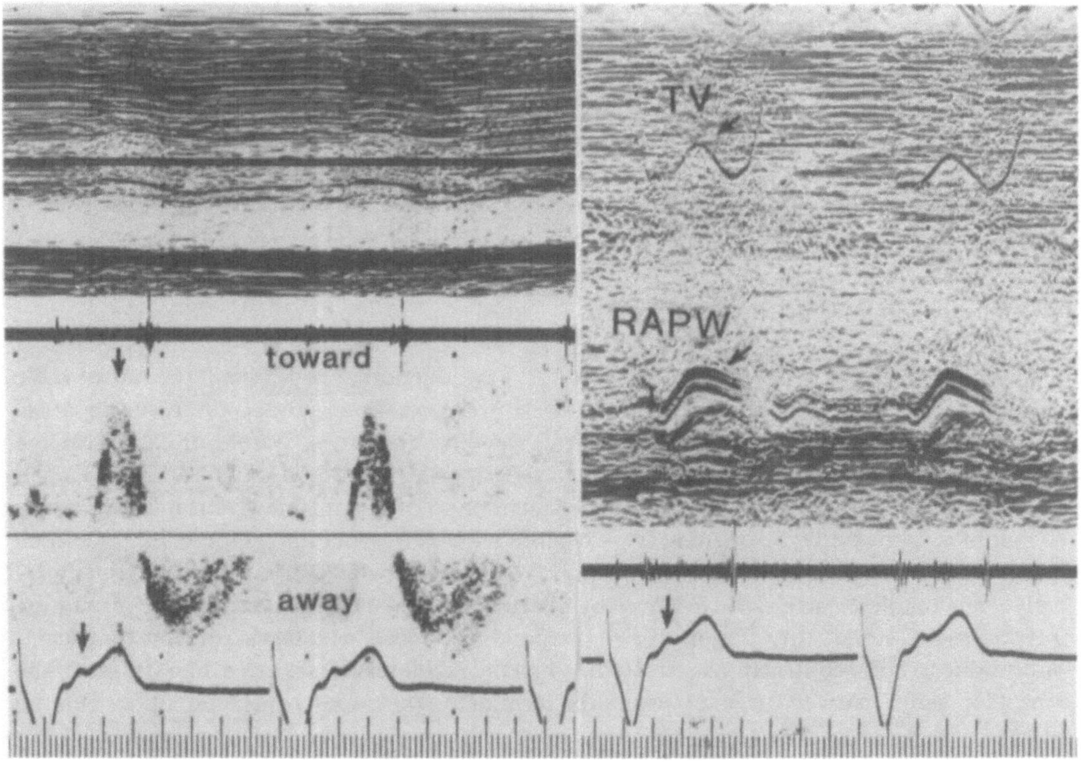

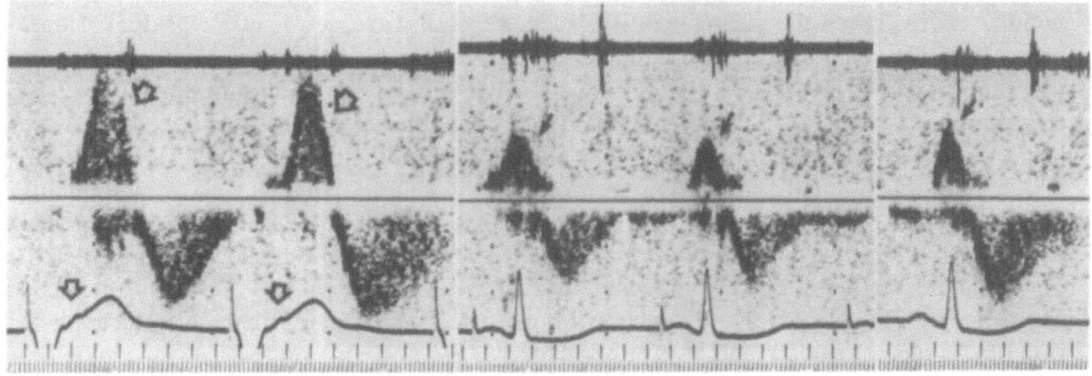

Figure 10.46. Pulsed Doppler and M-mode echocardiogram in a patient with VVI pacing and retrograde P waves. The retrograde flow from right atrium to hepatic vein is shown by arrow. In M-mode, systolic anterior displacement of tricuspid valve and right atrial posterior wall (RAPW) due to atrial contraction are also observed (arrow).

Figure 10.47. Pulsed Doppler echocardiogram of hepatic venous flow in a patient during VVI pacing with retrograde P wave, DDD pacing and sinus rhythm. The left-hand side illustrates the large retrograde venous flow due to a retrograde P wave (arrow). The middle and right-hand illustrations do not show this alteration due to the disappearance of the retrograde P wave.

induced VPCs, the relationship between coupling interval and hemodynamic changes is dynamic, and this arrythmia does not always introduce hemodynamic derangement in some patients (Figure 10.28).

During ventricular tachycardia, impairment of stroke volume is caused by interruption of diastolic filling (Figure 10.29), as also reflected by a reduction of left ventricular cavity size in the M-mode echocardiogram (Figure 10.30). These findings can be also observed in supraventricular tachycardia (Figure 10.31).

8. Abnormal atrio-ventricular conduction

In patients with prolonged atrio-ventricular (AV) conduction or A-V block, the mitral valve motion can be affected by the position of the P wave on the ECG and the resulting atrial contraction in the cardiac cycle. When the P wave occurs during systole, it can affect the motion of the tricuspid valve but the mitral valve motion is not altered (Figure 10.32). When P waves occur in early to mid diastole, the closing motion of the mitral valve is initiated and is sometimes followed by re-opening, resulting in 'shoulder formation' (Figure 10.33). When atrial contraction is not followed by a properly timed ventricular systole, closure of the mitral valve is incomplete and may be followed by a certain degree of presystolic mitral regurgitation (atriogenic diastolic reflux, Figure 10.34). Depending on the P-R interval, the left ventricular inflow due to atrial contraction is affected. When the P-R interval is shorter than 100 msec, the onset of ventricular contraction promptly terminates the atrial contraction flow (Figure 10.35).

9. Cardiac pacing

In ventricular demand (VVI) pacing, the contraction of ventricle and atrium is independent. Therefore, the atrial contribution to ventricular filling is different from beat to beat and stroke volume varies. When the pacing beat is preceded by a P wave, left ventricular dimensional enlargement and prolonged ejection time is sometimes demonstrated in the M-mode echocardiogram (Figure 10.36). These findings indicate increased left ventricular filling due to atrial contribution. Using pulsed Doppler echocardiography, the same hemodynamic changes are more directly evidenced (Figure 10.37). The dual-chamber, fully automatic (DDD) pacemaker permits automatic adaptation according to the sinus rhythm as well as maintaining atrioventricular (AV) synchrony. This temporal relationship between atrial and ventricular contraction is also an important determinant of ventricular performance, since this interval may influence both ventricular filling and atrioventricular valve closure. However, the need for invasive methods to evaluate LA contribution to left ventricular filling limits the application of this type of assessment. The pulsed Doppler method can noninvasively evaluate the LA contribution, independent of left ventricular filling, to assess beat-to-beat changes in stroke volume. In patients with a larger LA contribution to left ventricular filling, a greater increase in left ventricular filling volume was obtained by converting the pacing mode from VVI to AV sequential pacing, at the optimal AV interval (Figures 10.38, 39). Patients with a relatively small atrial contribution to ventricular filling show no definitive changes in stroke volume with variable pacing conditions (Figure 10.40, 41, 42). With shorter AV intervals the onset of ventricular contraction prematurely terminates atrial contraction, and with longer AV intervals atrial relaxation decelerates left ventricular inflow and sometimes produces a retrograde flow. The increment of left ventricular inflow volume from the least adequate to the optimal AV interval and VVI to DDD correlates positively with the degree of LA contribution to left ventricular filling (Figures 10.43, 44). Augmentation of LA contribution to left ventricular filling with aging has been reported recently and a similar result is also obtained in patients with DDD pacemakers (Figure 10.45). Physiological cardiac pacing should have, in general, more beneficial effects on elderly than younger patients, due to the decreased left ventricular compliance with aging. The optimal AV interval and its importance varies from patient to patient, therefore Doppler measurement of left ventricular inflow velocity would be useful in determining which patients might derive the greatest benefits from DDD pacing and also to determine the optimal AV interval. In patients with VVI pacing, sometimes a retrograde P wave can occur, generating a retrograde flow from the atrium to the venous system in this phase (Figure 10.46). However, if the VVI pacemaker is replaced by DDD, the retrograde P waves and the venous retrograde flow usually disappear (Figure 10.47).

CHAPTER 11

Color coded Doppler flow mapping

Color coded Doppler flow mapping (color flow mapping or color Doppler) is a newly developed technology which displays blood flow as color-coded information on the two-dimensional image. This method is an application of the pulsed Doppler method. The conventional FFT analysis takes too much time to analyze the blood flow information for color flow mapping. Moving target indication and autocorrelation methods are employed to process the spatial flow information in real time. In these methods, the pulses are transmitted several times in the same direction along a certain scan line for data processing. When the echo comes from a stationary target, the delay time from the transmission and reference signals is constant each time, while it varies when the target moves (Figure 11.1). The number of transmitted pulses in the same direction is called the 'packet size', which must contain at least three pulses for velocity evaluation. After obtaining data for one color scan line, the beam is steered to the next color scan line. To improve the color quality (velocity verification), it is necessary to enhance the autocorrelation by increasing the packet size. The packet size also affects the color frame rate: the larger the packet size, the lower the frame rate. The color frame rate is also affected by the number of the color scan lines related to the color angle of the sector: the wider the color angle, the lower the frame rate. A low frame rate can sometimes lose real time information about blood flow, especially in patients with higher heart rates. Therefore, the small packet size and narrower angle color presentation is required in such cases.

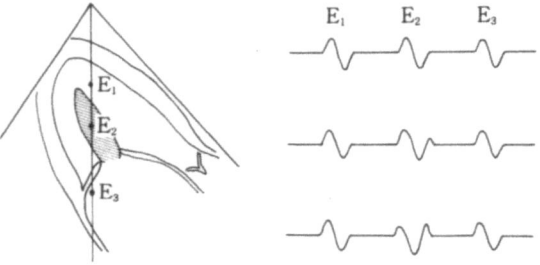

Figure 11.1. The concept of the moving target indicator in the measurement of the velocity. When the ultrasonic pulses are transmitted several times in same direction, the phase of the receiving signal from the stationary object (E_1) is always same as the previous echo. However, the phase of the received echo is shifted relative to that of the previous echo when the target is moving. (E_2). The magnitude of the phase shift is related to the velocity of the target.

Color coded flow mapping presents the flow direction, the mean velocity and the variance of the velocity. Blood flow toward the transducer was expressed as a reddish-orange shade and away from the transducer was a bluish hue, with the two-dimensional echocardiographic image gray scale. The mean velocity is demonstrated as the intensity change or the hue change, which is divided into 8 or more degrees. The first degree near the zero line in each direction is used as a wall filter and is not colored. The variance of the velocity is demonstrated by mixing 'green' with the original color according to the mean velocity (Figure 11.3). The packet size must be more than four pulses to obtain information about the variance. When the degree of variance is large such as in a stenotic, regurgitant or shunt flow, a characteristic yellow/cyan mosaic pattern appears in the appropriate area. In addition, color flow mapping can provide spatial information, such as the angle of incidence of the blood flow as it courses through the valves, alleviating one of the limitations of conventional pulsed or continuous Doppler echocardiography (see Figures 11.8, 14 and 23). The color flow gain should be adjusted to show maximal diameter or area throughout the cardiac cycle, without the appearance of a spontaneous color signal (noise).

When the blood flow velocity is faster than the maximum measurable velocity (Fd_{max}), aliasing occurs, which shows as the opposite color, similar to that of the pulsed Doppler. For example, color flow images of mitral stenosis are always accompanied by aliasing in the center of stenotic flow. The ultrasonic pulse is transmitted after receiving the echo from the maximum depth, according to the depth setting, of the previous pulse transmission. Thus, the depth setting limits the pulse repetition frequency. The transducer frequency also affects the occurrence of aliasing. In cases of stenotic, regurgitant or shunt flow, multiple aliasing frequently occurs and is sometimes accompanied by mosaic patterns, which can introduce some difficulty in the identification of the true characteristics of flow. The color-coded flow data are also displayed on the M-mode echocardiogram, which can provide the time sequence of color flow. Qualitatively, color flow mapping provides a rapid orientation to the presence and location of the flow in the cardiac structures and great vessels, which might be missed with conventional Doppler echocardiography. Because color Doppler method has relatively poor resolution with time, additional pulsed and/or CW Doppler examinations should be necessary to recognize the actual characteristics of flow.

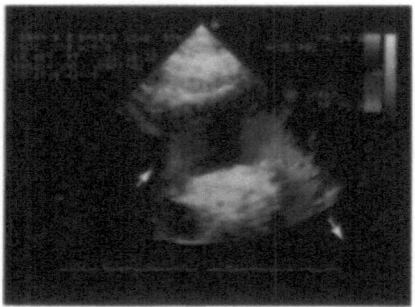

Figure 11.2.   Color flow mapping of aortic arch flow obtained from the suprasternal notch window. Ascending aortic flow is displayed as a red color (toward the transducer) and descending aortic flow is illustrated as a blue color (away from the transducer). In the center of the aortic arch, the flow is not colored as a result of the perpendicular Doppler angle to the blood flow.

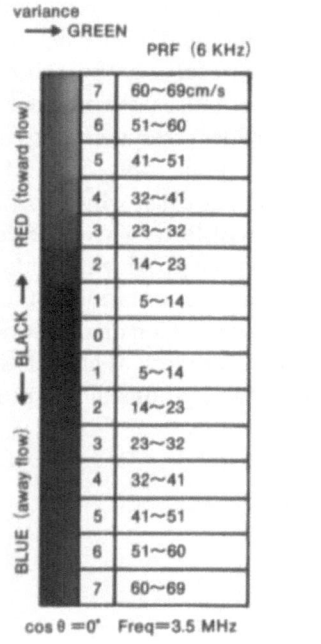

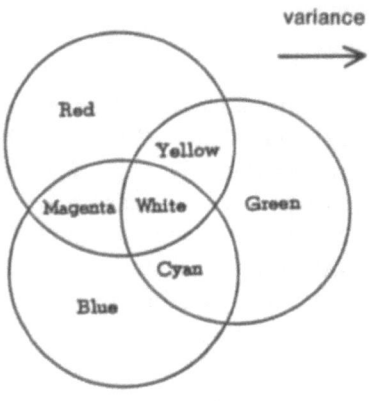

Figure 11.3.   The color-coded display of mean velocity, direction and variance. The blood flow directions are indicated in red as the flow toward the transducer, and in blue as flow away from the transducer. The mean velocity is demonstrated as the intensity change or the hue change, which is divided into 8 degrees in this equipment (Aloka SSD-880). One degree near the zero line in each direction is used as a wall filter and is not colored. The variance of the velocity is demonstrated by mixing 'green' with the original color according to the mean velocity.

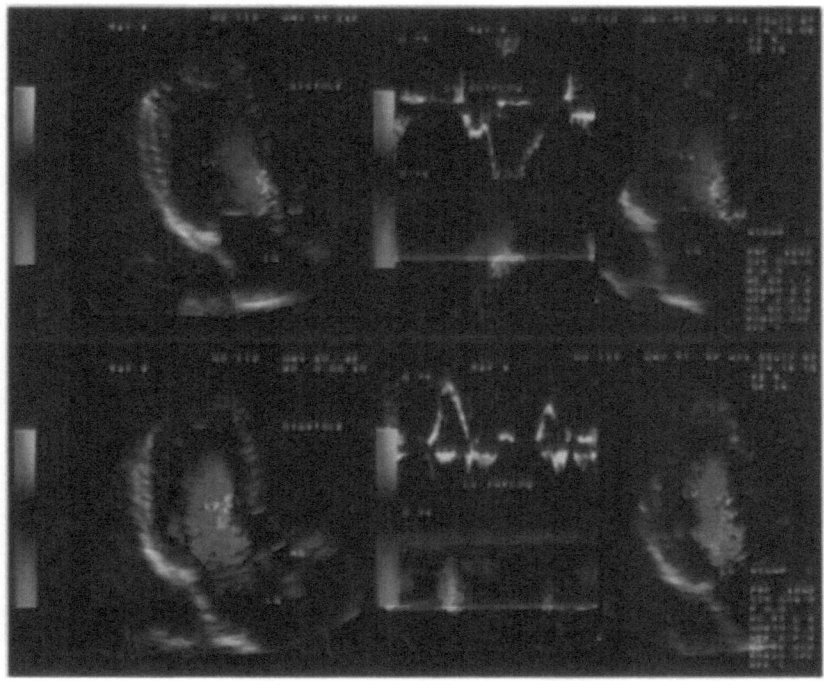

Figure 11.4.   Color flow mapping of left ventricular outflow and inflow using the apical long axis view in a 54 year-old healthy male. The left ventricular ejection flow is encoded in blue (away from the transducer) with aliasing in the center showing as red during systole in upper left panel. The color M-mode and pulsed Doppler echocardiogram of left ventricular outflow is also shown at the upper right. The lower left shows the left ventricular inflow as red (toward the transducer) during diastole. In the center of the inflow, aliasing is illustrated in blue. The color M-mode and pulsed Doppler echocardiogram of left ventricular inflow is also shown at the lower right.

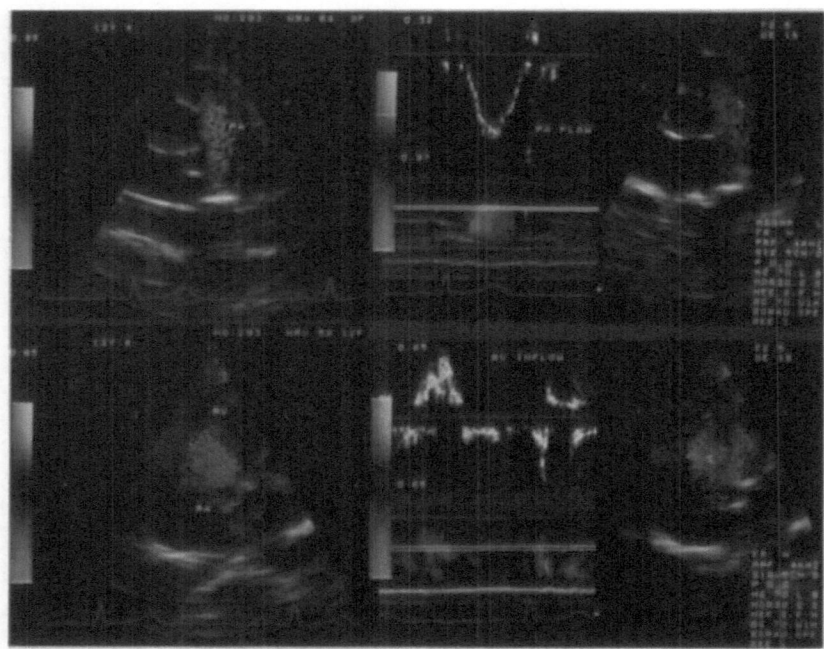

Figure 11.5. Color flow mapping of right ventricular outflow and inflow using the parasternal short axis view and parasternal right ventricular inflow view in a 13 year-old healthy boy. The upper left demonstrates the right ventricular ejection flow as blue during systole with aliasing in the center as a red color. The color M-mode and pulsed Doppler echocardiogram also demonstrate the right ventricular ejection flow away from the transducer at the upper right. The right ventricular inflow is encoded in red during diastole at the lower left. The color M-mode and pulsed Doppler echocardiogram also demonstrate the right ventricular inflow toward the transducer at the lower right.

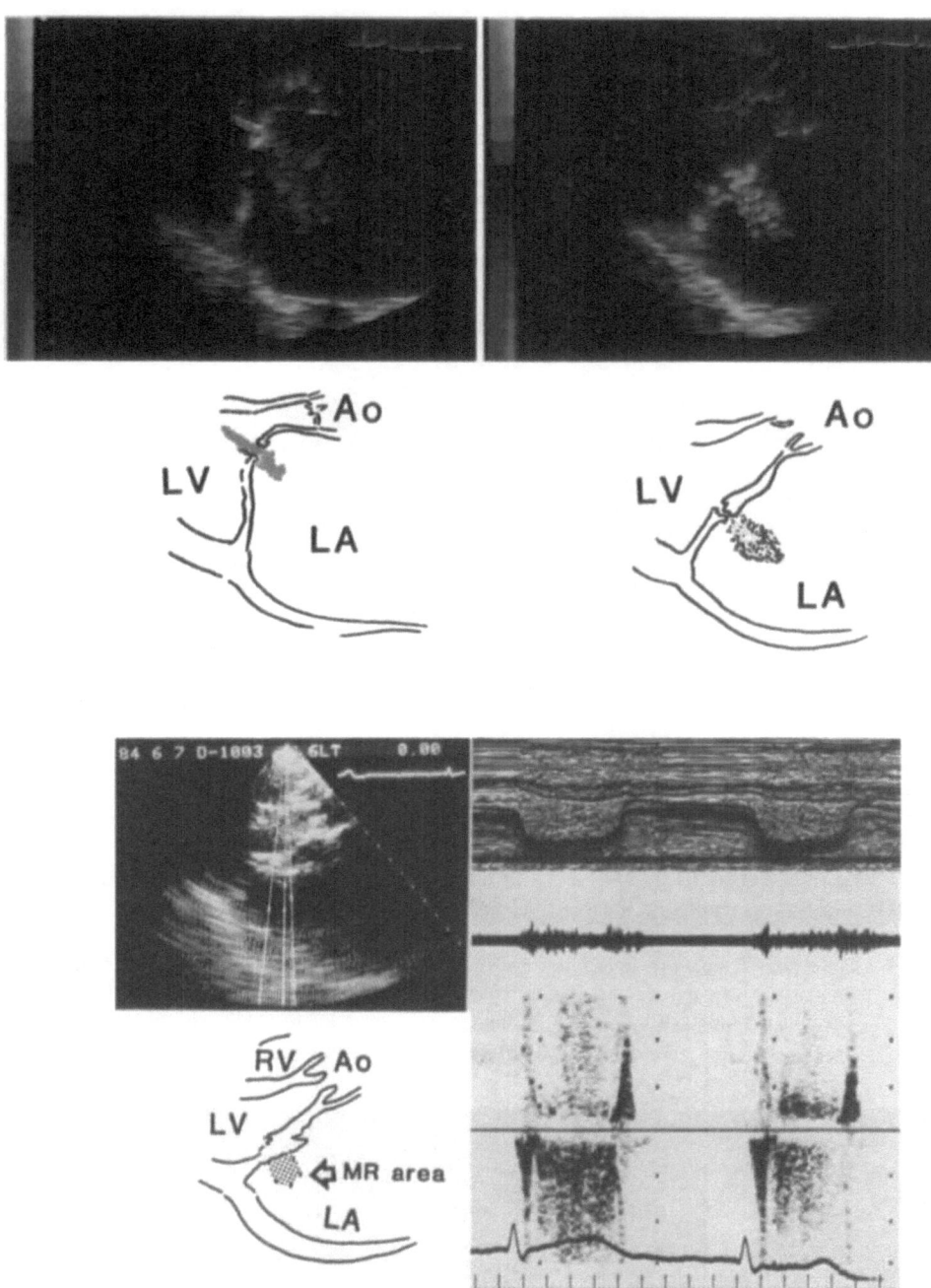

Figure 11.6. Color flow mapping of the transmitral flow using the parasternal long axis view in a patient with mitral stenosis and regurgitation. The upper left panel shows the left ventricular inflow through the stenotic mitral valve in red during diastole. The upper right demonstrates the regurgitant flow through the mitral valve as a mosaic pattern due to turbulence or spectral broadening. The lower panel shows a flow mapped area of mitral regurgitation obtained in the pulsed Doppler mode. This area is very similar to that obtained by color flow mapping.

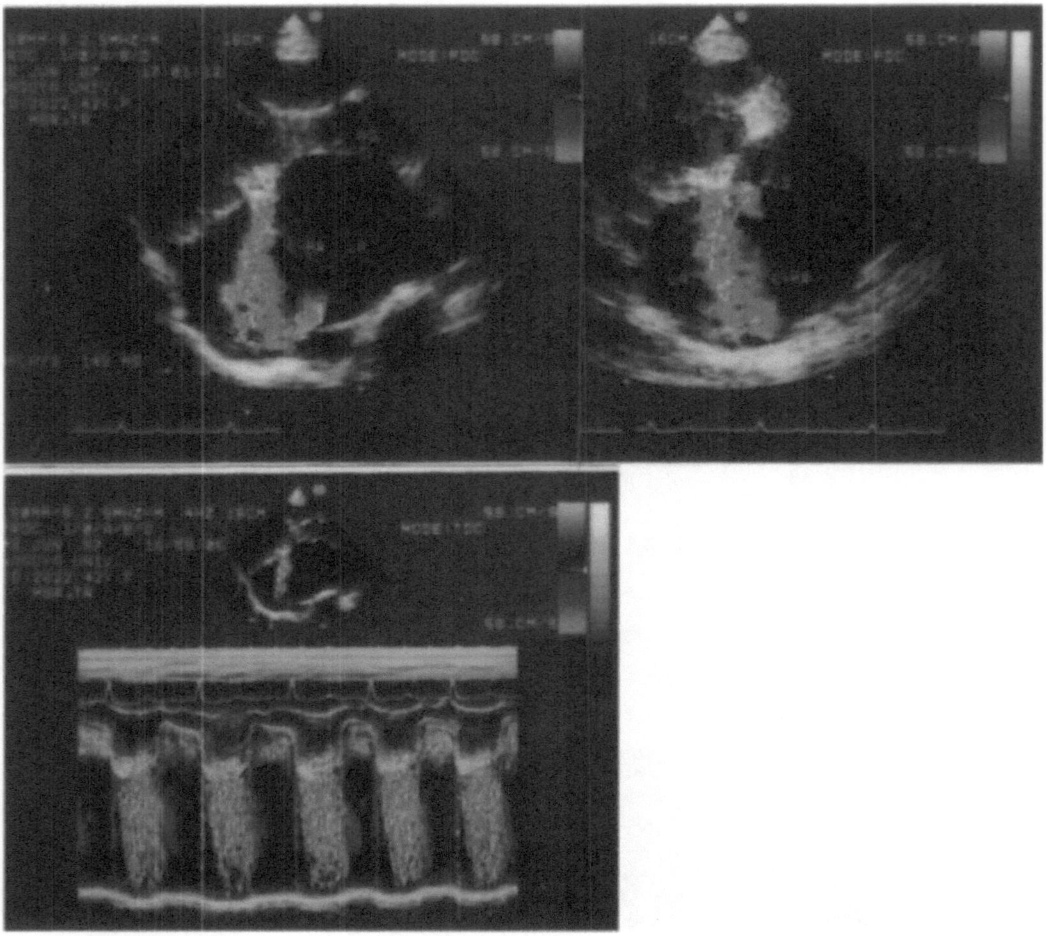

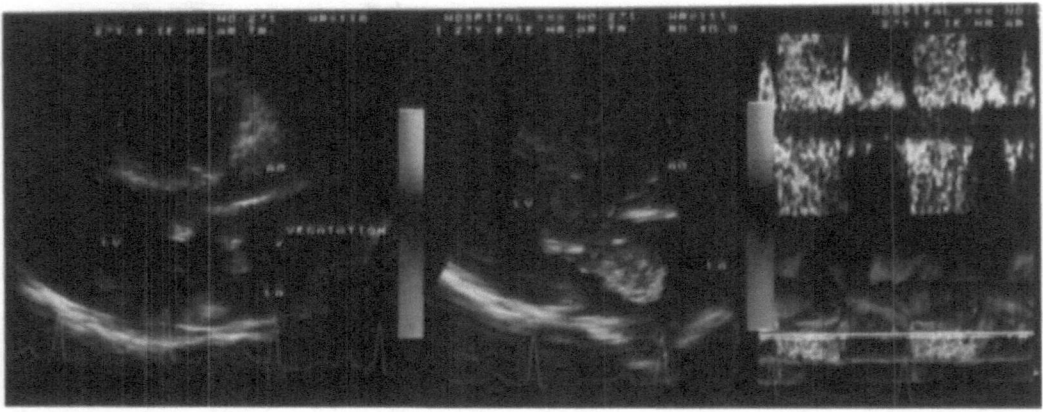

Figure 11.7. Color flow mapping of transmitral flow using the parasternal long and short axis view and color M-mode in a patient with severe mitral regurgitation. The upper panel demonstrates the transmitral regurgitant flow as mosaic pattern into the enlarged left atrium during systole. The color M-mode echocardiogram also clearly demonstrate this turbulent flow during systole.

Figure 11.8. Color flow mapping of the parasternal long axis view of a patient with vegetations on the mitral valve and mitral regurgitation. The transmitral regurgitant flow is encoded in a mosaic pattern in the left atrium during systole. Its relationship with the cardiac cycle is well illustrated in the color M-mode tracing below the mitral valve.

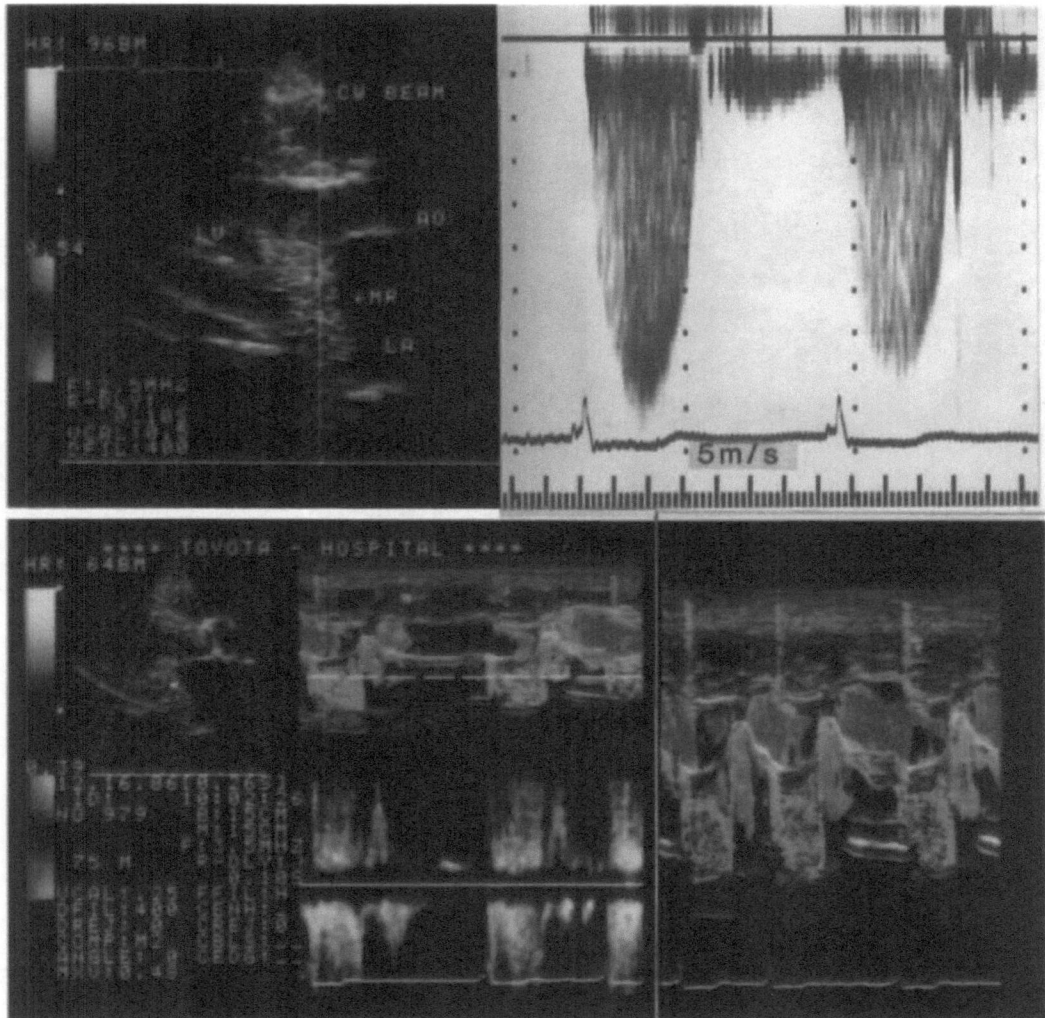

Figure 11.9. Color flow mapping and CW Doppler echocardiograms obtained from the parasternal long axis view in a patient with mitral regurgitation. The upper left panel shows the transmitral regurgitant flow as a mosaic pattern directed to the left atrial posterior wall. The peak velocity is measured using the CW Doppler in the upper right. The color M-mode and pulsed Doppler echocardiogram also clearly demonstrate this turbulent flow.

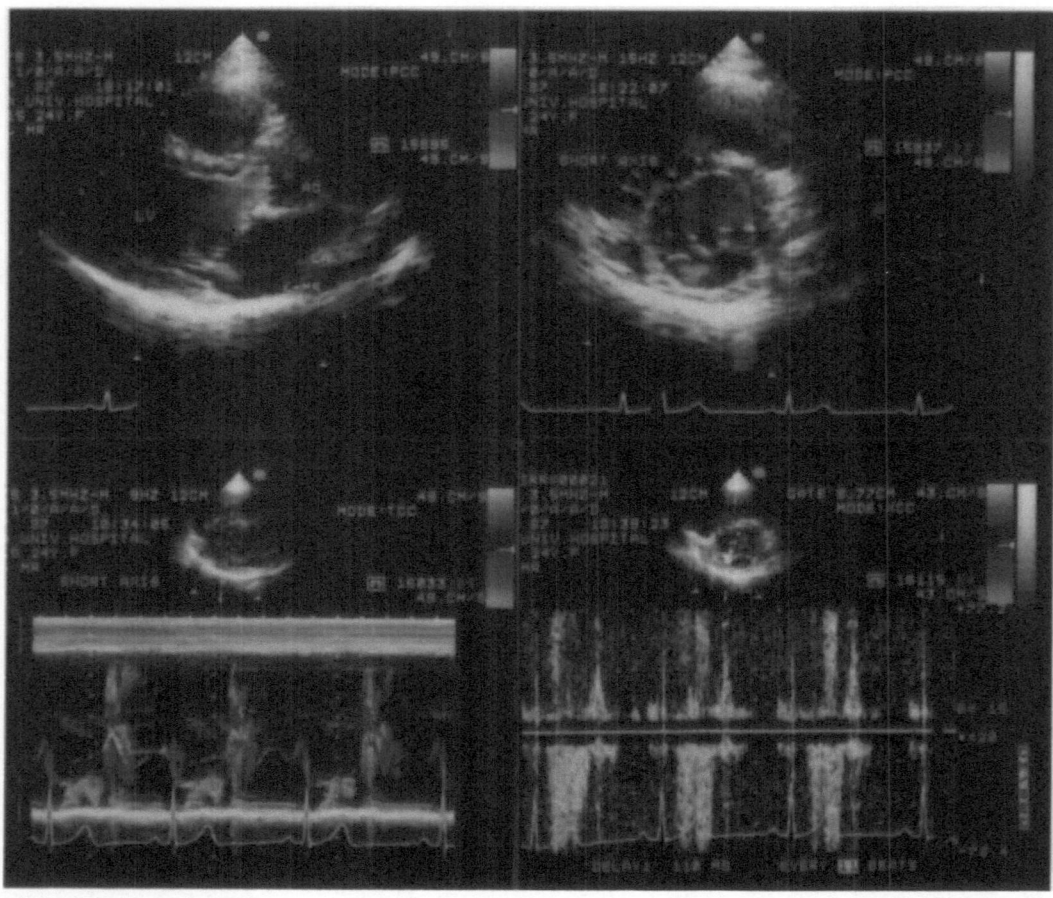

Figure 11.10. Color flow mapping of the parasternal long axis view in a patient with an anterior mitral valve prolapse and mitral regurgitation. The small regurgitant flow directed to left atrial posterior wall is shown in blue during late-systolic phase. The color M-mode and pulsed Doppler echocardiograms clearly demonstrate the time course of the regurgitant signal.

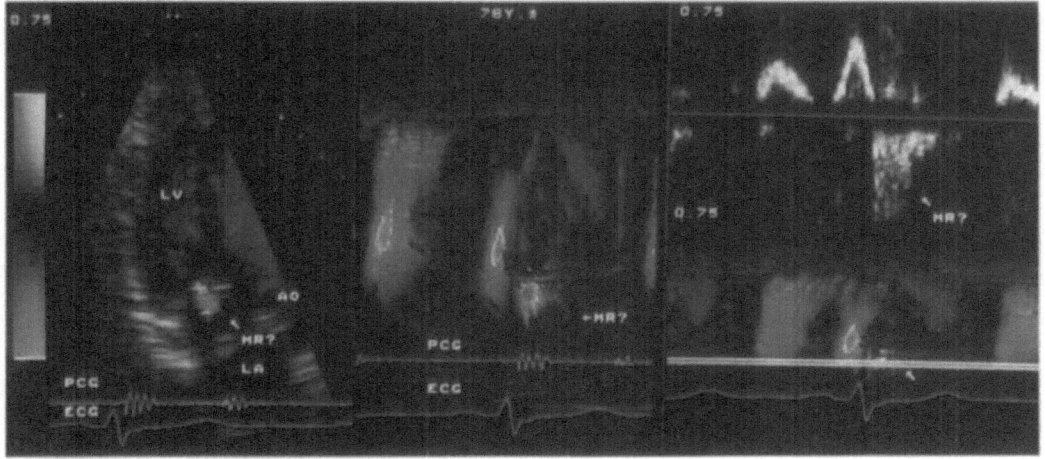

Figure 11.11.   Color flow mapping of the apical long axis view of mitral regurgitant flow pattern of a normal subject. The small mitral regurgitant signal is shown as a blue mosaic pattern. The color M-mode and pulsed Doppler echocardiograms demonstrate this regurgitant signal presented only at early diastole, where the flow pattern is clearly different from that of a well-established pathological regurgitation.

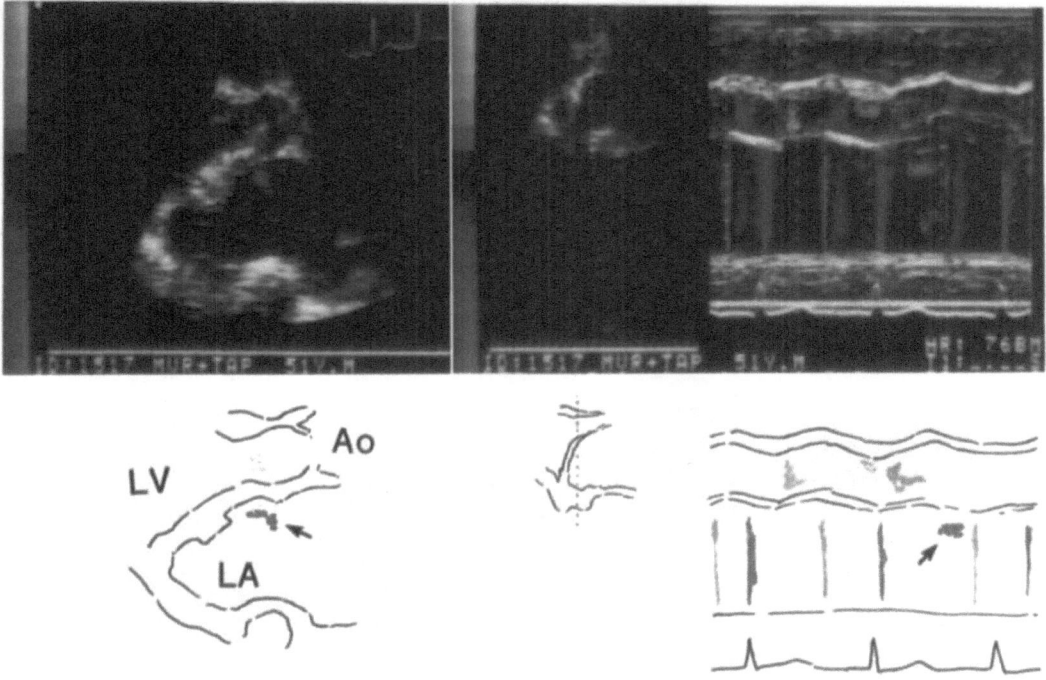

Figure 11.12.   Color flow mapping of the parasternal long axis view in a patient with prosthetic mitral valve and paravalvular leak. A small paravalvular leak is clearly evidenced as a blue color in the upper side of the left atrium (arrow).

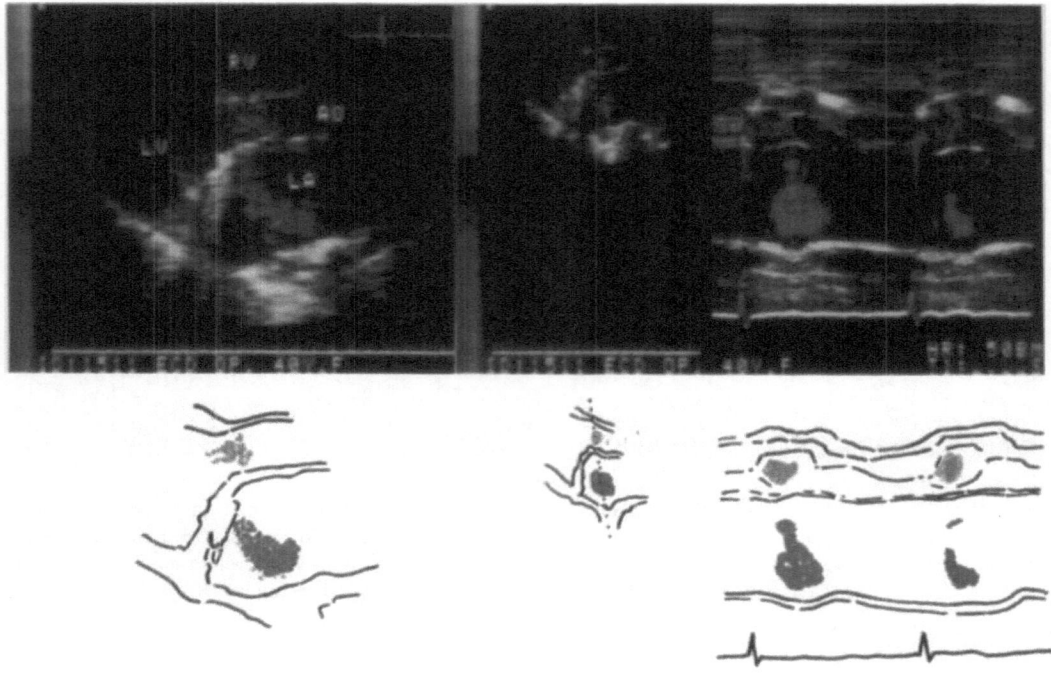

Figure 11.13. Color flow mapping of the parasternal long axis view in a patient with a prosthetic mitral valve and transvalvular regurgitation. A transprosthetic valvular regurgitation is illustrated as a blue color in the center part of the left atrium.

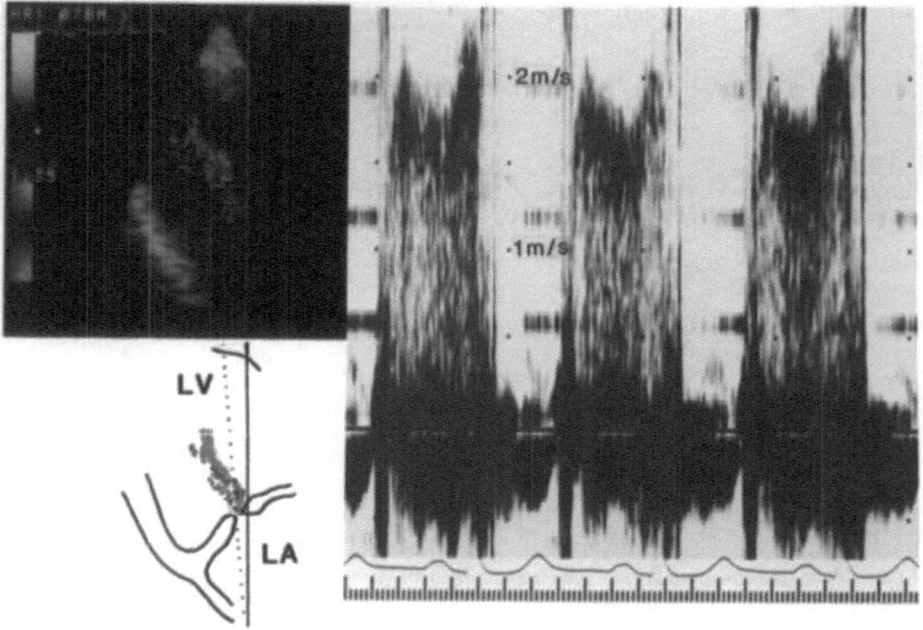

Figure 11.14. Color flow mapping and CW Doppler obtained from the apical long axis view in a patient with mitral stenosis. The left ventricular inflow through the stenotic valve is demonstrated as a mosaic pattern in the left ventricle. Its peak velocity using CW Doppler echocardiography is demonstrated on the right.

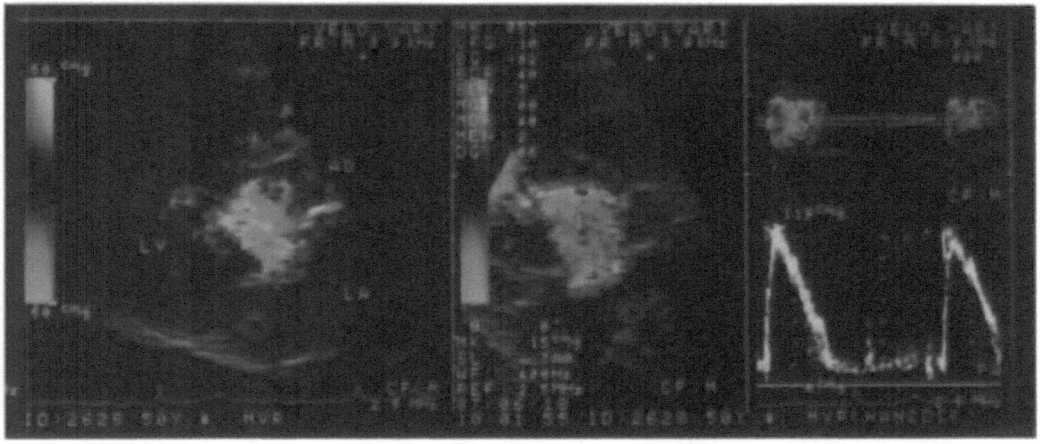

Figure 11.15. Color flow mapping of the parasternal long axis view in a patient with prosthetic mitral valve and normal function. The transprosthetic left ventricular inflow directed to the IVS is shown. Its peak velocity is increased resulting in aliasing (a blue color).

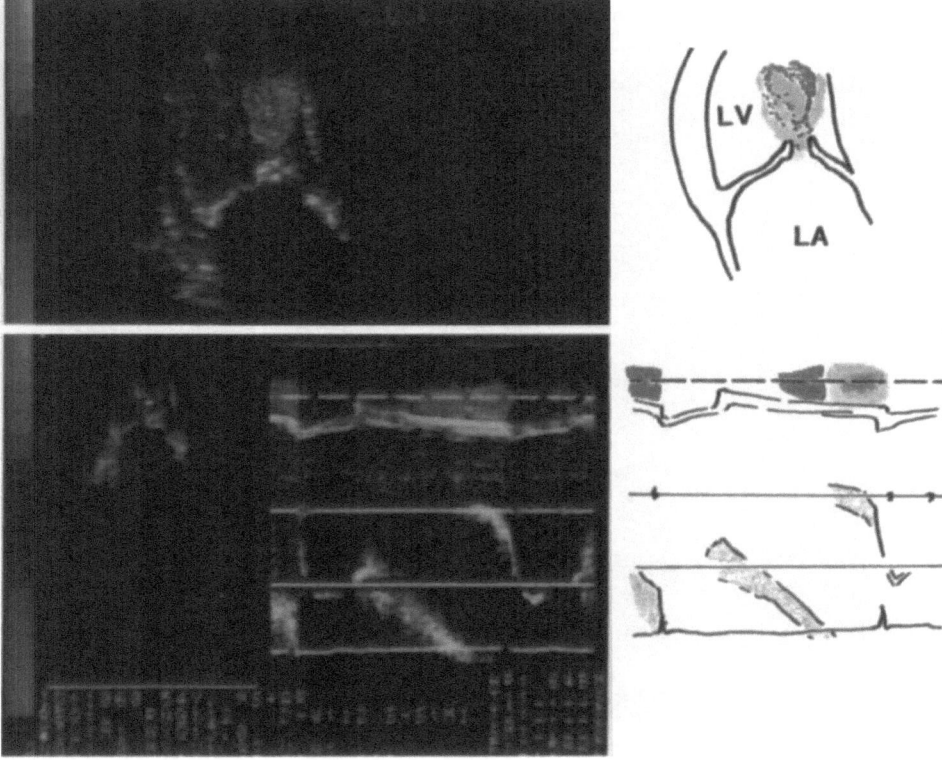

Figure 11.16. Color flow mapping obtained from the apical long axis view in a patient with mitral stenosis. The upper part shows turbulent flow in the left ventricle during diastole. The color M-mode tracing cannot demonstrate the early diastolic highest flow due to aliasing. Pulsed Doppler shows early diastolic left ventricular inflow near the baseline with aliasing. This may be an example of the relatively poor resolution of velocity in the color Doppler system.

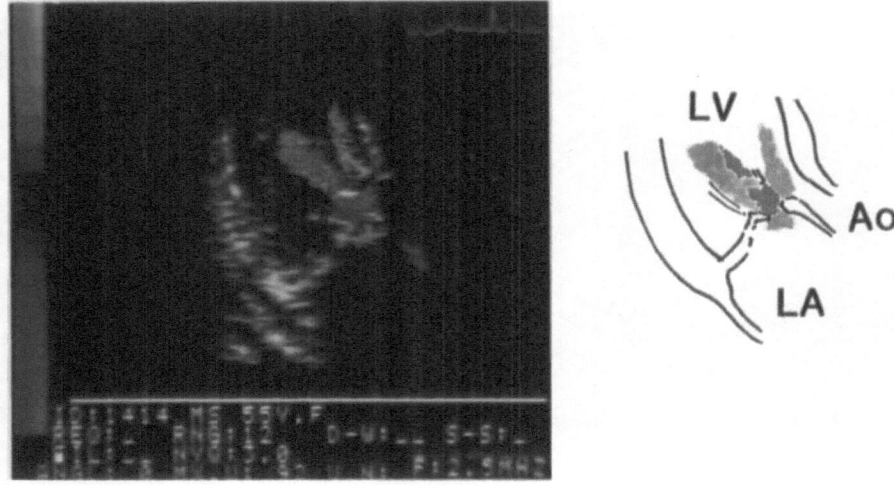

Figure 11.17.   Color flow mapping obtained from the apical long axis view in a patient with mitral stenosis and two distinct transmitral flows. The turbulent transmitral flow during diastole shows two different directions due to severe valvular and subvalvular deformities. Therefore, the evaluation of transmitral pressure gradient by continuous mode has some limitations in this case.

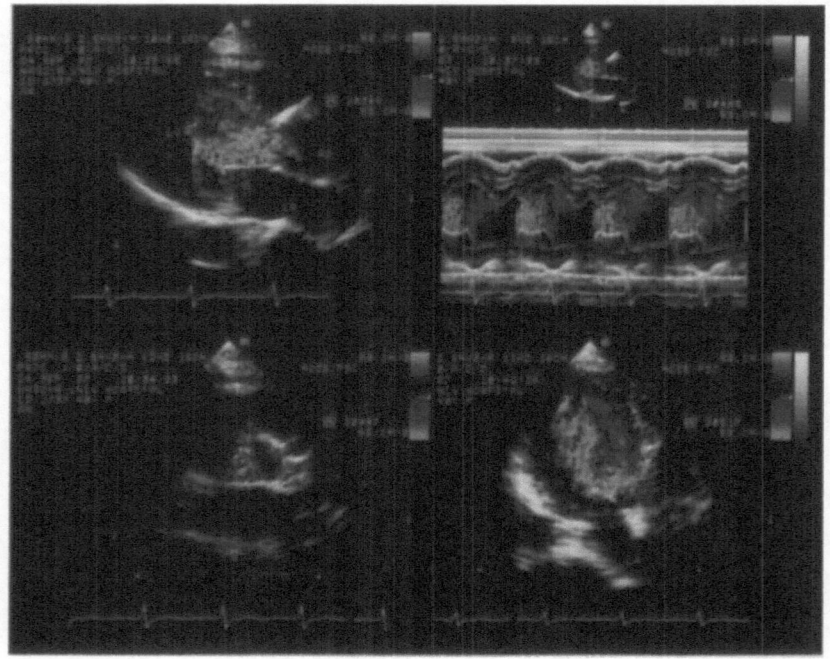

Figure 11.18.   Color flow mapping obtained from the parasternal long and short axis view, color M-mode and apical long axis view in a patient with severe aortic regurgitation. The turbulent regurgitant aortic flow is evidenced as a mosaic pattern in the left ventricular outflow tract during diastole. The color M-mode tracing clearly evidences aortic regurgitant signal in the left ventricular outflow tract during diastole.

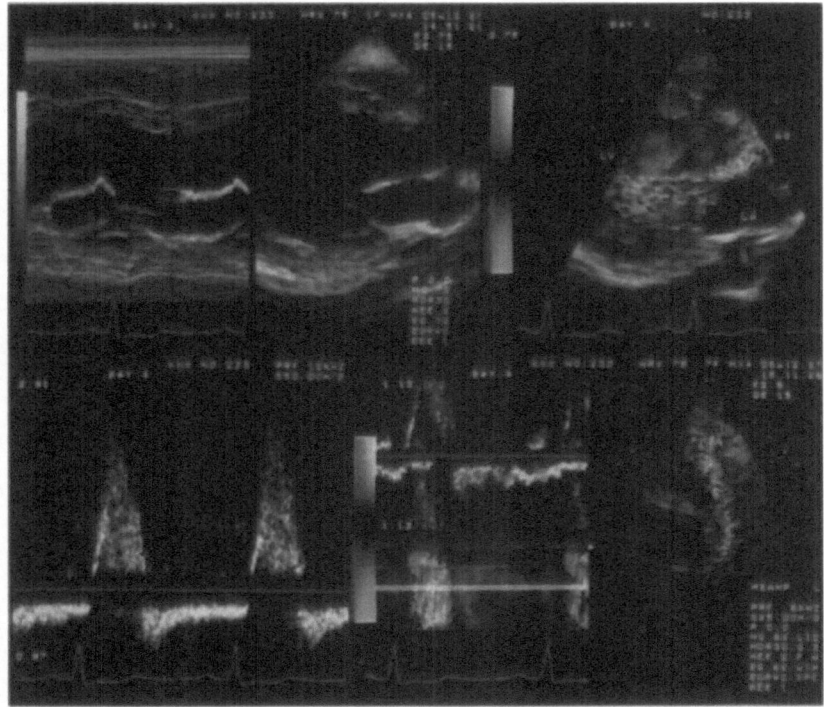

Figure 11.19. Color flow mapping of the parasternal long axis view and suprasternal approach in a patient with aortic stenosis and regurgitation. In this patient aortic regurgitant flow can be seen as mosaic pattern in the left ventricular outflow tract, above the mitral valve during diastole. It is quite easy to understand this regurgitant flow causing the mitral valve to flutter (upper panel). From the suprasternal approach (lower right panel) stenotic aortic flow is demonstrated as a mosaic pattern in the ascending aorta. Using continuous wave Doppler, the peak velocity of this stenotic flow can be measured in the lower left panel. Aortic reverse flow is also observed due to aortic regurgitation.

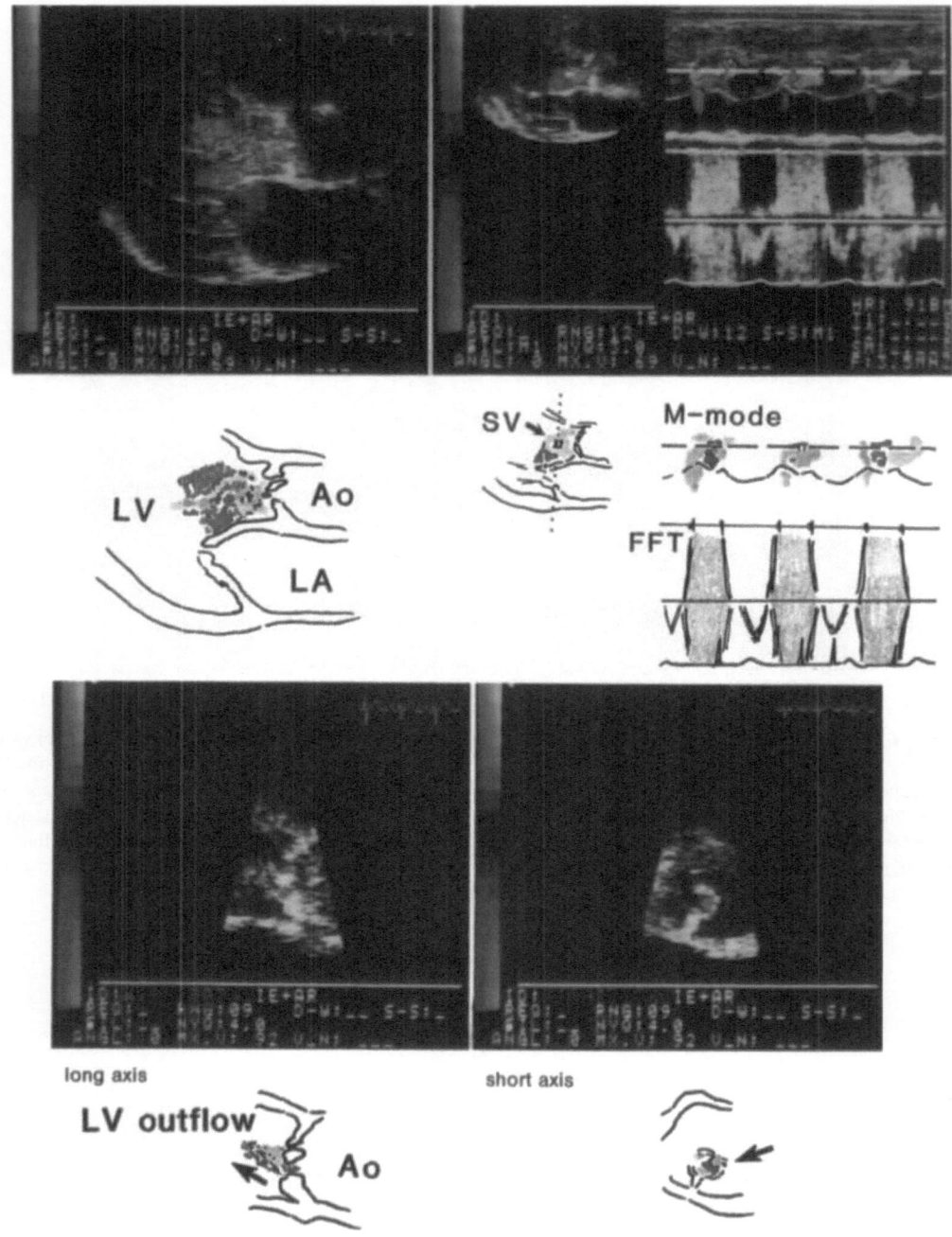

Figure 11.20.   Color flow mapping obtained from the parasternal long and short axis views in a patient with infective endocarditis and aortic regurgitation due to aortic valve perforation. The upper panel demonstrates the severe aortic regurgitation as a mosaic pattern during diastole. The lower part demonstrates the aortic regurgitant flow through the perforated area as a mosaic pattern using higher PRF (6 kHz to 8 kHz) and a faster frame rate (15 to 30 frames/sec).

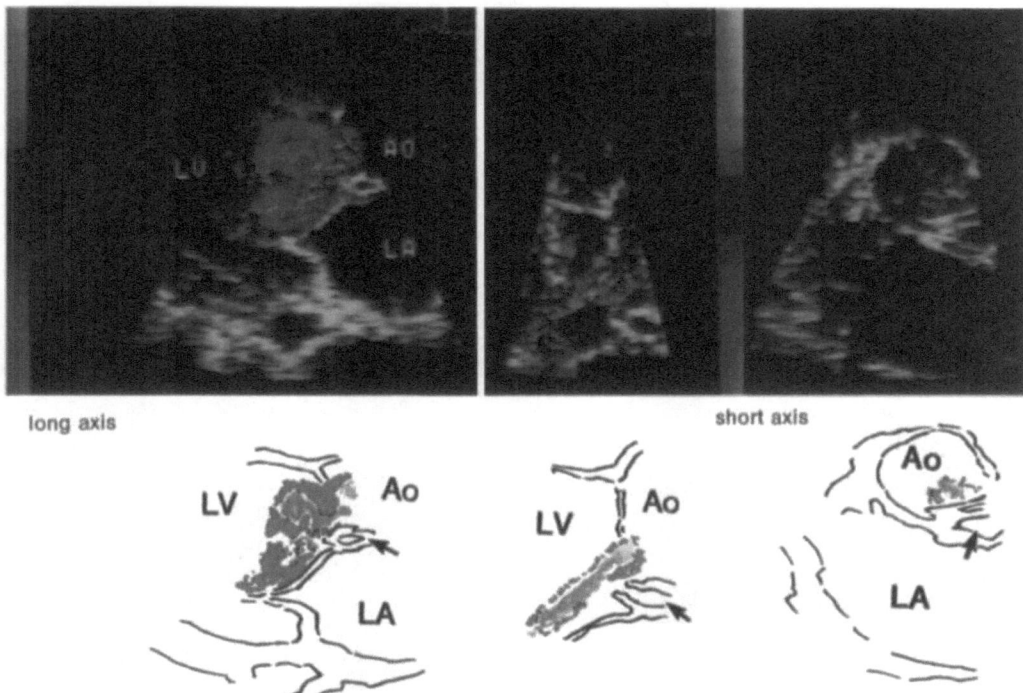

long axis   short axis

Figure 11.21.   Color flow mapping of the parasternal long and short axis views in a patient with infective endocarditis and aortic annular abscess. The left part shows the aortic regurgitant signal as a mosaic pattern in diastole. Premature closure of the mitral valve is also present due to severe aortic regurgitation. The right-hand side demonstrates the location of regurgitant flow (long and short axis view), but does not evidence this flow into the abscess (arrow).

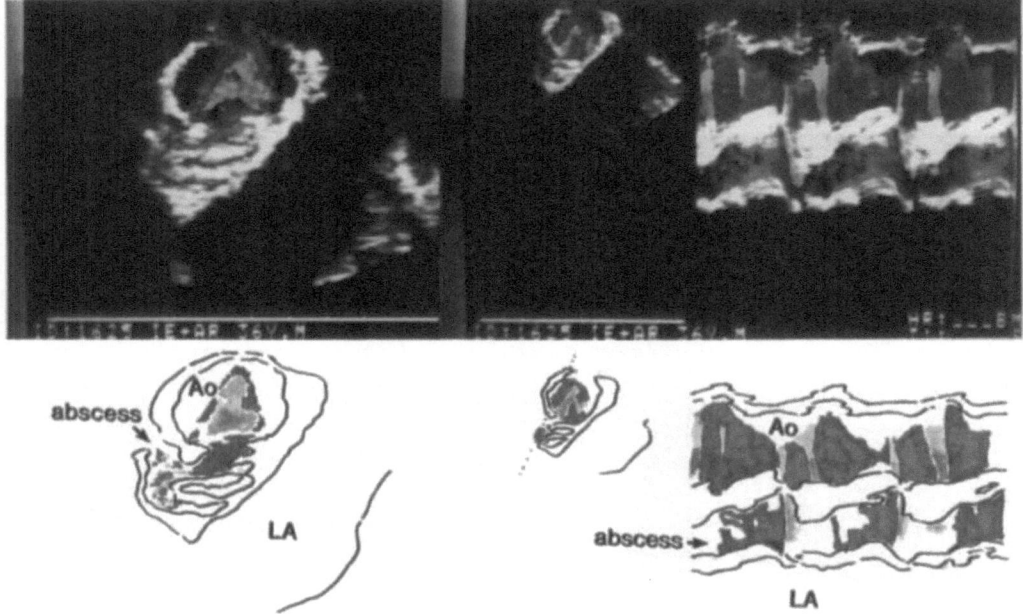

Figure 11.22.   Transoperatory color flow mapping of the parasternal short axis view and M-mode in the same patient with infective endocarditis and aortic annular abscess. Compared with the precordial recording (Figure 11.21), the flow into the abscess formation (arrow) can be detected because of the better acoustic window contacting the transducer directly with heart.

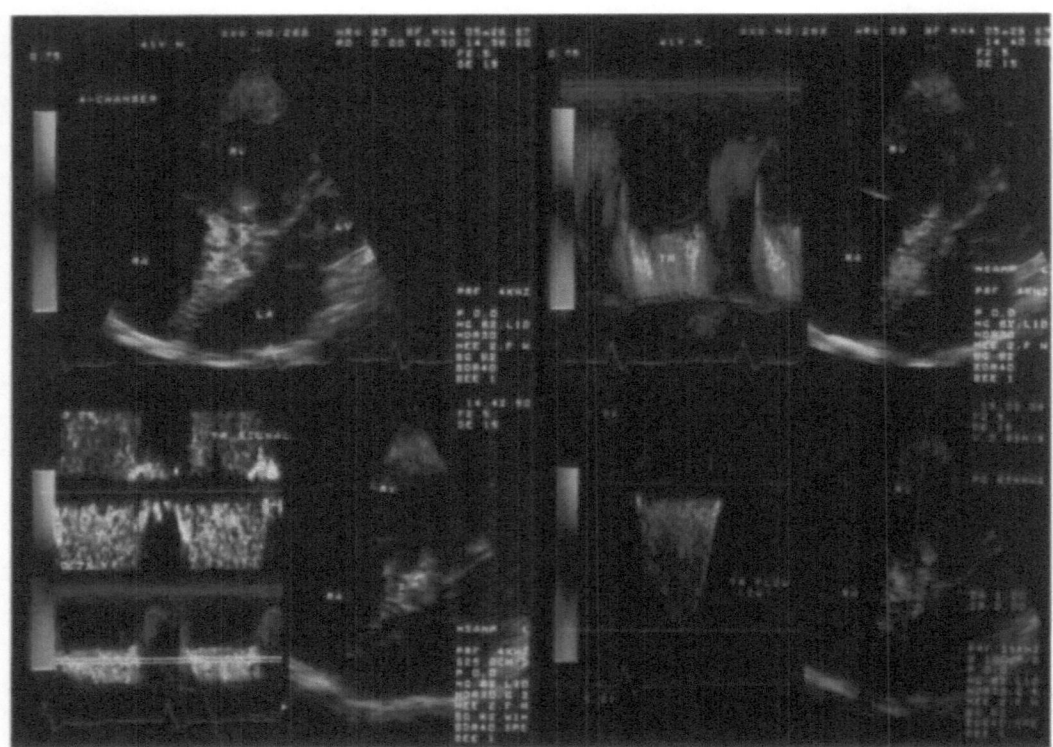

Figure 11.23. CW Doppler and color flow mapping evaluation of tricuspid regurgitation. The tricuspid regurgitant flow is shown as a bluish mosaic pattern in two-dimensional right ventricular inflow view (upper left). The color M-mode recording demonstrates the tricuspid regurgitant flow as a bluish mosaic pattern below the tricuspid valve (upper right). Pulsed Doppler shows a turbulent flow with multiple aliasing during systole, in which it is impossible to identify the peak velocity (lower left). CW Doppler indicates a high peak velocity (V) of 3.84 m/sec. The pressure gradient (PG) of 63 mm Hg is also calculated using the simplified Bernoulli equation (lower right).

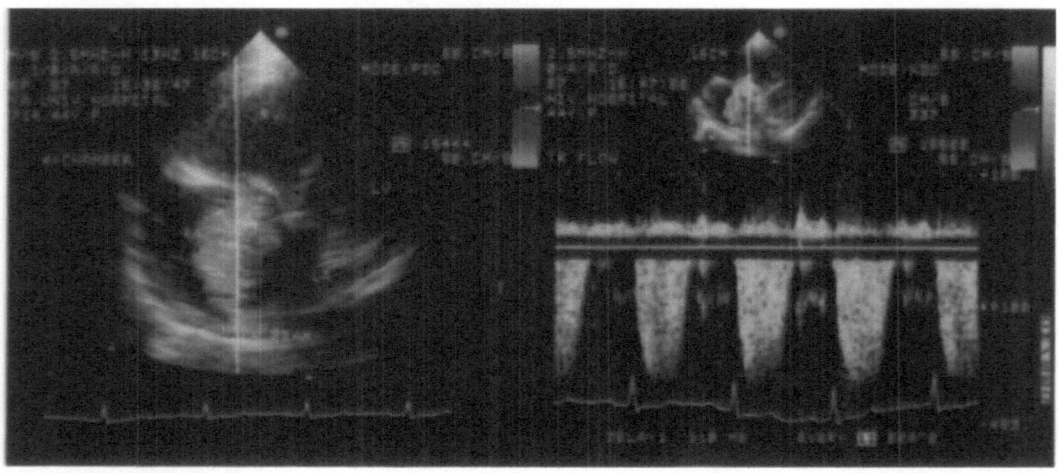

Figure 11.24. CW Doppler and color flow mapping evaluation of tricuspid regurgitation. The tricuspid regurgitant flow is shown as a bluish mosaic pattern in two-dimensional right ventricular inflow view (left). CW Doppler beam is also indicated as a bold white line in the color flow mapping. CW Doppler indicates an increased peak velocity of 337 cm/sec.

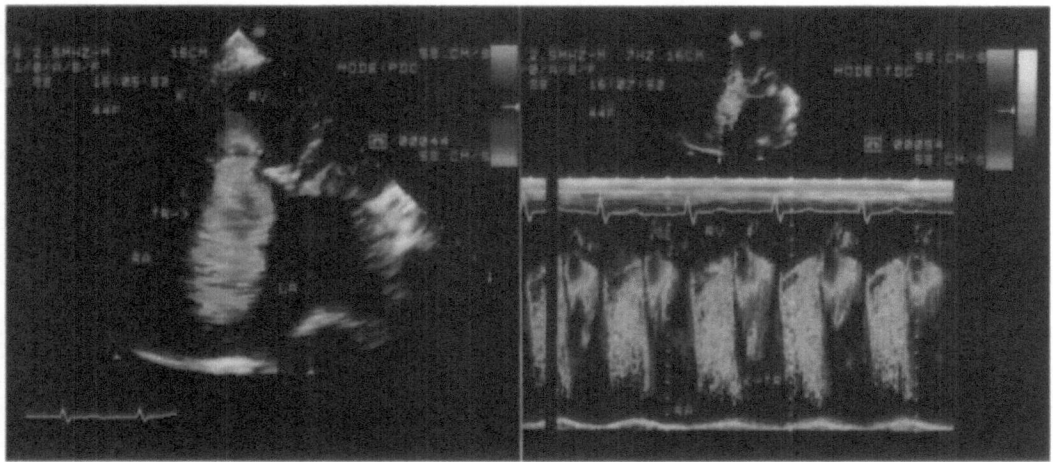

Figure 11.25. Color flow mapping of the parasternal right ventricular inflow view of a patient with severe tricuspid regurgitation. The tricuspid regurgitant flow is shown as a mosaic pattern directed toward the interatrial septum occupying a significant portion of right atrium. The color M-mode recording demonstrates the tricuspid regurgitant flow as a mosaic pattern below the tricuspid valve during systole.

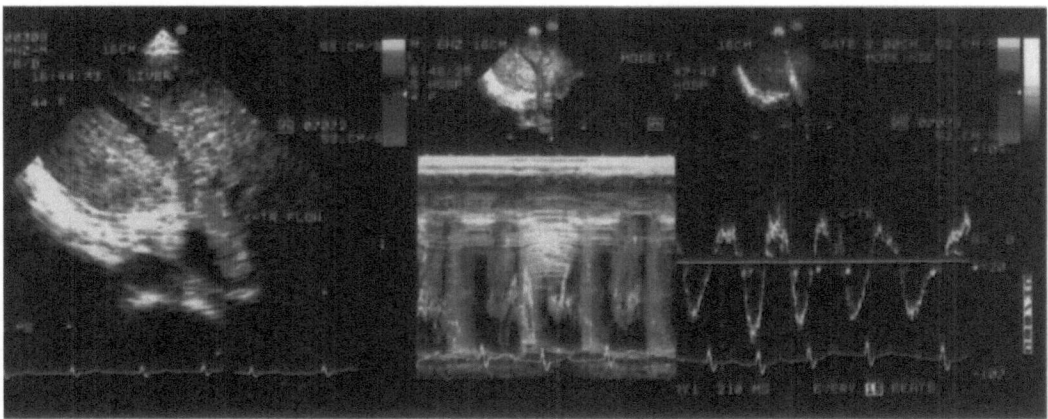

Figure 11.26. Color flow mapping obtained from the subcostal view in a patient with severe tricuspid regurgitation. The regurgitant flow is shown as red in the dilated hepatic vein. This finding is also evidenced by the color M-mode and pulsed Doppler recording in the hepatic vein.

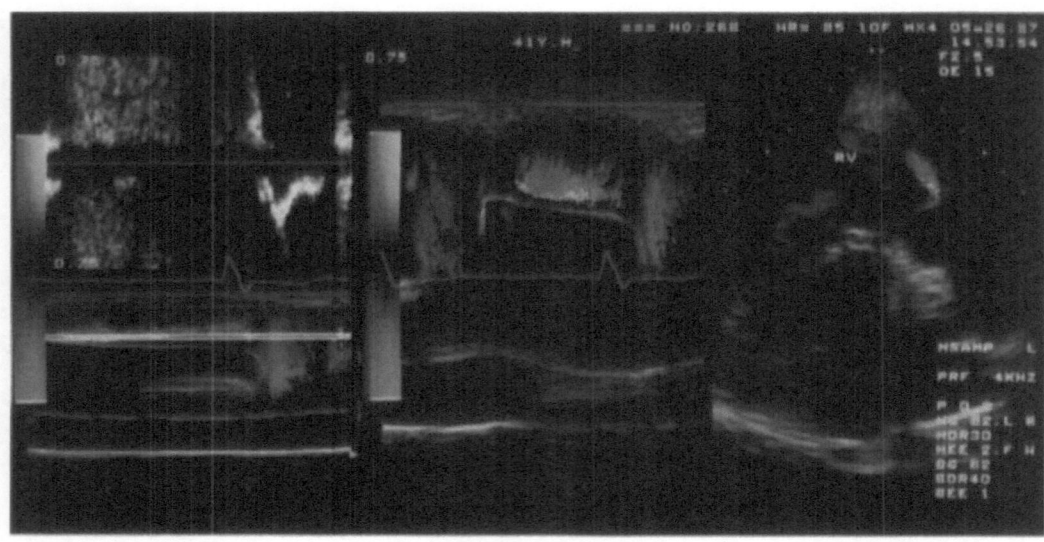

Figure 11.27. Color flow mapping obtained from the parasternal short axis view in a patient with mild PR. During diastole, pulmonary regurgitant flow is demonstrated as a red color in the right ventricular outflow tract (right). The color M-mode demonstrates the regurgitant flow as a mosaic pattern appearing above the pulmonic valve (middle). Pulsed Doppler shows diastolic turbulent flow (left).

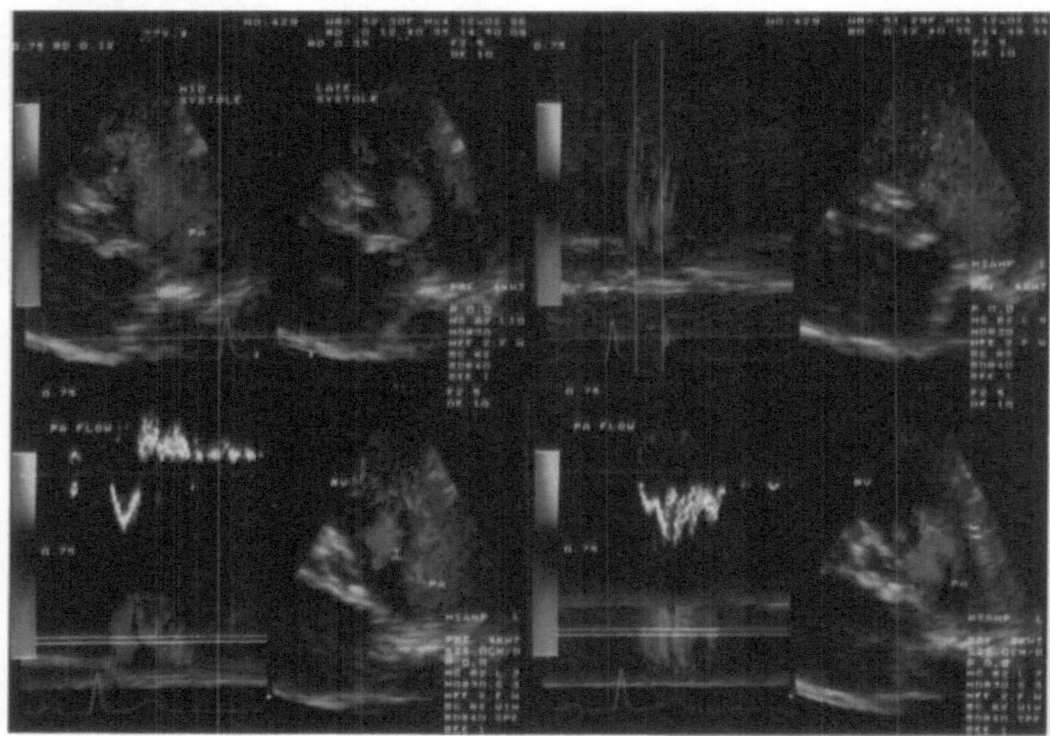

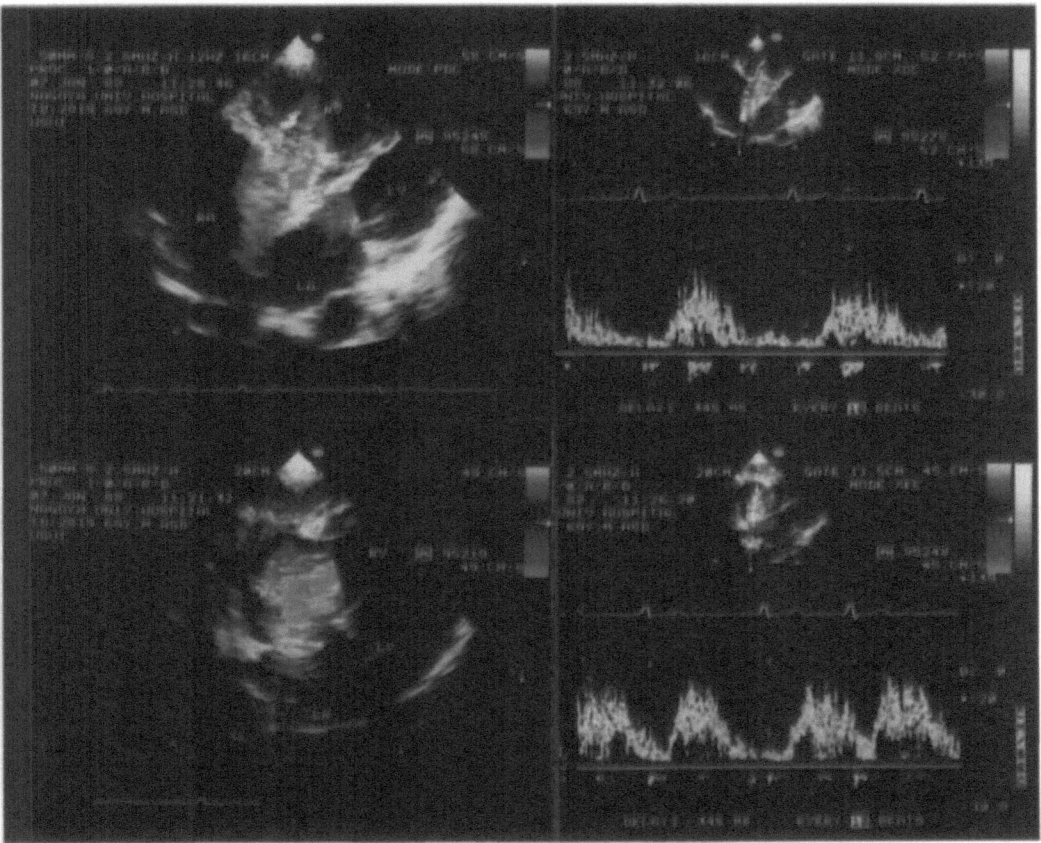

Figure 11.29. Color flow mapping of a four-chamber view recorded from parasternal (upper panel) and subcostal (lower panel) window in a patient with ostium secundum ASD. The left-to-right shunt flow through the atrial septal defect is demonstrated as a red color and is more parallel to the ultrasound beam from the subcostal approach. The pulsed Doppler recording shows left-to-right shunt flow having more laminar elements from the subcostal approach.

Figure 11.28. Color flow mapping of a patient with idiopathic pulmonary artery dilatation. Right ventricular ejection flow into the dilated pulmonary artery is shown as a blue color in mid-systole. However, a reverse flow (red color) is displayed on its internal side in late-systole. The upper right section shows a color M-mode recording, illustrating with a green line the timing of mid- and late-systole. The lower left shows the pulsed Doppler recording of the internal side of the dilated main pulmonary artery which demonstrates a late systolic reverse flow. The lower right demonstrates the pulsed Doppler recording obtained from the external portion of the dilated main pulmonary artery and an ejection flow through the systole is demonstrated. In this case, the dilated main pulmonary artery shows an abnormal distribution of pulmonary arterial flow velocity and also abnormal velocity changes through time. In this case, pulsed Doppler echocardiographic evaluation of pulmonary arterial pressure has some limitations. (See Chapter 9.)

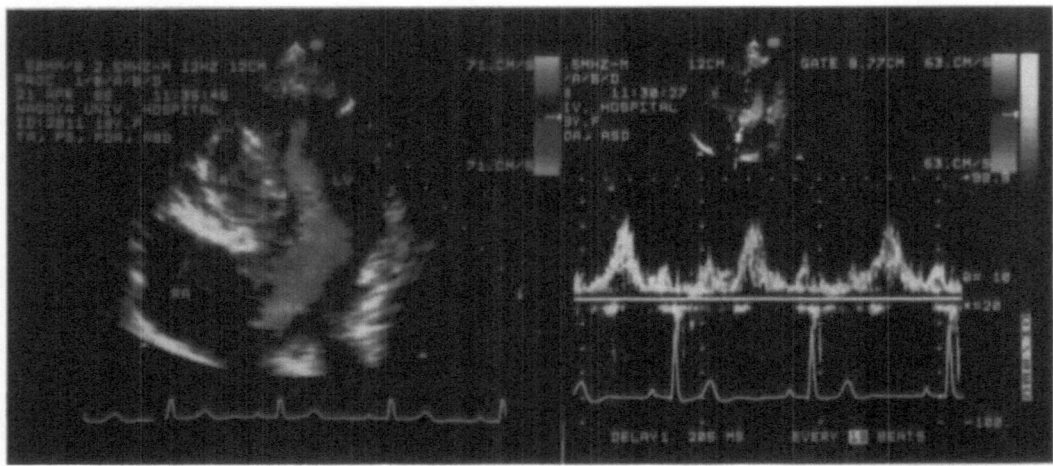

Figure 11.30. Color flow mapping of a parasternal four-chamber view in a patient with tricuspid atresia, ostium secundum ASD and PDA. The right-to-left shunt flow through the atrial septal defect is demonstrated as a red color. No right ventricular inflow can be observed. The pulsed Doppler recording shows right-to-left shunt flow during all cardiac cycles.

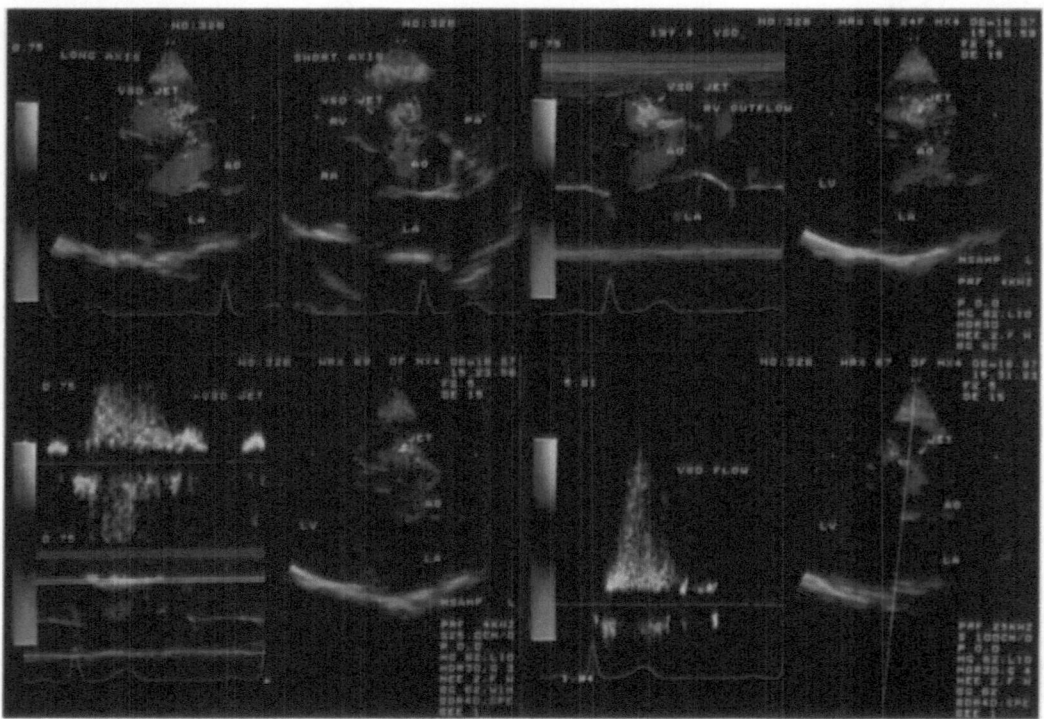

Figure 11.31. Color flow mapping obtained from the parasternal long and short axis views, color M-mode and pulsed and CW Doppler echocardiogram in a patient with membranous type VSD. The left-to-right shunt flow is clearly seen as a mosaic pattern through the septal defect. The color M-mode and pulsed Doppler recording show its time course, and CW Doppler evidences the peak velocity.

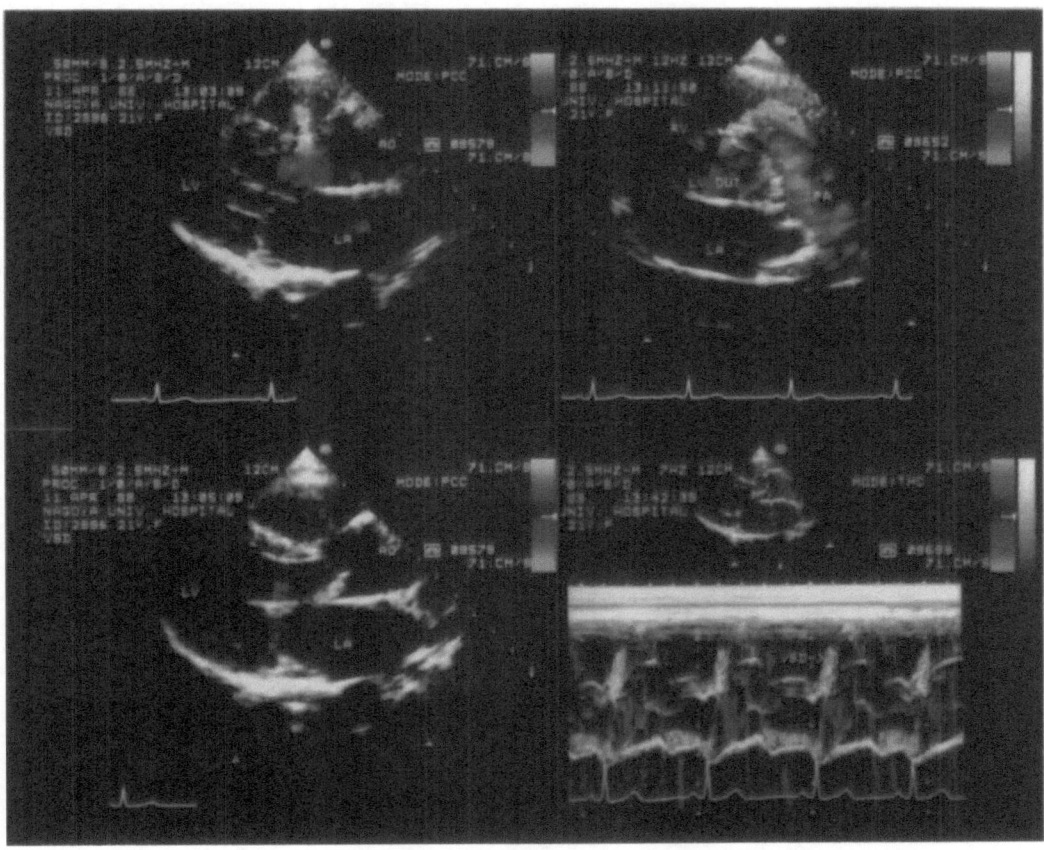

Figure 11.32. Color flow mapping of a patient with subpulmonary supracristal type VSD and mild aortic regurgitation due to aortic valve prolapse. The upper left shows the VSD jet as a mosaic pattern in a long axis view. The upper right shows the VSD jet as a mosaic pattern just below the pulmonic valve (supracristal). The lower left demonstrates a very mild aortic regurgitant flow during diastole. The lower right clearly evidences both the VSD jet during systole and aortic regurgitant flow during diastole in the color M-mode.

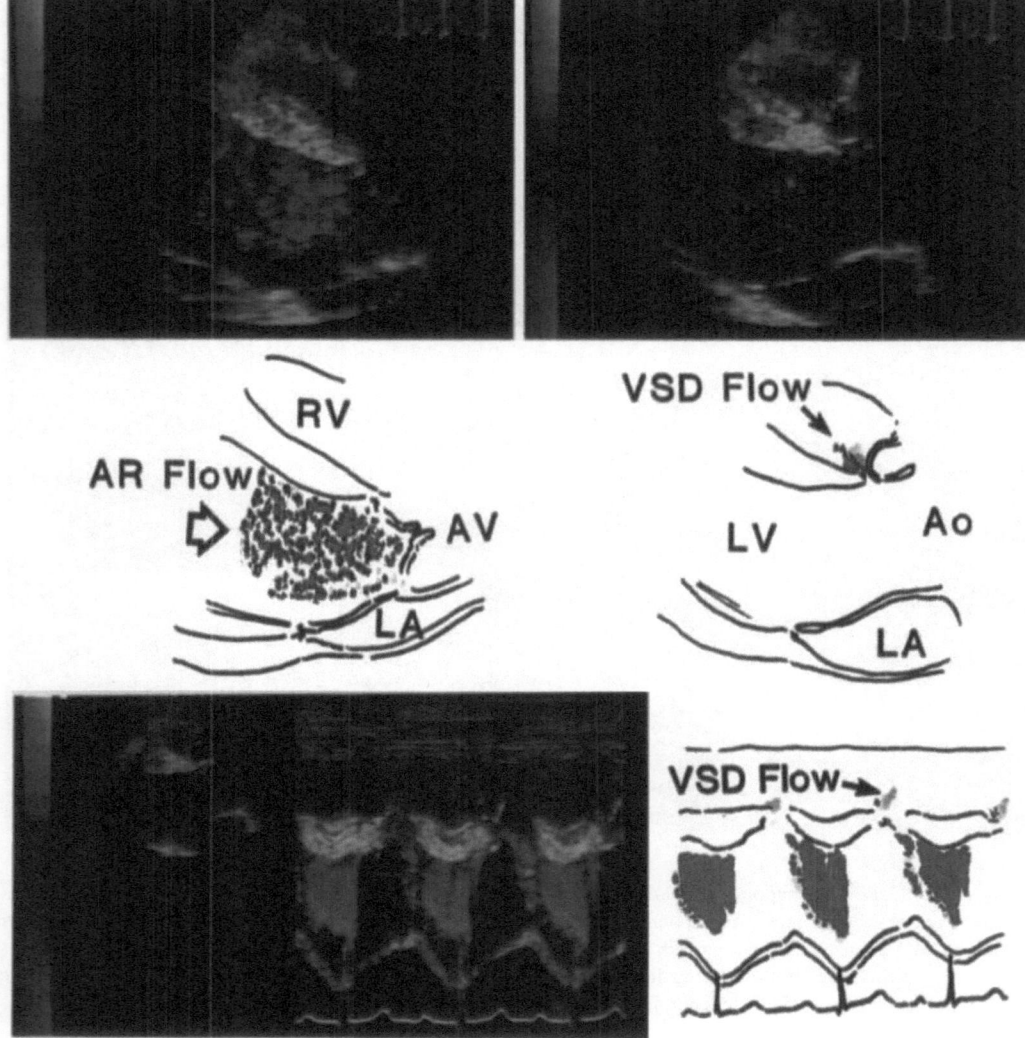

Figure 11.33.   Color flow mapping of a patient with membranous type VSD and severe aortic regurgitation (aortic valve prolapse). The upper left shows aortic regurgitant flow during diastole. The upper right clearly evidences the small shunt across the ventricular septal defect during systole. We can appreciate the same finding in the color M-mode recording.

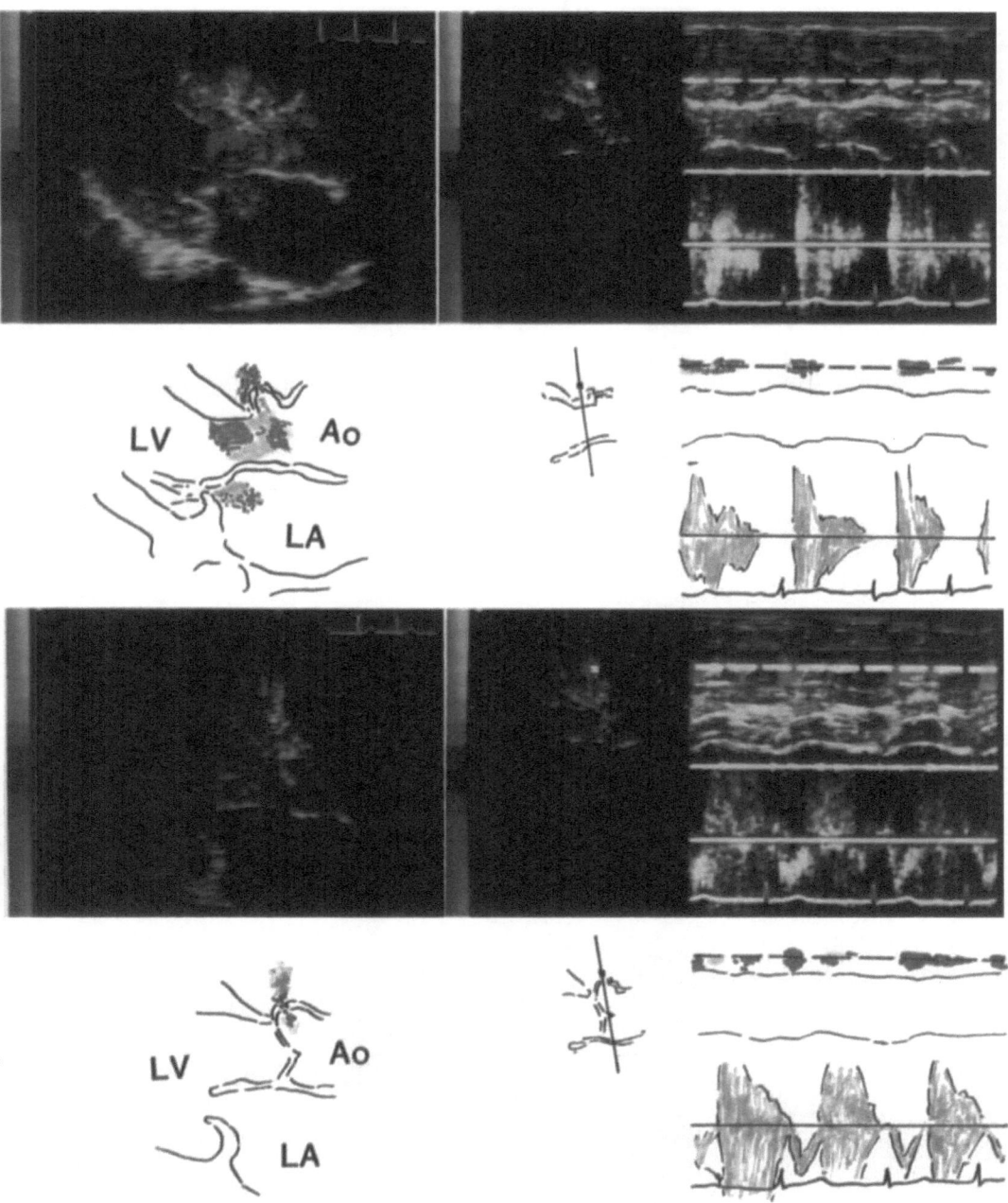

Figure 11.34. Color flow mapping obtained from the parasternal long axis view of a patient with ruptured Valsalva sinus aneurysm. Upper left shows the left-to-right shunt through the ruptured Valsalva sinus aneurysm in systole (arrow). During diastole (lower left), the shunt is also evidenced. However, the pulsed Doppler recordings could not demonstrate the shunt flow during the entire cardiac cycle because, in this patient, the shunt had two different directions in systole and diastole.

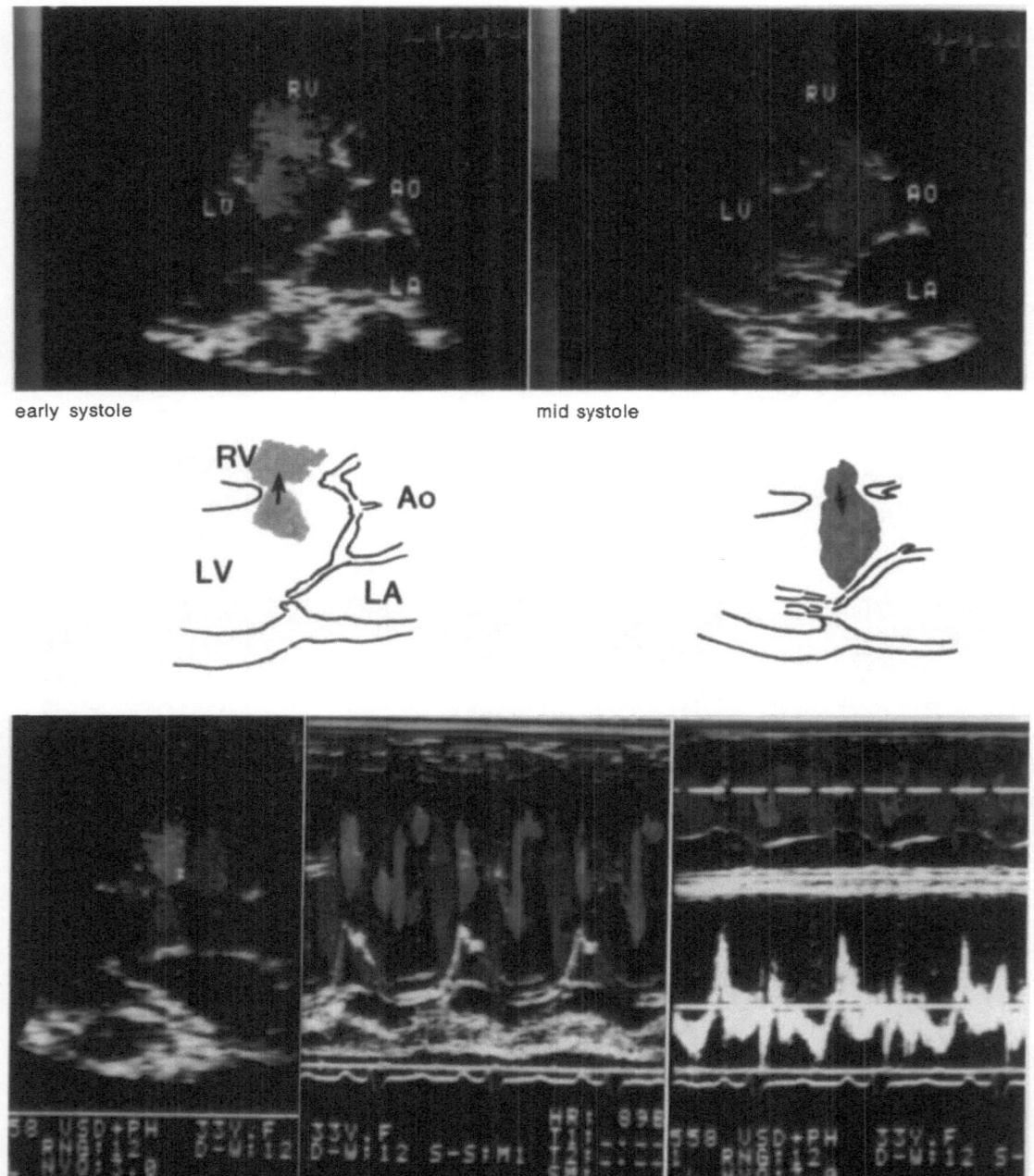

Figure 11.35. Color flow mapping of the parasternal long axis view in a patient with large VSD and Eisenmenger complex. In early systole, we can see the left-to-right shunt (red color) through the defect and, in mid systole, that the shunt becomes right-to-left (blue color). This time course is more clearly demonstrated by the color M-mode and pulsed Doppler recordings.

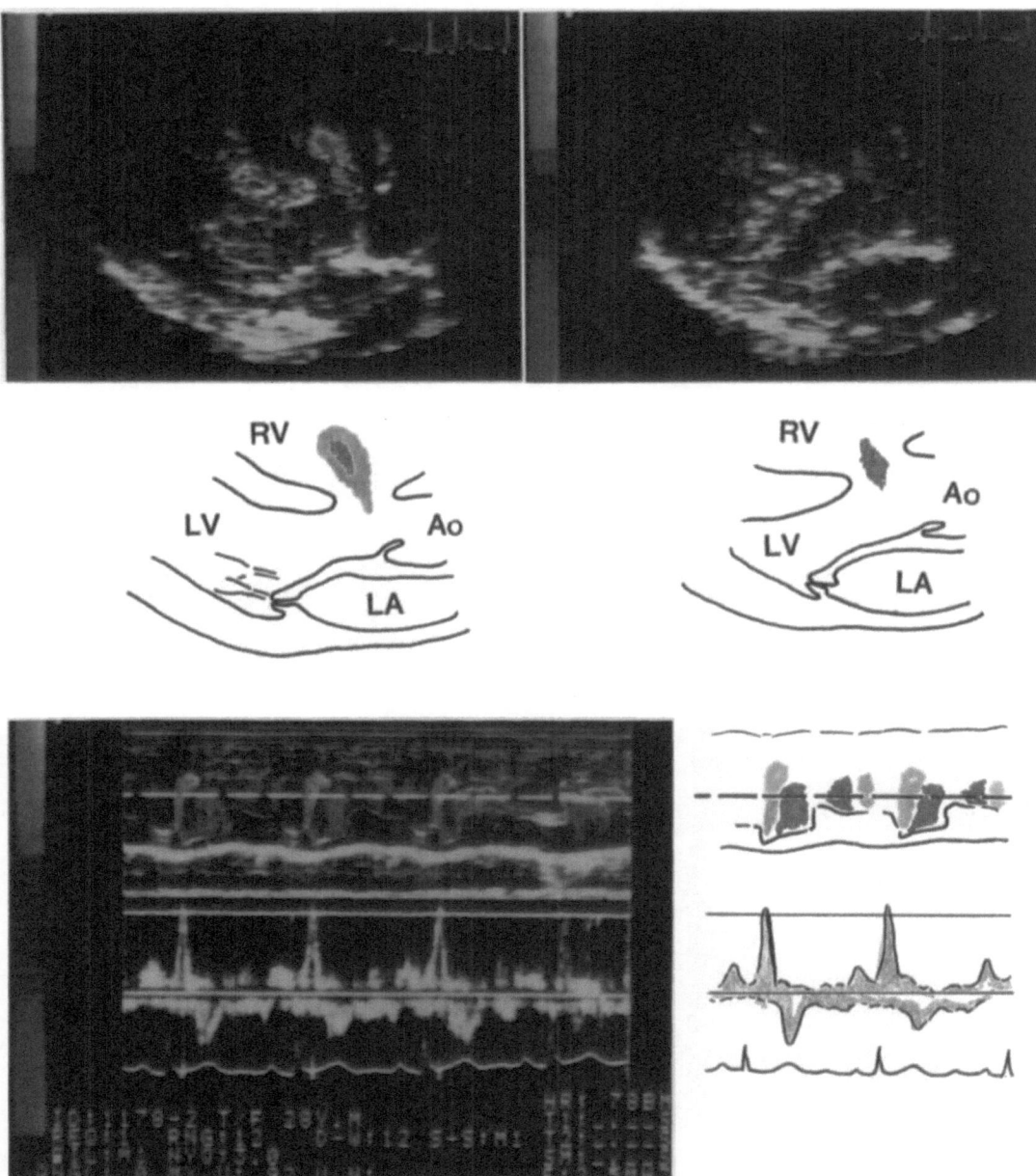

Figure 11.36. Color flow mapping of the parasternal long axis view in a patient with tetralogy of Fallot. The left-to-right shunt through the large VSD is illustrated as a red color in early systole and the right-to-left shunt is shown as a blue color in mid systole. This time course is more clearly demonstrated by the color M-mode and pulsed Doppler recordings.

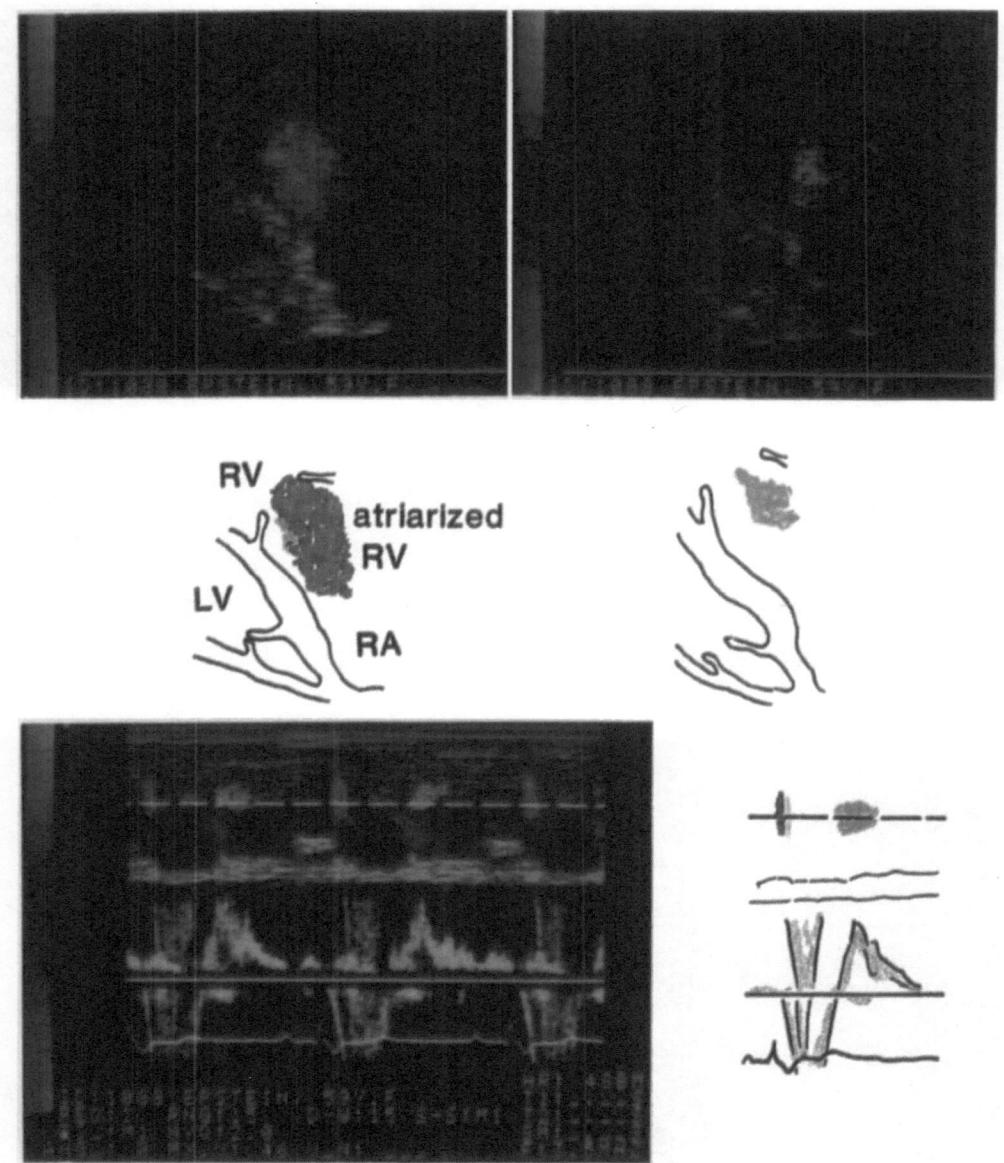

Figure 11.37. Color flow mapping of the right ventricular inflow view of a patient with Ebstein's anomaly. In systole, a regurgitant tricuspid flow is illustrated as a blue color. This regurgitant flow is also evidenced by pulsed Doppler recording.

$\longrightarrow$

Figure 11.39. Color flow mapping of four-chamber view and pulsed Doppler echocardiogram of a patient with coronary arterio-venous fistula. The upper left shows fistular flow draining into the right atrium as a red color, and the upper right demonstrates its time course. The lower left shows a dilated right coronary artery and the increased flow in it as a blue color. The lower right demonstrates intracoronary flow as being away from the transducer during all cardiac cycles.

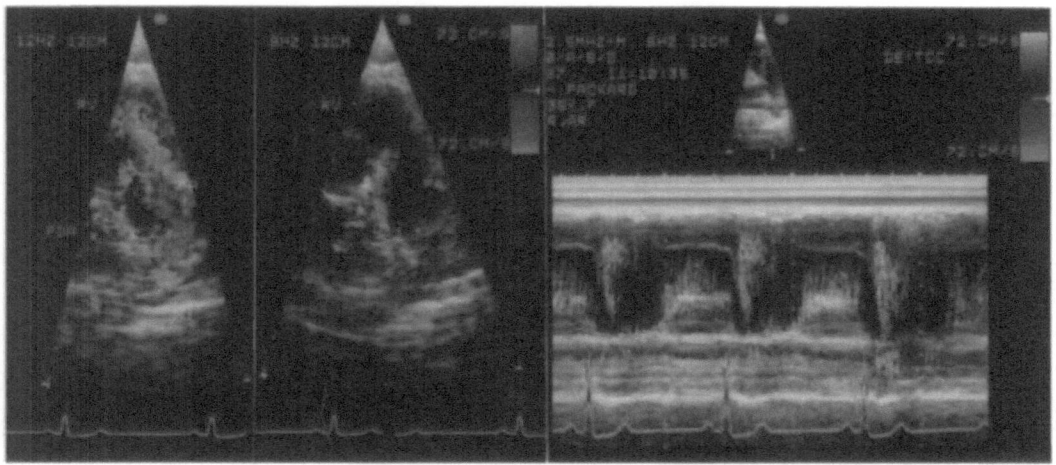

Figure 11.38. Color flow mapping of the parasternal short axis view in a patient with patent ductus arteriosus (PDA). The shunt flow is illustrated as an orange color with aliasing during systole (left) and diastole (middle). In systole, right ventricular ejection flow is also illustrated as a blue color in the main pulmonary artery (PA). In color M-mode, the shunt flow is shown as an orange color during all cardiac cycles, and right ventricular ejection flow is shown as a blue color in systole.

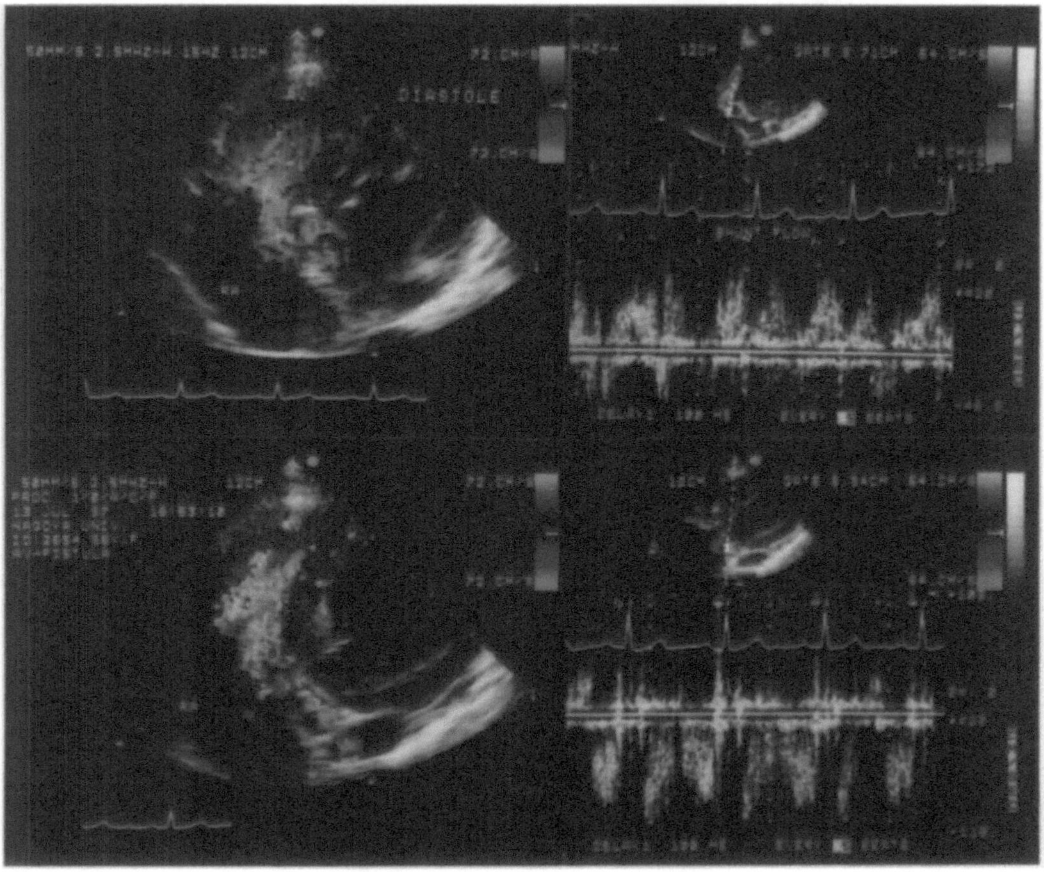

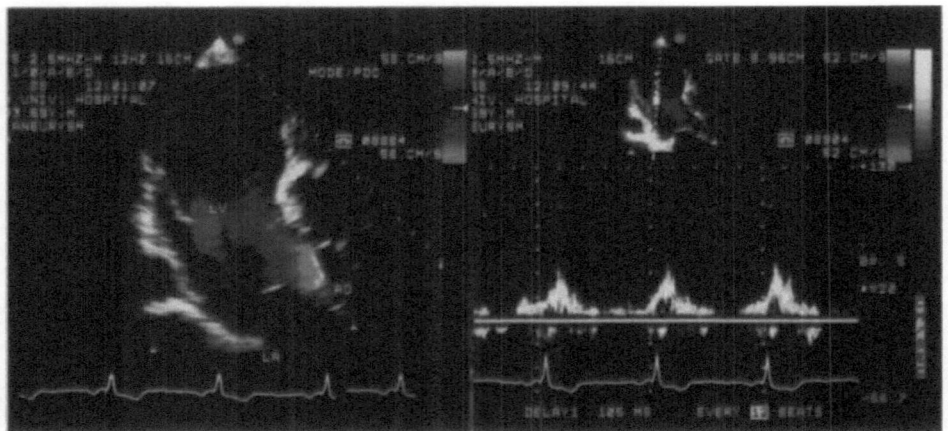

Figure 11.40.   Color flow mapping of the apical long axis view and pulsed Doppler echocardiogram of a patient with apical aneurysm. Near the aneurysmatic portion, systolic reversal flow can be observed as a red color. When the pulsed Doppler sample volume is placed into the aneurysmatic portion, a systolic reversal flow can be demonstrated (right panel).

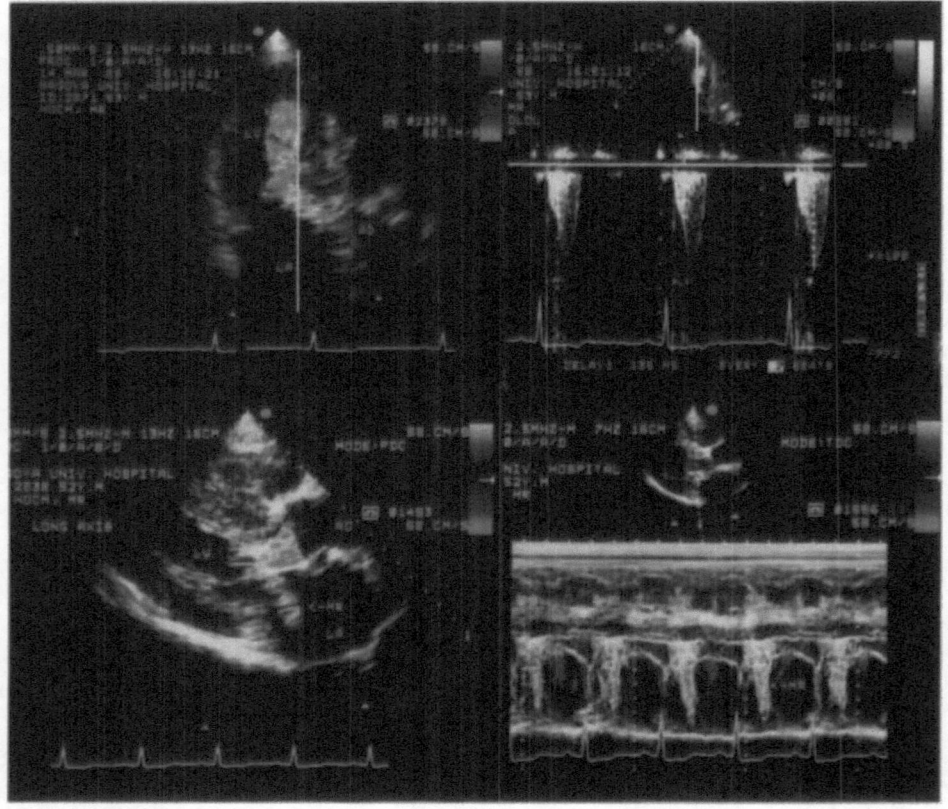

Figure 11.41.   Color flow mapping and CW Doppler evaluation from the apical and the parasternal approach in a patient with hypertrophic obstructive cardiomyopathy and mitral regurgitation. The upper left panel demonstrates a mosaic pattern ejection flow due to obstruction in the left ventricular outflow tract. CW Doppler demonstrates the increased peak flow velocity (406 cm/sec) in the upper right. The lower panels demonstrate the mitral regurgitant flow into the left atrium and the obstructed outflow jet as a mosaic pattern in long axis view and color M-mode.

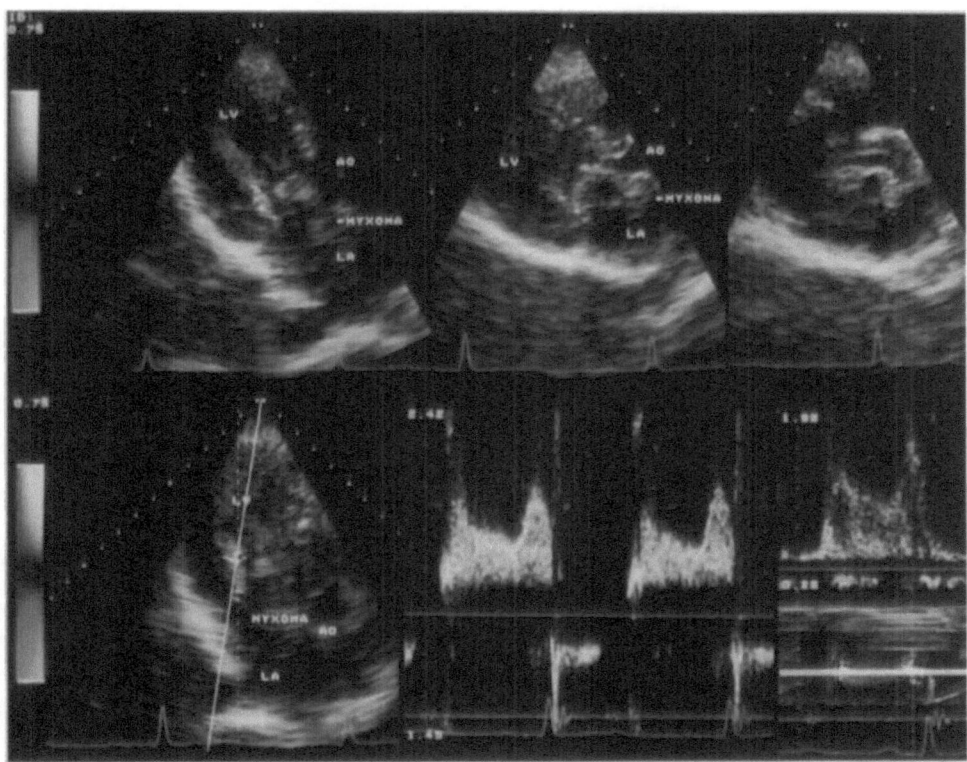

Figure 11.42. Color flow mapping, CW and pulsed Doppler echocardiogram of a patient with medium-sized prolapsing left atrial myxoma. During diastole, the tumor prolapses into the mitral orifice, producing stenotic flow between the tumor and posterior mitral leaflet in color flow mapping (upper panel). The time course of this flow, which is very similar to those in mitral stenosis, is clearly appreciated by CW and pulsed Doppler recordings (lower panel).

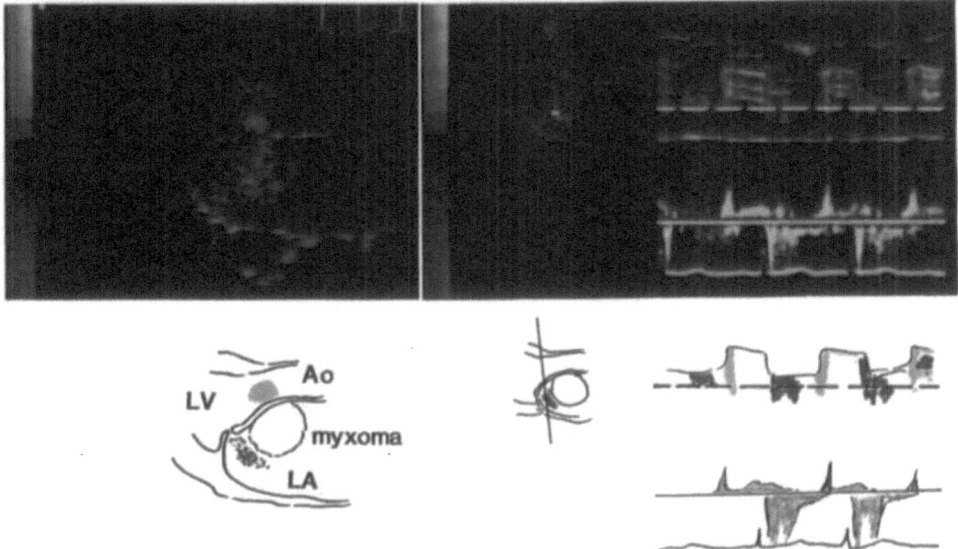

Figure 11.43. Color flow mapping of a patient with medium sized prolapsing left atrial myxoma. During systole, the tumor returns to the left atrium and a mild regurgitant flow into the left atrium (blue color) is demonstrated.

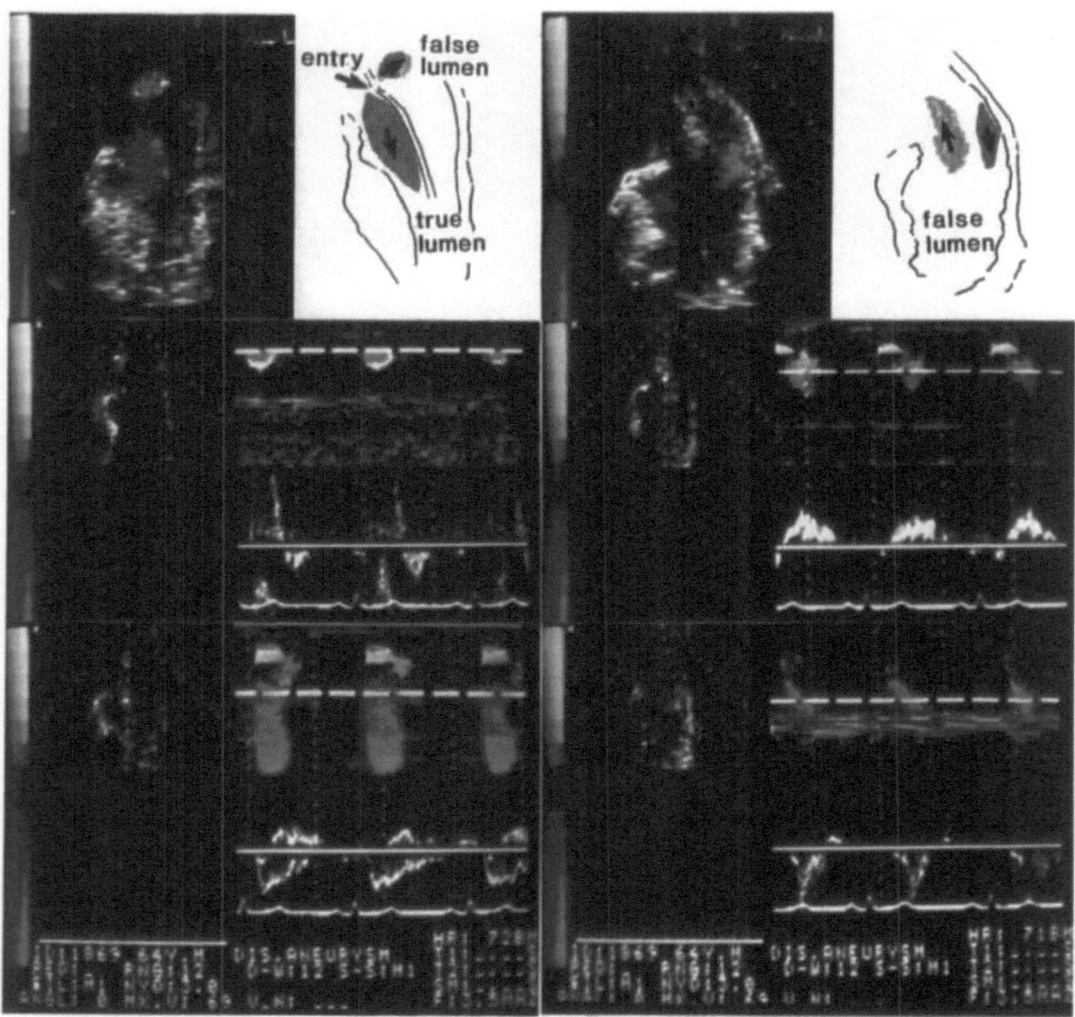

Figure 11.44. Color flow mapping obtained from the suprasternal notch of a patient with a dissected aortic aneurysm. The upper left panel shows the flow through the entry of the dissection (arrow). The middle left one evidences the high peak velocity (aliasing) through the entry. In the descending aorta (lower left), the flow velocity is relatively low. The upper right panel demonstrates the rotating flow in the false lumen (arrow), which is still more clearly identified by pulsed Doppler echocardiography (mid and lower right).

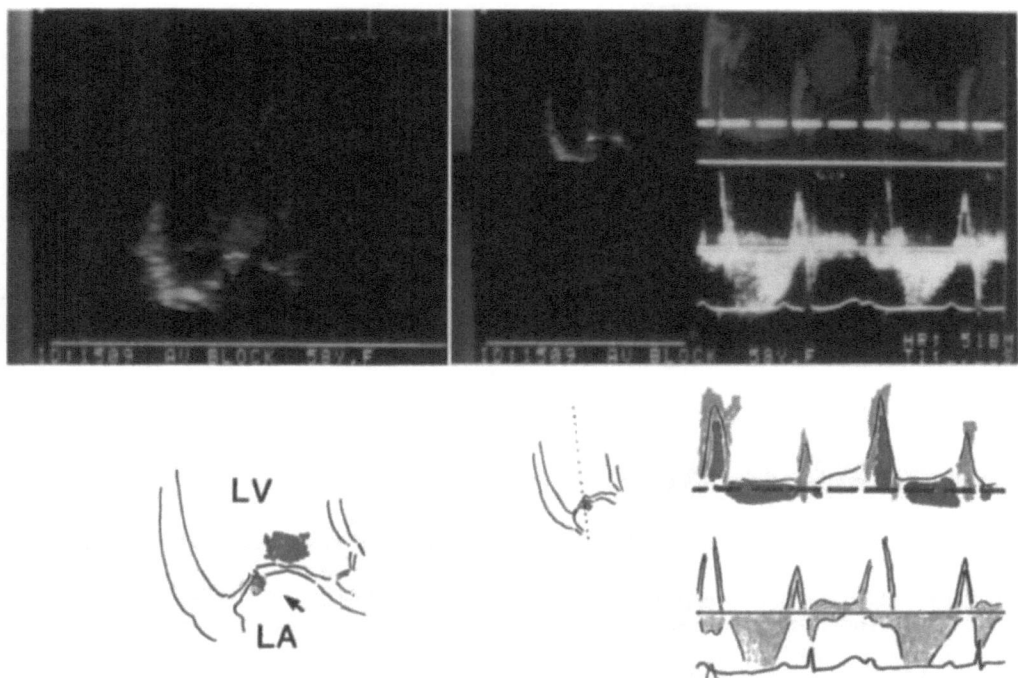

Figure 11.45. Color flow mapping illustrating atriogenic diastolic reflux as a mosaic pattern (small area) in the left atrium.

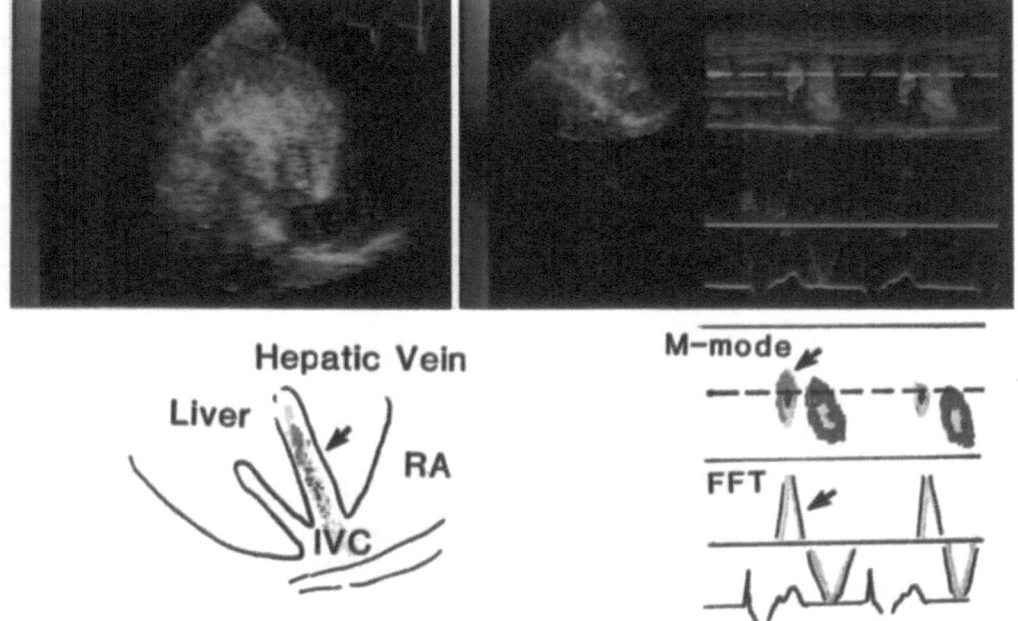

Figure 11.46. Color flow mapping obtained from the subcostal view of a patient with retrograde P wave in ECG. After the P wave, a reversed flow into the hepatic vein is observed as a mosaic pattern (arrow).

References*

1. Basics and methodology of echocardiography

1. Edler I, Gustafson A, Karlefors T, Christensson B: Ultrasound cardiography Acta Med Scand (suppl) 1961; 68: 370.
2. Ebina T, Oka S, Tanaka M, Kosaka S, Terasawa Y, Unno K, Kikuchi D, Uchida R: The ultrasonotomography of the heart and great vessels in living human subjects by means of the ultrasonic reflection technique. Jpn Heart J 1967; 8: 331.
3. Light LH: Noninjurous ultrasonic technique for observing flow in the human aorta. Nature 1969; 224: 1119.
4. Benchimol A, Desser KB, Gartlan JL: Bidirectional blood flow velocity in the cardiac chambers and great vessels studied with the Doppler ultrasonic flometer. Am J Med 1973; 52: 467.
5. Bom N, Lancee CT, Van Zwieten G, Kloster FE, Roeland J: Multi-scan echocardiography. I. Technical description. Circulation 1973; 48: 1066.
6. Griffith JM, Henry WL: A sector scanner for real time two-dimensional echocardiography. Circulation 1974; 49: 1147.
7. Kalmanson D, Bernier A, Veyrate C, Witchitz S, Savier CH, Chiche P: Normal pattern and physiological significance of mitral valve flow velocity recorded using transseptal directional Doppler ultrasound catheterization. Br Heart J 1975; 37: 249.
8. Roeland J, Vandorp WG, Bom N, Laird JD, Hugenholtz PG: Resolution problems in echocardiography: a source of interpretation errors. Am J Cardiol 1976; 37: 256.
9. vonRamm OT, Thurston FL: Cardiac imaging using a phased array ultrasound system. Circulation 1976; 53: 258.
10. Matsuo H, Kitabatake A, Haayashi T, Asao M, Terao Y, Senda S, Hamanaka Y, Matsumoto M, Nimura Y, Abe H: Intracardiac flow dynamics with bi-directional ultrasound pulsed Doppler technique. Jap Circ J 1977; 41: 515.
11. Matsumoto M, Matsuo H, Kitabatake A, Inoue M, Hamanaka Y, Tamura S, Tanaka K, Abe H: Three-dimensional echocardiographic images at desired planes by a computerized system. Ultrasound Med Biol 1977; 3: 163.
12. Baker DW, Rubenstein SA, Lorch GS: Pulsed Doppler echocardiography; Principles and applications. Am J Med 1977; 63: 69.
13. Sahn DJ, DeMaria AN, Kisslo J, Weyman A: The committee on M-mode standardization of the American society of echocardiography; recommendations regarding quantitation in M-mode echocardiography. Circulation 1978; 58: 1072.
14. Brinkley JF, Moritz WE, Baker DW: Ultrasonic three-dimensional imaging and volume from a series of arbitrary sector scan. Ultrasound Med Biol 1978; 4: 317.
15. Popp RL, Macovski A: Ultrasonic diagnostic instruments. Science 1980; 210: 268.
16. Henry WL, DeMaria AN, Gramiak R, King DL, Kisslo JA, Popp RL, Sahn DJ, Schiller NB, Tajik A, Teichholz LE, Weyman AE: Report of the American society of echocardiography committee on nomenclature and standards in two-dimensional echocardiography. Circulation 1980; 62: 212.
17. Kotler MN, Mintz GS, Segal BL, Party WR: Clinical uses of two-dimensional echocardiography. Am J Cardiol 1980; 45: 1061.

---

* See also the additional references on pp. 296ff.

18. Popp RL, Rubenson DS, Tucker CR, French JW: Echocardiography: M-mode and two-dimensional methods. Ann Intern Med 1980; 93: 844.
19. Popp RL, Fortuin NJ, Johnson ML, Kisslo JA: Optimal resources for ultrasonic examination of the heart. Echocardiography Study Group. Circulation 1982; 65: 423.
20. Joynt L, Popp RL: The concept of three dimensional resolution in echocardiographic imaging. Ultrasound Med Biol 1982; 8: 237.
21. DeMaria AN, Bommer W, Takeda P, Mason DT, Kwan OL, Resor J: Value and limitation of contrast echocardiography in cardiac diagnosis. J Cardiography 1983; 13: 1.
22. Bommer WJ, Shah PM, Allen H, Meltzer R, Kisslo J: The safety of contrast echocardiography. Report of the committee on contrast echocardiography for the American society of echocardiography. J Am Coll Cardiol 1984; 3: 6.
23. Berman W, Alverson D: Assessment of hemodynamic function with pulsed Doppler ultrasound. J Am Coll Cardiol 1985; 5: 104.
24. Stewart WJ, Galvin KA, Gillam LD, Guyer DE, Weyman AE: Comparison of high pulse repetition frequency and continuous wave Doppler echocardiography in the assessment of high flow velocity in patients with valvular stenosis and regurgitation. J Am Coll Cardiol 1985; 6: 565.
25. Teirstein PS, Yock PG, Popp RL. The accuracy of Doppler ultrasound measurement of pressure gradients across irregular, dual and tunnel-like obstructions to blood flow. Circulation 1985; 72: 577.
26. Gussenhoven EJ, Taams MA, Roelandt JRTC, Ligtvoet KM, McGhie J, Herwerden LA, Cahalan MK: Transesophageal two-dimensional echocardiography: its role in solving clinical problems. J Am Coll Cardiol 1986; 8: 975.
27. Valdes-Cruz LM, Yoganathan AP, Tamura T, Tomizuka F, Woo YR, Sahn DJ: Studies in vitro of the relationship between ultrasound and laser Doppler velocimetry and applicability of the simplified Bernoulli relationship. Circulation 1986; 73: 300.
28. Come PC: The optimal Doppler examination: pulsed, continuous wave or both? J Am Coll Cardiol 1986; 7: 886.
29. DeMaria AN, Crawford MH, Feigenbaum H, Popp RL, Tajik AJ: Task Force IV: Training in Echocardiography. J Am Coll Cardiol 1986; 7: 1207.
30. Meltzer RS, Gramiak R. Safety considerations related to ultrasonic energy exposure during echocardiographic examinations. Am J Cardiol 1986; 58: 1268.
31. Perlman AS, Gardin JM, Martin RP, Parisi AF, Popp RL, Quinones MA, Stevenson GS: Guidelines for optimal physical training in echocardiography: Recommendations of the American society of echocardiography committee for physician training in echocardiography. Am J Cardiol 1987; 60: 158.
32. Appleton CP, Hatle LK, Popp. RL: Superior vena cava and hepatic vein Doppler echocardiography in healthy adults. J Am Coll Cardiol 1987; 10: 1032.

2. Valvular heart disease

1. Edler I: Ultrasound cardiogram in mitral valve disease. Acta Chir Scand III 1956; 230.
2. Edler I. Ultrasoundcardiography in mitral valve stenosis. Am J Cardiol 1967; 17: 19.
3. Dillon JC, Haine CL, Change S, Feigenbaum H: Use of echocardiography in patients with prolapsed mitral valve. Circulation 1971; 43: 503.
4. Kerber RE, Isaeff DM, Hancock EW: Echocardiographic patterns in patients with the syndrome of systolic click and late systolic murmur. N Engl J Med 1971; 284: 691.
5. Sigger DC, Srivongse SA, Deuchar D: Analysis of dynamics of mitral Starr-Edwards valve prosthesis using reflected ultrasound. Br Heart J 1971; 33: 401.
6. Duchak JM Jr, Chang S, Feigenbaum H: The posterior mitral valve echo and the echocardiographic diagnosis of mitral stenosis. Am J Cardiol 1972; 29: 628.
7. Nimura Y, Wada O, Mochizuki S, Matsuo H, Aoki K, Kimura H, Izumi T, Kato K, Abe H: The ultrasound cardiogram of the tricuspid valve in healthy subjects. Jpn Heart J 1972; 13: 394.
8. Burgess J, Clark R, Kamigaki M, Cohn K: Echocardiographic findings in different types of mitral regurgitation. Circulation 1973; 48: 97.
9. Johnson ML, Holmes JH, Paton BC: Echocardiographic determination of mitral disc valve excursion. Circulation 1973; 47: 97.
10. DeMaria AN, King JF, Bogren HG, Lies JE, Mason DT: The variable spectrum of echocardiographic manifestation of the mitral valve prolapse syndrome. Circulation 1973; 50: 33.
11. Douglas JE, Williams GD: Echocardiographic evaluation of the Bjork-Shiley prosthetic valve. Circulation 1974; 50: 52.

12. Mary DAS, Pakrashi BC, Catchpole RW, Ionescu MI: Echocardiographic studies of stented fascia lata grafts in the mitral position. Circulation 1974; 49: 237.

13. Laniado S, Yellin E, Kotler M, Levy L, Stadler J, Terdiman R: A study of the dynamic relations between the mitral valve echogram and phasic mitral flow. Circulation 1975; 51: 104.

14. Henry WL, Griffith JM, Michaelis LL, McIntoch CL, Morrow AG, Epstein SE: Measurement of mitral orifice area in patients with mitral valve disease by real-time, two-dimensional echocardiography. Circulation 1975; 51: 827.

15. Mann T, McLaurin L, Grossman W, Craige E: Assessing the hemodynamic severity of acute regurgitation due to infective endocarditis. N Engl J Med 1975; 293: 108.

16. Weyman AE, Feigenbaum H, Dillon JC, Change S: Cross-sectional echocardiography in assessing the severity of valvular aortic stenosis. Circulation 1975; 52: 828.

17. Chandratna P, Samet P, Robinson MJ, Byrd C: Echocardiography of the 'floppy' aortic valve. Circulation 1975; 52: 959.

18. Gilbert BW, Schatz RA, VonRamm OT, Behar VS, Kisslo JA: Mitral valve prolapse. Two-dimensional echocardiographic and angiographic correlation. Circulation 1976; 42: 716.

19. Markiewicz W, Stoner J, London E, Hunt SA, Popp RL. Mitral valve prolapse in one hundred presumably healthy young females. Circulation 1976; 53: 464.

20. Berndt TB, Goodman DJ, Popp RL: Echocardiographic and phonocardiographic confirmation suspected caged mitral valve malfunction. Chest 1976; 70: 221.

21. Horowitz MS, Goodman DJ, Hancock EW, Popp RL. Noninvasive diagnosis of complication of the mitral bioprosthesis. J Thorac Cardiovasc Surg 1976; 45: 71.

22. Horowitz MS, Tecklenbereg PL, Goodman DJ, Harrison DC, Popp RL: Echocardiographic evaluation of the stent mounted aortic bioprosthetic valve in the mitral position; in vitro and in vivo studies. Circulation 1976; 54: 91.

23. Laniado S, Yeillin E, Tediman R, Meytes I, Stadler J: Hemodynamic correlates of the normal aortic valve echogram. A study of sound, flow, and motion. Circulation 1976; 54: 729.

24. Child JS, Skorton DJ, Taylor RD, Krivokapich J, Abbasi AS, Wong M, Shah PM: M-mode and cross-sectional echocardiographic features of mitral leaflets. Am J Cardiol 1977; 39: 499.

25. Nichol PM, Gilbert BW, Kisslo JA: Two-dimensional echocardiographic assessment of mitral stenosis. Circulation 1977; 55: 120.

26. Kalmanson D, Veyrat C, Bouchareine F, Degroote A: Non-invasive recording of mitral valve flow velocity patterns using pulsed Doppler echocardiography. Application to diagnosis and evaluation of mitral valve disease. Br Heart J 1977; 39: 517.

27. Gilbert BW, Haney RS, Crawiord F, McClellan J, Gallis HA, Johnson ML, Kisslo JA: Two-dimensional echocardiographic assessment of vegetative endocarditis. Circulation 1977; 55: 346.

28. Mintz GS, Kotler MN, Segal BL, Parry WR: Two-dimensional echocardiographic recognition of ruptured chordae tendineae. Circulation 1978; 57: 244.

29. Hatle L, Brubakk A, Tromsdal A, Angelsen B: Noninvasive assessment of pressure drop in mitral stenosis by Doppler ultrasound. Br Heart J 1978; 40: 131.

30. Lieppe W, Behar US, Scallion R, Kisssolo JA: Detection of tricuspid regurgitation with two-dimensional echocardiography and peripheral vein injections. Circulation 1978; 57: 128.

31. Martin RP, Rakowski H, Kleinman JH, Beaver W, London E, Popp RL: Reliability and reproducibility of two-dimensional echocardiographic measurement of the stenotic mitral valve orifice area. Am J Cardiol 1979; 43: 560.

32. Mikell FL, Asinger RW, ROurke T, Hodges M, Sharma B, Francis GS: Two-dimensional echocardiographic demonstration of left atrial thrombi in patients with prosthetic mitral valve. Circulation 1979; 60: 1183.

33. Schapira JN, Martin RP, Fowles RE, Rakowski H, Stinson EB, French JW, Shumway NE, Popp RL: Two-dimensional echocardiographic assessment of patients with bioprosthetic valves. Am J Cardiol 1979; 43: 510.

34. Holen J, Simonsen S, Froysker T: An ultrasound Doppler technique for the noninvasive determination of the pressure gradient in the Bjork-Shiley mitral valve. Circulation 1979; 59: 436.

35. Mintz GS, Kotler MN, Segal BL, Parry WR: Comparison of two-dimensional and M-mode echocardiography in the evaluation of patients with infective endocarditis. Am J Cardiol 1979; 43: 59.

36. Barlow JB, Pocock WA: Mitral valve prolapse, the specific billowing mitral leaflet syndrome, or an insignificant non-ejection systolic click. Am Heart J 1979; 97: 277.

37. Mintz GS, Kotler MN, Segal BL, Parry WR: Two-dimensional echocardiographic evaluation of patients with mitral insufficiency. Am J Cardiol 1979; 44: 670.

38. Yokota Y, Kawanishi H, Ohmori K, Oda A, Inoh T, Fukuzaki H: Studies on systolic anterior motion (SAM) pattern in idiopathic mitral valve prolapse by echocardiography. J Cardiography 1979; 9: 259.
39. Hatle L, Angelsen B, Tromsdal A: Noninvasive assessment of atrioventricular pressure half-time by Doppler ultrasound. Circulation 1979; 60: 1096.
40. Miyatake, Kinoshita N, Nagata S, Beppu S, Park Y, Sakakibara H, Nimura Y: Intracardiac flow pattern in mitral regurgitation studied with combined use of the ultrasonic pulsed Doppler technique and cross-sectional echocardiography. Am J Cardiol 1980; 45: 155.
41. Waggoner AD, Quinones MA, Young JB, Nelson JG, Winters WL, Peterson PK, Miller RP: Echocardiographic evaluation of obstraction of prosthetic mitral valve. Chest 1980; 78: 60.
42. DeMaria AN, Bommer W, Joye J, Lee G, Bouteller J, Bason DT: Value and limitations of cross-sectional echocardiography of the aortic valve in the diagnosis and quantification of valvular aortic stenosis. Circulation 1980; 62: 304.
43. Henry WL, Borer JS, Ware JH, Kent KM, Redwood DR, Morrow AG, Epstein SE: Observations on the optimum time for operative intervention in aortic regurgitation. I. Evaluation of the results of aortic valve replacement in symptomatic patients. Circulation 1980; 61: 471.
44. Krivokapich J, Child JS, Skorton DJ: Flail aortic valve leaflets: M-mode and two-dimensional echocardiography. Am Heart J 1980; 99: 425.
45. Mardelli TJ, Morganroth J, Naito M, Chen CC: Cross-sectional echocardiographic detection of aortic valve prolapse. Am Heart J 1980; 100: 295.
46. Stewart JA, Silimperi D, Harris P, Wise NK, Fraker TD, Kisslo JA: Echocardiographic documentation of vegetative lesions in infective endocarditis: clinical implications. Circulation 1980; 61: 374.
47. Schweizer P, Bardos P, Erbel R, Meyer J, Merx W, Messmer BJ, Effert S: Detection of left atrial thrombi by echocardiography. Br Heart J 1981; 45: 148.
80. Mardelli EJ, Morganroth J, Chen CC, Naito M, Vegal J: Tricuspid valve prolapse diagnosed by cross-sectional echocardiography. Chest 1981; 79: 201.
49. Amann FW, Durckhardt D, Hasse J, Gradel E: Echocardiographic features of the correctly functioning St. Jude medical valve prosthesis. Am Heart J 1981; 101: 45.
50. Ormiston JA, Shah PM, Tei C, Wong M: Size and motion of the mitral valve annulus in man. I. A two-dimensional echocardiographic method and findings in normal subjects. Circulation 1981; 64: 113.
51. Tei C, Pilgrim JP, Shah PM, Ormiston JA, Wong M: The tricuspid valve annulus: study of size and motion in normal subjects and in patients with tricuspid regurgitation. Circulation 1982; 66: 665.
52. Stamm RB, Martin RP: Quantification of pressure gradients across stenotic valves by Doppler ultrasound. J Am Coll Cardiol 1983; 2: 707.
53. Shrestha NK, Moreno F, Narciso FV, Torres L, Calleja HB: Two-dimensional echocardiographic diagnosis of left atrial thrombus in rheumatic heart disease: a clinicopathologic study. Circulation 1983; 67: 341.
54. Yock PG, Popp RL: Noninvasive estimation of right ventricular systolic pressure by Doppler ultrasound in patients with tricuspid regurgitation. Circulation 1984; 70: 149.
55. Pennestri F, Loperfido F, Salvatori MP, et al. Assessment of tricuspid regurgitation by pulsed Doppler ultrasonography of the hepatic veins. Am J Cardiol 1984; 54: 363.
56. Currie PJ, Seward JB, Reeder GS, Vietstra RE, Bresnahan DR, Bresnahan JF, Smith HC, Hagler DJ, Tajik AJ: Continuous-wave Doppler echocardiographic assessment of severity of calcific aortic stenosis: a stimultaneous Doppler-catheter correlative study in 100 adult patients. Circulation 1985; 71: 1162.
57. Cannon SR, Richards KL, Crawford M: Hydraulic estimation of stenotic orifice area: a correction of the Gorlin formula. Circulation 1985; 71: 1170.
58. Ascah KJ, Stewart WJ, Jiang L, Guerrero JL, Newell JB, Gillam LD, Weyman AE. A Doppler two-dimensional echocardiographic method for quantitation of mitral regurgitation. Circulation 1985; 72: 377.
59. Kitabatake A, Ito H, Inoue M, Tanouchi J, Ishihara K, Morita T, Fujii K, Yoshida Y, Masuyama T, Yoshima H, Hori M, Kamada T: A new approach to noninvasive evaluation of aortic regurgitant fraction by two-dimensional Doppler echocardiography. Circulation 1985; 72: 523.
60. Skjaerpe T, Hegrenaes L, Hatle L: Noninvasive estimation of valve area in patients with aortic stenosis by Doppler ultrasound and two-dimensional echocardiography. Circulation 1985; 72: 810.
61. Stewart WJ, Galvin KA, Gillam LD, Guyer DE, Weyman AE: Comparison of high pulse repetition frequency and continuous wave Dopper echocardiography in the assessment of high flow velocity in patients with valvular stenosis and regurgitation. J Am Coll Cardiol 1985; 6: 565.
62. Beppu S, Nimura Y, Skakibara H, Nagata S, Park YD, Izumi S: Smoke like echo in the left atrial cavity in mitral valve disease: Its features and significance. J Am Coll Cardiol 1985; 6: 744.
63. Iliceto S, Antonelli G, Sorino M, Biasco G, Rizzon P: Dynamic intracavitary left atrial echoes in mitral stenosis. Am J Cardiol 1985; 55: 603.

64. Williams GA, Labovitz AJ, Nelson JG, Kennedy HL: Value of multiple echocardiographic views in the evaluation of aortic stenosis in adults by continuous-wave Doppler. Am J Cardiol 1985; 55: 445.

65. Hickey AJ, Wilcken DEL, Wright JS, Warren BA: Primary (spontaneous) chordal rupture: relation to myxomatous valve disease and mitral valve prolapse. J Am Coll Cardiol 1985; 5: 1341.

66. Smith MD, Handshoe R, Handshoe S, Kwan OL, DeMaria AN: Comparative accuracy of two-dimensional echocardiography and Doppler pressure half-time method in assessing severity of mitral stenosis in patients with and without prior commissurotomy. Circulation 1986; 73: 100.

67. Hsu TL, Chen CC, Chen CY, Hsiung MC, Chiang BN: Two-dimensional echocardiographic features of floating left atrial thrombus. Am J Cardiol 1986; 57: 701.

68. Takenaka K, Dabestani A, Gardin JM, Russell D, Clark S, Allfie A, Henry WL: A simple Doppler echocardiographic method for estimating severity of aortic regurgitation. Am J Cardiol 1986; 57: 1340.

69. Alpert MA, Carney RJ, Munuswamy K, Ruder MA, Kapoor AS, Webel RR, Sanfelippo JF, Haikal M, Perkins SK, Kelly DL: Observer variation in the echocardiographic diagnosis of mitral valve prolapse. Am Heart J 1986; 111: 1123.

70. Miyatake K, Izumi S, Okamoto M, Kinoshita N, Asonuma H, Nakagawa H, Yamamoto K, Takamiya M, Sakakibara H, Nimura Y: Semiquantitative grading of severity of mitral regurgitation by real-time two-dimensional Doppler flow imaging technique. J Am Coll Cardiol 1986; 7: 82.

71. Currie PJ, Hagler DJ, Seward JB, Reeder GS, Fyfe DA, Bove AA, Tajik AJ: Instantaneous pressure gradient: A stimultaneous Doppler and dual catheter correlative study. J Am Coll Cardiol 1986; 7: 800.

72. Richards KL, Cannon SR, Miller JF, Carawford MH. Calculation of aortic valve area by Doppler echocardiography: a direct application of the continuity equation. Circulation 1986; 73: 964.

73. Blumlein S, Bouchard A, Schiller NB, Dae M, Byrd III BF, Ports T; Botvinick EH: Quantitation of mitral regurgitation by Doppler echocardiography. Circulation 1986; 74: 306.

74. Masuyama T, Kodama K, Kitabatake A, Sato H, Nanto S, Inoue M: Continuous-wave Doppler echocardiographic detection of pulmonary regurgitation and its application to noninvasive estimation of pulmonary artery pressure. Circulation 1986; 74: 484.

75. Wilkins GT, Gillam LD, Kritzer GL, Levine RA, Palacios IF, Weyman AE. Validation of continuous-wave Doppler echocardiographic measurements of mitral and tricuspid prosthetic valve gradients: a stimultaneous Doppler-catheter study. Circulation 1986; 74: 876.

76. Czer LS, Gray RJ, Bateman TM, DeRobertis MA, Resser K, Chaux A, Matloff JM: Hemodynamic differentiation of pathologic and physiologic stenosis of mitral porcine bioprostheses. J Am Coll Cardiol 1986; 7: 284.

77. Waller BF, Moriarty AT, Eble JN, Davey DM, Hawley DA, Pless JE: Etiology of pure tricuspid regurgitation based on annular circumference and leaflet area: analysis of 45 necropsy patients with clinical and morphologic evidence of pure tricuspid regurgitation. J Am Coll Cardiol 1986; 7: 1063.

78. Devereux RB, Kramer-Fox R, Brown WB, Shear K, Hartman N, Kligfield P, Lutas EM, Spitzer M, Litwin SD: Relation between clinical features of mitral prolapse syndrome and echocardiographically documented mitral valve prolapse. J Am Coll Cardiol 1986; 8: 763.

79. Mann DL, Gillam LD, Marshall JE, King ME, Weyman AE: Doppler and two-dimensional echocardiographic diagnosis of Bjork-Shiley prosthetic valve malfunction: Importance of interventricular septal motion and timing of onset of valve flow. J Am Coll Cardiol 1986: 8: 971.

80. Teirstein P, Yeager M, Yock PG, Popp RL: Doppler echocardiographic measurement of aortic valve area in aortic stenosis: A noninvasive application of the Gorlin formula. J Am Coll Cardiol 1986; 8: 1059.

81. Kostucki W, Vandenbossche JL, Friart A, Englert M: Pulsed Doppler regurgitant flow patterns of normal valves. Am J Cardiol 1986; 58: 309.

82. Rashtian MY, Stevenson DM, Allen DT, Yoganathan AP, Harrison EC, Edmiston A, Faughan P, Rahimtoola SH: Flow characteristics of four commonly used mechanical heart valves. Am J Cardiol 1986; 58: 743.

83. Lutas EM, Roberts R, Devereux RB, Prieto LM: Relation between the presence of echocardiographic vegetations and the complication rate in infective endocarditis. Am Heart J 1986; 112: 107.

84. Panidis IP, Mintz GS, Ross J: Value and limitations of Doppler ultrasound in the evaluation of aortic stenosis: A statistical analysis of 70 consecutive patients. Am Heart J 1986; 112: 150.

85. Iwase M, Yokota M, Aoki T, Jing HX, Takagi S, Kawai N, Hayashi H, Sotobata I, Uozumi Z, Mizuno Y: Assessment of the severity of mitral regurgitation in patients with mitral valve prolapse by pulsed Doppler echocardiography. J Cardiovasc Ultrason 1986; 5: 245.

86. Labovitz AJ, Ferrara RP, Kern MJ, Bryg RJ, Williams GA: Quantitative evaluation of aortic insufficiency by continuous wave Doppler echocardiography. J Am Coll Cardiol 1986; 8: 1341.

87. Come PC, Riley MF, Carl LV, Nakao S: Pulsed Doppler echocardiographic evaluation of valvular regurgitation in patients with mitral valve prolapse: comparison with normal subjects. J Am Coll Cardiol 1986; 8: 1355.

88. Barzilai B, Eisen HJ, Saffitz JE, Perez JE: Detection of thrombotic obstruction of a Bjork-Shiley prosthesis by Doppler echocardiography. Am Heart J 1986; 112: 1088.
89. Buda AJ, Zotz RJ, LeMire MS, Bach DS: Prognostic significance of vegetations detected by two-dimensional echocardiography in infective endocarditis. Am Heart J 1986; 112; 1291.
90. Beyer RW, Ramirez M, Josephson MA, Shah PM: Correlation of continuous-wave Doppler assessment of chronic aortic regurgitation with hemodynamics and angiography. Am J Cardiol 1987; 60: 852.
91. Reid CL, McKay CR, Chandratna PAN, Kawanishi DT, Rahimtoola SH: Mechanisms of increase in mitral valve area and influence of anatomic features in double-balloon, catheter balloon valvuloplasty in adults with rheumatic mitral stenosis: A Doppler and two-dimensional echocardiographic study. Circulation 1987; 76: 628.

3. Congenital heart disease

1. Weyman AE, Feigenbaum H, Hurwitz RA, Girod DA, Dillon JC, Cang S: Cross-sectional echocardiography in evaluating patients with discrete subaortic stenosis. Am J Cardiol 1976; 37: 358.
2. Beppu S, Nimura Y, Nagata S, Tamai M, Matsuo H, Matsumoto M, Kawashima Y, Sakakibara H, Abe H: Diagnosis of endocardial cushion defect with cross-sectional and M-mode scanning echocardiography. Br Heart J 1976; 38: 911.
3. Henry WL, Maron BJ, Griffith JM. Cross-sectional echocardiography in the diagnosis of congenital heart disease. Circulation 1977; 56: 267.
4. Sahn DJ, Allen HD, Macdonalda G, Goldberg SJ: Real-time cross-sectional echocardiographic diagnosis of coarctation of the aorta. A prospective study of echocardiographic-angiographic correlations. Circulation 1977; 56: 762.
5. Sahn DJ, Allen HD: Real-time cross-sectional echocardiographic imaging and measurement of the patent ductus arteriosus in infants and children. Circulation 1978; 58: 343.
6. Stevenson JG, Kawabori I, Dooley T, Gunteroth WG: Diagnosis of ventricular septal defect by pulsed Doppler echocardiography: sensitivity, specificity and limitations. Circulation 1978; 58: 322.
7. Beppu S, Nimura Y, Tamai M, Nagata S, Matsuo H, Kawashima Y, Kozuka T, Sakakibara H: Two-dimensional echocardiography in diagnosing tricuspid atresia: differentiation from other hypoplastic right heart syndromes and common atrioventricular canal. Br Heart J 1978; 40: 1174.
8. Houston AB, Gregory NL, Coleman EN: Echocardiographic identification of aorta and main pulmonary artery in complete transposition. Br Heart J 1978; 40: 377.
9. Ports TA, Silverman NH, Schiller NB. Two-dimensional echocardiographic assessment of Ebstein's anomaly. Circulation 1978; 58: 336.
10. Stevenson JG, Kawabori I, Gunteroth WG: Noninvasive detection of pulmonary hypertention in patent ductus arteriosus by pulsed Doppler echocardiography. Circulation 1979; 59: 920.
11. Aziz KU, Cole RB, Paul MH: Echocardiographic features of supracristal ventricular septal defect with prolapsed aortic valve leaflet. Am J Cardiol 1979; 43: 854.
12. Fraker TD, Harris PJ, Behar VS, Kisslo JA: Detection and exclusion of interatrial shunts by two-dimensional echocardiography and peripheral venous injection. Circulation 1979; 59: 379.
13. Weyman AE, Wann LS, Caldwell RL, Hurwitz RA, Dillon JC, Feigenbaum H: Negative contrast echocardiography: a new method for detecting left-to-right shunts. Circulation 1979; 59: 498.
14. Snider AR, Silverman NH, Schiller NB, Ports TA: Echocardiographic evaluation of ventricular septal aneurysms. Circulation 1979; 59: 498.
15. Lange LW, Sahn DJ, Allen HD, GOldberg SJ: Subxiphoid cross-sectional echocardiography in infants and children with congenital heart disease. Circulation 1979; 59: 513.
16. Bierman FZ, William RG: Subxiphoid two-dimensional imaging of the interatrial septum in infants and neonates with congenital heart disease. Circulation 1979; 60: 80.
17. Snider AR, Silverman NH, Schiller NB: Two-dimensional echocardiographic evaluation of ventricular septal aneurysms. Circulation 1979; 60: 355.
18. Satomi G, Komatsu Y, Takao A: Echocardiographic identification of aorta and main pulmonary aretry in complete transposition. Br Heart J 1979; 41: 356.
19. Schreiber TL, Feigenbaum H, Weyman AE: Effect of atrial septal defect repair on left ventricular geometry and degree of mital valve prorapse. Circulation 1980; 61: 88.
20. Gussenhoven WJ, Spitaels SEC, Bom N, Becker AE. Echocardiographic criteria for Ebstein's anomaly of tricuspid valve. Br Heart J 1980; 43: 31.
21. Yoshikawa J, Katao H, Yanagihara K, Takagi Y, Okumachi F, Yoshida K, Tomita Y, Fukaya T, Baba K:

Noninvasive visualization of dilated main coronary arteries in coronary artery fistulas by cross-sectional echocardiography. Circulation 1982; 65: 600.

22. Sutherland G, Godman MJ, Smallhorn JF, Guiterras P, Anderson RH, Hunter S: Ventricular septal defects: two-dimensional echocardiographic and morphologic correlations. Br Heart J 1982; 47: 316.

23. Huhta JC, Smallhorn JF, Macartney FJ, Anderson RH, de Leval M: Cross-sectional echocardiographic diagnosis of systemic venous return. Br Heart J 1982; 388: 48.

24. Ueda T, Nishioka K, Mitawa H, Minami K, Konishi Y, Tatsuta N, Hikasa Y: Echocardiographic evaluation of aortic cusp prolapse in children with ventricular septal defect. Jap Circ J 1983; 47: 1359.

25. Beppu S, Minura Y, Sakakibara H, Nagata S, Park YD, Nambu S, Yamamota A: Supravalvular aortic stenosis and coronary ostial stenosis in familial hypercholesterolemia: two-dimensional echocardiographic assessment. Circulation 1983; 67: 878.

26. Oliveira LC, Sahn DJ, Valdes-Cruz LM, Goldberg SJ, Vargas BJ, Allen HD, Grenadier E: Noninvasive prediction of transvalvular pressure gradient in patients with pulmonary stenosis by quantitative two-dimensional echo Doppler studies. Circulation 1983; 67: 866.

27. Shub C, Dimopoulos IN, Seward JB, et al: Sensitivity of two-dimensional echocardiography in the direct visualization of atrial septal defect utilizing the subcostal approach: experience with 154 patients. J Am Coll Cardiol 1983; 127: 2.

28. Sanders SP, Yeager S, Williams RG: Measurements of systemic and pulmonary blood flow and Qp/Qs ratio using Doppler and two-dimensional echocardiography. Am Heart J 1984; 107: 257.

29. Beerman LB, Park SC, Fisher DR, Fricker FJ, Mathews RA, Neches WH, Lenox CC, Zuberbuhler JR: Ventricular septal defects associated with aneurysm of membranous septum. J Am Coll Cardiol 1985; 5: 118.

30. Ortiz E, Robinson PJ, Deanfield JE, Franklin R, Macartney FJ, Wyse RKH: Localization of ventricular septal defects by simultaneous display of superimposed color Doppler and cross sectional echocardiographic images. Br Heart J 1985; 54: 53.

31. Hagler DJ, Edwards WD, Seward JB, Tajik AJ. Standardized nomenclature of the ventricular septum and ventricular septal defects, with applications for two-dimensional echocardiography. Mayo Clin Proc 1985; 60: 741.

32. Shub C, Tajik AJ, Seward JB, Hagler DJ, Danielson GK: Surgical repair of uncomplicated atrial septal defect without 'routine' preoperative cardiac catheterization. J Am Coll Cardiol 1985; 6: 49.

33. Ramaciotti C, Keren A, Silverman NH: Importance of (perimembranous) ventricular septal aneurysm in the natural history of isolated perimembranous ventricular septal defect. Am J Cardiol 1986; 57: 268.

34. Murphy DJ, Ludomirsky A, Huhuta JC: Continuous-wave Doppler in children with ventricular septal defect: noninvasive estimation of interventricular pressure gradient. Am J Cardiol 1986; 57: 428.

35. Swensson RE, Valdes-Cruz LM, Sahn DJ, Sherman Sherman FS, Chung KJ, Scagnelli S, Hagen-Ansert S: Real-time Doppler color flow mapping for detection of patent ductus arteriosus. Am Coll Cardiol 1986; 8: 1105.

36. Feneley M, Gavaghan T: Paradoxical and pseudoparadoxical interventricular septal motion in patients with right ventricular volume overload. Circulation 1986; 74: 230.

37. Craig B, Smallhorn JF, Burrows P, Trusler GA, Rowe RD: Cross-sectional echocardiography in the evaluation of aortic valve prolapse associated with ventricular septal defect. Am Heart J 1986; 112: 800.

38. Albolias ET, Seward JB, Hagler DJ, Danielson GK, Puga FJ, Tajik AJ: Impact of two-dimensional and Doppler echocardiography on care of children aged two years and younger. Am J Cardiol 1988; 61: 166.

39. Schmidt KG, Cooper MJ, Silverman NH, Stanger P: Pulmonary artery origin of the left coronary artery: Diagnosis by two-dimensional echocardiography, pulsed Doppler ultrasound and color flow mapping. J Am Coll Cardiol 1988; 11: 396.

40. Frantz EG, Silverman NH: Doppler ultrasound evaluation of valvar pulmonary stenosis from multiple transduver positions in children requiring pulmonary valvuloplasty. Am J Cardiol 1988; 61: 844.

4. Coronary artery disease

1. Kerber RE, Abboud FM: Echocardiographic detection of regional myocardial infarction. Circulation 1973; 47: 997.

2. Jacobs JJ, Feigenbaum H, Corya BC, Phillips JF: Detection of left ventricular asynergy by echocardiography. Circulation 1973; 48: 263.

3. Yoshikawa J, Owaki T, Kato H, Tanaka K: Ultrasonic diagnosis of ventricular aneurysm. Jpn Heart J 1975; 16: 394.

4. Corya BC, Rasmussen S, Knoebel SB, Feigenbaum H. Echocardiography in acute myocardial infarction. Am J Cardiol 1975; 36: 1.

5. Weyman AE, Peskoe SM, Williams ES, Dillon JC, Feigenbaum H: Detection of left ventricular aneurysms by cross-sectional echocardiography. Circulation 1976; 54: 936.

6. Weyman AE, Feigenbaum H, Dillon JC, Johnston KW, Eggleton RC: Noninvasive visualization of the left main coronary artery by cross-sectional echocardiography. Circulation 1976; 54: 169.

7. Rasmussen S, Corya BC, Feigenbaum H, Knoebel SB: Detection of myocardial scar tissue by M-mode echocardiography. Circulation 1978; 57: 230.

8. Kisslo JA, Robertson D, Gilbert BW, von Ramm OT, Behar VS: A comparison of real-time, two-dimensional echocardiography and cineangiography in detecting left ventricular asynergy. Circulation 1977; 55: 134.

9. Eaton LW, Weiss JL, Bulkley BH, Garrison JB, Weisfeldt ML: Regional cardiac dilatation after acute myocardial infarction. N Engl J Med 1979; 300: 57.

10. Meltzer RS, Woythaler JN, Buda AJ, Griffin JC, Harrison WD, Martin RP, Harrison DC, Popp RL. Two-dimensional echocardiographic quantification of infarct size alteration by pharmacologic agents. Am J Cardiol 1979; 44: 257.

11. Wann LS, Faris JV, Childress RH, Dillon JC, Weyman AE, Feigenbaum H: Exercise cross-sectional echocardiography in ischemic heart disease. Circulation 1979; 60: 1300.

12. Heger JJ, Weyman AE, Wann LS, Dillon JC, Feigenbaum H: Cross-sectional echocardiography in acute myocardial infarction: detection and localization of regional left ventricular asynergy. Circulation 1979; 60: 531.

13. Ogawa S, Hubbard FE, Mardelli TJ, Dreifus LS: Cross-sectional echocardiographic spectrum of papillary muscle dysfunction. Am Heart J 1979; 97: 312.

14. DeMaria AN, Bommer W, Neumann A, Grehl T, Weinart L, Denard S, Amsterdam EA, Mason DT: Left ventricular thrombi identified by cross-sectional echocardiography. Ann Int Med 1979; 42: 261.

15. Meltzer RS, Guthaner D, Rakowski H, Popp RL, Martin RP: Diagnosis of left ventricular thrombi by two-dimensional echocardiography. Br Heart J 1979; 42: 261.

16. Hiraishi S, Yashiro K, Kusano S: Noninvasive visualization of coronary arterial aneurysm in infants and young children with mucocutaneous lymph node syndrome. Am J Cardiol 1979; 43: 1225.

17. Yoshikawa J, Yanagihara K, Owaki T, Kato H, Takagi Y, Okumachi F, Fukaya T, Tomita Y, Baba K. Cross-sectional echocardiographic diagnosis of coronary artery aneurysms in patients with the mucocutaneous lymph node syndrome. Circulation 1979; 59: 133.

18. Farcot JC, Boisante L, Rigaud M, Bardet J, Bourdarias JP: Two-dimensional echocardiographic visualization of ventricular septal rupture after acute anterior myocardial infarction. Am J Cardiol 1980; 370: 45.

19. Heger JJ, Weyman AE, Wann LS, Rogers EW, Killon JC, Feigenbaum H: Cross-sectional echocardiographic analysis of the extent of left ventricular asynergy in acute myocardial infarction. Circulation 1980; 61: 1113.

20. Come PC, Markis LE, Vine HS, Sacks B, Martin CE, Zelis RF: Echocardiographic diagnosis of left ventricular thrombi. Am Heart J 1980; 100: 523.

21. Weiss JL, Bulkley BH, Hutchins GM, Mason SJ: Two-dimensional echocardiographic recognition of myocardial injury in man: comparison with postmortem studies. Circulation 1981; 63: 401.

22. Godley RW, Wann LS, Rogers EW, Feigenbaum H, Weyman AE: Incomplete mitral leaflet closure in patients with papillary muscle dysfunction. Circulation 1981; 63: 565.

23. Parisi AF, Moynihan PF, Folland ED, Feldman CL. Quantitative detection of regional left ventricular contraction abnormalities by two-dimensional echocardiography. II Accuracy in coronary artery disease. Circulation 1981; 63: 761.

24. Horowitz RS, Morganorth J, Parrotto C, Cher CC, Soffer J, Pauletto FJ: Immediate diagnosis of acute myocardial infarction by two-dimensional echocardiography. Circulation 1982; 65: 323.

25. Armstrong WF, Mueller TM, Kinney EL, Tickner EG, Dillon JC, Feigenbaum H: Assessment of myocardial perfusion abnormalities with contrast enhanced two-dimensional echocardiography. Circulation 1982; 66: 166.

26. Nieminen M, Parisi AF, O'Boyle JE, Folland ED, Khuri S, Kloner RA: Serial evaluation of myocardial thickening and thinning in acute experimental infarction: identification and quantification using two-dimensional echocardiography. Circulation 1982; 66: 174.

27. Gibson RS, Bishop HL, Stamm RB, Crampton RS, Beller GA, Martin RP: Value of early two-dimensional echocardiography in patients with acute myocardial infarction. Am J Cardiol 1982; 49: 1110.

28. Rink LD, Feigenbaum H, Godley RW, Weyman AE, Dillon JC, Phillips JF, Marshall JE. Echocardiographic detection of left main coronary artery obstruction. Circulation 1982; 65: 719.

29. Visser CA, Kan G, David GK, Lie KI, Durrer D. Echocardiographic-cineangiographic correlation in detecting left ventricular aneurysm: a prospective study of 422 patients.

30. Mikell FL, Asinger RW, Elsperger KJ, Anderson WR, Hodges M: Tissue acoustic prosperities of fresh left ventricular thrombi and visualization by two-dimensional echocardiography: experimental observations. Am J Cardiol 1982; 49: 1157.

31. Stratton JR, Lighty GW jr, Pearlman AS, Ritchie JL: Detection of left ventricular thrombus by two-dimensional echocardiography: sensitivity, specificity and causes of uncertainty. Circulation 1982; 66: 156.
32. Nishimura RA, Tajik AJ, Shub C, Miller FA, Ilstrup DM, Harrison CE: Role of two-dimensional echocardiography in the prediction of in-hospital complications after acute myocardial infarction. J Am Coll Cardiol 1984; 4: 1080.
33. Recusani F, Raisdaro A, Sgalambro A, Tronconi L, Venco A, Salerno J, Ardissino D: Ventricular septal rupture after myocardial infarction: Diagnosis by two-dimensional and pulsed Doppler echocardiography. Am J Cardiol 1984; 54: 277.
34. Sharkey SW, Shelley W, Carlyle PF, Rysavy J, Cohn JN: M-mode and two-dimensional echocardiographic analysis of the septum in experimental right ventricular infarction: correlation with hemodynamic alterations. Am Heart J 1985; 110: 1210.
35. Chen Y, Sherrid MV, Dwyer EM: Value of two-dimensional echocardiography in evaluating coronary artery disease: a randomized blinded analysis. J Am Coll Cardiol 1985; 5: 911.
36. Bellamy GR, Rasmussen HH, Nasser FN, Wiseman JC, Cooper RA: Value of two-dimensional echocardiography, electrocardiography and clinical signs in detecting right ventricular infarction. Am Heart J 1986; 112: 304.
37. Loperrefido F, Biasucci LM, Pennestri' F, Laurenzi F, Gimigliand F, Vigna C, Rossi E, Favuzzi A, Santarelli P, Manzoli U. Pulsed Doppler echocardiographic analysis of mitral regurgitation after myocardial infarction. Am J Cardiol 1986; 58: 692.
38. Sharkey SW, Asinger WS, Elsperger KJ, Siegel J: Two-dimensional echocardiographic detection of left ventricular posterior wall motion abnormalities using an inferior angulation view. Am J Cardiol 1986; 58: 704.
39. Saner H, Asinger RW, Daniel JA, Olson J: Two-dimensional echocardiographic identification of left ventricular pseudoaneurysm. Am Heart J 1986; 112: 977.
40. Kloner RA, Parisi AF: Acute myocardial infarction: diagnostic and prognostic application of two-dimensional echocardiography. Circulation 1987; 75: 521.
41. Izumi S, Miyatake K, Beppu S, Park YD, Nagata S, Kinoshita N, Sakakibara H, Nimura Y: Mechanism of mitral regurgitation in patients with myocardial infarction: A study using real-time two-dimensional Doppler flow imaging and echocardiography. Circulation 1987; 76: 777.

5. Myocardial diseases

1. Shah PM, Gramiak R, Kramer DH: Ultrasound localization of left ventricular outflow obstruction in hypertrophic obstructive cardiomyopathy. Circulation 1969; 40: 3.
2. Popp RL, Harrison DC: Ultrasound in the diagnosis and evaluation of therapy of idiopathic hypertrophic subaortic stenosis. Circulation 1969; 40: 905.
3. Henry WL, Clark CE, Epstein SE: Asymmetric septal hypertrophy (ASH): echocardiographic identification of the pathognomonic anatomic abnormality of IHSS. Circulation 1973; 47: 1153.
4. Corya BC, Feigenbaum H, Rasmussen S, Black MJ: Echocardiographic features of congestive cardiomyopathy compared with normal subjects and patients with coronary artery disease. Circulation 1974; 49: 1153.
5. Henry WL, Clark CE, Roberts WC, Morrow AG, Epstein SE: Differences in distribution of myocardial abnormalities in patients with obstructive and nonobstractive asymmetric septal hypertrophy (ASH). Circulation 1974; 50: 447.
6. Henry WL, Clark CE, Griffith JM, Epstein SE: Mechanism of left ventricular outflow obstructive asymmetric septal hypertrophy (Idiopathic hypertrophic subaortic stenosis). Am J Cardiol 1975; 35: 337.
7. Child JS, Levisman JA, Abbasi AS, MacAlpin RN: Echocardiographic manifestations of infiltrative cardiomyopathy: a report of seven cases due to amyloid. Chest 1976; 70: 184.
8. Borer JS, Henry WJ, Epstein SE: Echocardiographic observations in patients with systemic infiltrative disease involving the heart. Am J Cardiol 1977; 39: 184.
9. Henry WL, Nienhuis AW, Wiener M, Miller DR, Canale VC, Piomelli S: Echocardiographic abnormalities in patients with transfusion-dependent anemia and secondary myocardial iron deposition. Am J Med 1978; 64: 547.
10. Shimada H, Inoue M, Tamura T, Ishihara T, Kanemitsu H, Ishikawa K: Echocardiograms in progressive muscular dystrophy. J Cardiography 1978; 64: 547.
11. Martin RP, Rakowski H, Frenth J, Popp RL: Idiopathic hypertrophic subaortic stenosis viewed by wide-angle, phased-array echocardiography. Circulation 1979; 59: 206.
12. Giltert BS, Pollic C, Adelman AG, Wigle ED: Hypertrophic cardiomyopathy: Subclassification by M-mode echocardiography. Am J Cardiol 1980; 45: 861.
13. Dol YL, McKenna WJ, Gehrke J, Oakley CM, Goodwin JF: M-mode echocardiography in hypertrophic cardiomyopathy. Diagnostic criteria and prediction of obstruction. Am J Cardiol 1980; 45: 6.

14. Siqueria-Filho AG, Cunha CLP, Tajik AJ, Seward JB, Schattenberg TT, Giuliani ER: M-mode and two-dimensional echocardiographic features of cardiac amyloidosis. Circulation 1981; 63: 188.
15. Pollick C, Pittman M, Filly K, Fitzgerald PJ, Popp RL: Mitral and aortic valve orifice area in normal subjects and in patients with congestive cardiomyopathy: determination by two-dimensional echocardiography. Am J Cardiol 1982; 49: 1191.
16. Callahan JA, Wroblewski EM, Reeder GS, Edwards WD, Seward EM, Tajik AJ: Echocardiographic features of carcinoid heart disease. Am J Cardiol 1981; 50: 762.
17. Pollick C, Rakowski H, Wigle ED: Muscular subaortic stenosis: the quantitative relationship between systolic anterior motion and the pressure gradient. Circulation 1984; 69: 43.
18. Maron BJ, Gottdiener JS, Arce J, Rosing DR, Wesley YE, Epstein SE: Dynamic subaortic obstruction in hypertrophic cardiomyopathy:-analysis by pulsed Doppler echocardiography. J Am Coll Cardiol 1985; 6: 1.
19. Gartin JM, Dabestani A, Glasgow GA, Butman S, Burn CS, Henry WL: Echocardiographic and Doppler flow observations in obstructed and nonobstracted hypertrophic cardiomyopathy. Am J Cardiol 1985; 56: 546.
20. Spirito P, Maron BJ, Chiarella F, Bellotti P, Tramarin R, Pozzoli M, Vecchio C: Diastolic abnormalities in patients with hypertrophic cardiomyopathy: relation to magnitude of left ventricular hypertrophy. Circulation 1985; 72: 310.
21. Takenaka K, Dabestani A, Gardin JM, Russell D, Clark S, Allfie A, Henry WL: Pulsed Doppler echocardiographic study of left ventricular filling in dilated cardiomyopathy. Am J Cardiol 1986; 58: 143.
22. Goldman ME, Cantor R, Schwartz MF, Barker M, Desnick RJ: Echocardiographic abnormalities and disease severity in Fabry's disease. J Am Coll Caediol 1986; 7: 1157.
23. Hongo M, Ikeda S. Echocardiographic assessment of the evolution of amyloid heart disease: a study with familial amyloid polyneuropathy. Circulation 1986; 73: 249.
24. Falk RH, Plehn JF, Deering T, Schick EC, Boinay P, Rubinow A, Skinner N, Cohen AS: Sensitivity and specificity of the echocardiographic features of cardiac amyloidosis. Am J Cardiol 1987; 59: 418.
25. Wigle ED: Hypertrophic cardiomyopathy: a 1987 viewpoint. Circulation 1987; 75: 311.
26. Sasson Z, Yock PG, Hatle LK, Alderman EL, Popp RL: Doppler echocardiographic determination of the pressure gradient in hypertrophic cardiomyopathy. J Am Coll Cardiol 1988; 11: 752.

6. Other cardiac diseases

1. Effert S, Domaning E: The diagnosis of intraatrial tumor and thrombi by the ultrasonic echo method. Dtsch Med Wochenschr 1959; 84: 6
2. Feigeman H, Waldhausen JA, Hyde LP: Ultrasound diagnosis of pericardial effusion. JAMA 1965; 191: 107.
3. Wolfe SB, Popp, RL, Feigenbaum H: Diagnosis of atrial tumors by ultrasound. Circulation 1969; 39: 615.
4. Nasser WK, Davis RH, Dillon JC, Tavel ME, Helmen CH, Feigenbaum H, Fisch C: Atrial myxoma. II. Phonocardiographic, echocardiographic, hemodynamic and angiographic features in nine cases. Am Heart J 1972; 83: 810.
5. Harbold NB Jr, Gau GTJ: Echocardiographic diagnosis of right atrial myxoma. Mayo Clin Proc 1973; 48: 284.
6. Nasser WK, Gramiak R, Shah PM: Diagnosis of aortic dissection by echocardiography. Circulation 1973; 48: 506.
7. Horowitz MS, Schulz CS, Stinson EB, Harrison DC, Popp RL: Sensitivity and specificity of echocardiographic diagnosis of pericardial effusion. Circulation 1974; 50: 239.
8. D'Cruz IA, Cohen HC, Prabhu R, Glick G: Diagnosis of cardiac tamponade by echocardiography: changes in mitral valve motion and ventricular dimensions, with special reference to paradoxical pulse. Circulation 1975; 52: 460.
9. Pool EP, Seagren SC, Abbasi AS, Dharuzi Y, Kraus R: Echocardiographic manifestations of constrictive pericarditis. Chest 1975; 68: 684.
10. Levisman JA, MacAlpin RN, Abbasi AS, Ellis N, Eber LM: Echocardiographic diagnosis of a mobile, pedunculated tumor in the left ventricular cavity. Am J Cardiol 1975; 36: 17.
11. Brown OR, Popp RL, Kloster FE: Echocardiographic criteria for aortic root dissection. Am J Cardiol 1975; 36: 17.
12. Meller J, Techholz LE, Pichard AD, Matta R, Litwak R, Herman MV, Massie KF: Left ventricular myxoma. Echocardiographic diagnosis and review of the literature. Am J Med 1977; 63: 816.
13. Morgan DL, Palazola J, Reed W, Bell HH, Kindred LH, Beauchamp GD: Left heart myxomas. Am J Cardiol 1977; 40: 611.
14. Schnittger I, Bowden RE, Abram J, Popp RL: Pericardial thickening and constractive pericarditis. Am J Cardiol 1978; 42: 388.

15. Martin RP, Rakowski H, French J, Popp RL: Localization of pericardial effusion with wide angle phased array echocardiography. Am J Cardiol 1978; 42: 904.

16. Ports TA, Cogan J, Schiller NB, Rapaport E: Echocardiography of left ventricular mass. Circulation 1978; 58: 528.

17. Yoshikawa J, Sabah I, Yanagihara K, Owaki T, Kato H, Tanemoto K: Cross-sectional echocardiographic diagnosis of large left atrial tumor and extracardiac tumor compressing the left atrium. Am J Cardiol 1978; 42: 853.

18. Horowitz MS, Rossen R, Harrison DC: Echocardiographic diagnosis of pericardial disease. Am Heart J 1979; 97: 420.

19. Lappe DL, Bulkley BH, Weiss JL: Two-dimensional echocardiographic diagnosis of left atrial myxoma. Chest 1978; 74: 55.

20. Shiina S, Yaginuma T, Kondo K, Kawai N, Hosoda S: Echocardiographic evaluation of impeding cardiac tamponade. J Cardiography 1979; 9: 555.

21. D'Cruz I, Panetta F, Cohen H, Glock G: Submitral calcification or sclerosis in elderly patients. M-mode and two-dimensional echocardiography in mitral annulus calcification. Am J Cardiol 1979; 44: 31.

22. DeMaria AN, Bommer W, Neumann A, Weinert L, Borgen H, Mason DT: Identification of aneurysms of the ascending aorta by cross-sectional echocardiography. Circulation 1979; 59: 755.

23. Mintz GS, Kotler MN, Segal BL, Parry WR: Two-dimensional echocardiographic recognition of the descending thoracic aorta. Am J Cardiol 1979; 44: 232.

24. Fulkerson PK, Beaver BM, Auseon JC, Graber HL: Calcification of the mitral annulas. Etiology, clinical associations, complications and therapy. Am J Med 1979; 66: 967.

25. Matsuo H, Matsumoto M, Hamanaka Y, Ohara T, Senda S, Inoue M, Abe H: Rotational excursion of heart in massive pericardial effusion studied by phased-array echocardiography. Br Heart J 1979; 41: 513.

26. Haaz WS, Mintz GS, Kotler MN, Parry W, Segal BL: Two-dimensional echocardiographic recognition of the descending thoracic aorta: value in differentiating pericardial from pleural effusions. Am J Cardiol 1980; 46: 739.

27. Martin RP, Bowden R, Filly K, Popp RL: Intrapericardial abnormalities in patients with pericardial effusion: findings by two-dimensional echocardiography. Circulation 1980; 61: 568.

28. DePace NL, Soulen RL, Kotler MN, Mintz GS: Two-dimensional echocardiographic detection of intraatrial masses. Am J Cardiol 1981; 48: 1155.

29. Victor MF, Mintz GS, Kotler MN, Wilson AR, Segal BL. Two-dimensional echocardiographic diagnosis of aortic dissection. Am J Cardiol 1981; 46: 374.

30. Shapiro LM, Mackinnon J, Beevers DG: Echocardiographic features of malignant hypertension. Br Heart J 1981; 46: 374.

31. Cohn A, Hagan AD, Watkins J, Mitas J, Schwartzman M, Mazzolen A, Cohen IM, Warren SE, Vieweg WR: Clinical correlations in hypertensive patients with left ventricular hypertrophy diagnosed with echocardiogram. Am J Cardiol 1981; 47: 334.

32. Perry B, King J, Zeft H, Manley J, Gross C, Wann L: Two-dimensional echocardiography in the diagnosis of left atrial myxoma. Br Heart J 1981; 43: 667–71.

33. Donaldson RM, Emanuel RW, Earl CJ: The role of two-dimensional echocardiography in the detection of potentially embolic intra-cardiac masses in patients with cerebral ischemia. J Neurol Neurosurg Psychiatry 1981; 44: 803–9.

34. Niederle P, Stepanek Z, Grospic A, et al: Character of mitral valve flow in left atrial tumor. Eur J Cardiol 1981; 12: 357.

35. Armstrong WFW, Schilt BF, Helper DJ, Dillon JC, Feigenbaum H: Diastolic collapse of the right ventricle with cardiac tamponade: an echocardiographic study. Circulation 1982; 65: 1491.

36. Hiceto S, Antonelli G, Biasco G, Rizzon P: Two-dimensional echocardiographic evaluation of aneurysms of the descending thoracic aorta. Circulation 1982; 66: 1045.

37. Panidis IP, Kotler MN, Mintz GS, Ross J: Clinical and echocardiographic features of right atrial masses. Am Heart J 1984; 107: 745.

38. Iwase M, Yokota M, Takagi S, Koide M, Hu XJ, Kawai N, Hayashi H, Sotobata I, Tanaka M: The disturbance of left ventricular inflow by prolapsing and non-prolasping left atrial myxoma: estimation with pulse Doppler echocardiography. In Cardiac Doppler Diagnosis ed. by Spencer MP. Martinus Nijhoff Publishers, Boston. 1984; 205.

39. Kutalek SP, Panidis IP, Kotler MN, Mintz GS, Carver J, Ross JJ: Metastatic tumors of the heart detected by two-dimensional echocardiography. Am Heart J 1985; 109: 343.

40. Fyke III FE, Seward JB, Edwards WD, Miller FA, Reeder GS, Schattenberg TT, Clarence S, Callahan JA, Tajik AJ. Primary cardiac tumors: experience with 30 consecutive patients since the introduction of two-

dimensional echocardiography. J Am Coll Cardiol 1985; 5: 1465.

41. Engle PJ, Fowler NO, Tei C, Shah PM, Driedger HJ, Shan PM, Driedger HJ, Shabetao R, Haebin AD, Franch RH: M-mode echocardiography in constrictive pericarditis. J Am Coll Cardiol 1985; 6: 471.
42. Bass JL, Breningstall GN, Swaiman KF: Echocardiographic incidence of cardiac rhabdomyoma in tuberous sclerosis. Am J Cardiol 1985; 55: 1379.
43. Luetmer PH, Edwards WD, Seward JB, Tajik AJ: Incidence and distribution of left ventricular false tendons: an autopsy study of 483 normal human hearts. J Am Coll Cardiol 1986; 8: 179.
44. Kasper W, Meinertz T, Henkel B, Eissner D, Hahn K, Hofman T, Zeiher A, Just H: Echocardiographic findings in patients with proved pulmonary embolism. Am Heart J 1986; 112: 1284.
45. Vargas-Barron J, Lacy-Niebla MC, Keirns C, Gonzalez-Medina AR, Bassa-Kury R, Dubach P: Pulsed Doppler echocardiographic analysis of atrioventricular flow changes in patients with atrial myxomas. Am Heart J 1986; 112: 850.
46. Goli V, Thadani U, Thomas SR, Voyles W, Teague SM. Doppler echocardiographic profiles in obstructive right and left atrial myxomas. J Am Coll Cardiol 1987; 9: 701.

7. Left ventricular function

1. Feigenbaum H, Zaky A, Nasser WK. Use of ultrasound to measure left ventricular stroke volume. Circulation 1967; 35: 1092.
2. Popp RL, Wolfe SB, Hirata T, Feigenbaum H: Estimation of right and left ventricular size by ultrasound. Am J Cardiol 1969; 24: 523.
3. Pombo JF, Troy BL, Russel RO Jr: Left ventricular volumes and ejection fraction by echocardiography. Circulation 1971; 43: 26.
4. Fortuin NJ, Hood WP Jr, Craige E: Evaluation of left ventricular function by echocardiography. Circulation 1972; 46: 26.
5. Konecke LL, Feigenbaum H, Chang S, Corya BC, Fischer JC: Abnormal mitral valve motion in patients with elevated left ventricular diastolic pressures. Circulation 1973; 47: 989.
6. Grossman W, McLaurin LP, Moss SP, Stefadouros M, Young DT: Wall thickness and diastolic properties of the left ventricle. Circulation 1974; 49: 129.
7. Teichholz LE, Cohen MV, Sonnenblock EH, Gorlin R: Study of left ventricular geometry and function by B-scan ultrasonography in patients with and without asynergy. N Engl J Med 1974; 291: 1220.
8. Grossman W, Jones D, McLaurin LP: Wall stress and patterns of hypertrophy. J Clin Invest 1975; 56: 56.
9. Linhart JW, Mintz GS, Segal BL, Kawai N, Kotler MN: Left ventricular volume measurement by echocardiography: fact or fiction? Am J Cardiol 1976; 37: 7.
10. Teichholz LE, Kreulen T, Herman M, Gorlin R: Problems in echocardiographic volume determinations: echocardiographic-angiographic correlations in the presence or absence of asynergy. Am J Cardiol 1976; 37: 7.
11. Upton MT, Gibson DG, Brown DJ: Echocardiographic assessment of abnormal left ventricular relaxation in man. Br Heart J 1976; 38: 1001.
12. Devereux RB, Reichek N: Echocardiographic determination of left ventricular mass in man. Circulation 1977; 55: 613.
13. Massie BM, Schiller NB, Ratshin RA, Parmley WW. Mitral-septal separation: a new echocardiographic index of left ventricular function. Am J Cardiol 1977; 39: 1008.
14. Fortuin NJ, pawsey CGK. The evaluation of left ventricular function by echocardiography. Am J Cardiol 1977; 63: 1.
15. Parkash R: Determination of right ventricular wall thickness in systole and necropsy correlation in 32 patients. Br Heart J 1978; 40: 1257.
16. Trail TA, Gilson DG, Brown DJ: Study of left ventricular wall thickness and dimension changes using echocardiography. Br Heart J 1978; 40: 1257.
17. Bommer W, Weinert L, Neumann A, Neef J, Mason DT, DeMaria AN: Determination of right atrial and right ventricular size by two-dimensional echocardiography. Circulation 1979; 60: 320.
18. Eaton LW, Maughan WL, Shoukas AA, Weiss JL: Accurate volume determination in the isolated ejecting canine left ventricle by two-dimensional echocardiography. Circulation 1979; 320: 60.
19. Folland ED, Parisi AF, Moynihan PF, Jones DR, Feldman CL, Tow DE: Assessment of left ventricular ejection fraction and volumes by real-time, two-dimensional echocardiography. A comparison of cineangiographic and radionuclide techniques. Circulation 1979; 60: 760.
20. Gibson DG, Brown DJ: Assessment of left ventricular systolic function in man from simultaneous echocar-

diographic and pressure measurements. Br Heart J 1979; 38: 8.

21. Kronik G, Slany J, Mosslacher H: Comparative value of eight M-mode echocardiographic formulas for determining left ventricular stroke volume. Circulation 1979; 60: 1308.

22. Schiller NB, Axquatella H, Ports TA, Drew D, Goerke J, Ringertz H, Silverman NH, Brundage B, Botvinck EH, Boswell R, Carlsson E, Parmley WW: Left ventricular volume from paired biplane two-dimensional echocardiography. Circulation 1979; 60: 547.

23. Sugishita Y, Koseki S: Dynamic exercise echocardiography. Circulation 1979; 60: 743.

24. Clark RD, Korcuska K, Cohn K: Serial echocardiographic evaluation of left ventricular function in valvular disease, including reproducibility guidelines for serial studies. Circulation 1980; 62: 564.

25. Stalling MR, Crawford MH, Sorensen SG, Levi B, Richards KL, O'Rourke RA: Comparative accuracy of apical biplane cross-sectional echocardiography and gated equilibrium radionuclide angiography for estimating left ventricular size and performance. Circulation 1981; 63: 1075.

26. Popp RL: M-mode echocardiographic assessment of left ventricular function. Am J Cardiol 1982; 49: 1312.

27. Schnittger I, Fitzgerald PJ, Daughter GT, Ingels NB, Krantrowitz NE, Schwarzkopf A, Mead CW, Popp RL: Limitations of comparing left ventricular volumes by two-dimensional echocardiography, myocardial markers and cinéangiography. Am J Cardiol 1982; 50: 512.

28. Staring MR, Crawford MH, Sorensen SG, O'Rourke RA: A new two-dimensional echocardiographic technique for evaluating right ventricular size and performance in patients with obstructive lung disease. Circulation 1982; 66: 612.

29. Elkayam U, Gardin JM, Berkley R, Hughes CA, Henry WL: The use of Doppler flow velocity measurement to assess the hemodynamic response to vasodilators in patients with heart failure. Circulation 1983; 67: 377.

30. Tortoledo FA, Quinones MA, Fernandez GC, Waggoner AD, Winters WL: Quantification of left ventricular volumes by two-dimensional echocardiography: a simplified and accurate approach. Circulation 1983; 67: 579.

31. Huntsman LL, Stewart DK, Barnes SR, Franklin SB, Colocousis JS, Hessel EA. Noninvasive Doppler determination of cardiac output in man, clinical validation. Circulation 1983; 67: 872.

32. Fisher DC, Sahn DJ, Friedman MJ, Larson D, Lillian M, Cruz V, Horowitz S, Goldbery SJ, Allen HD: The mitral valve orifice method for noninvasive two-dimensional echo Doppler determinations of cardiac output. Circulation 1983; 67: 872.

33. Iwase M, Yokota M, Takagi S, Koide M, Kawai N, Yoshida R, Hayashi H, Sotobata I: Analysis of diastolic behavior of the left ventricle on dynamic exercise by pulse Doppler combined with 2-D echocardiograph. Cardiac Doppler Diagnosis ed. by Spencer MP. Martinus Nijhoff, Publishers, Boston. 1983; 121.

34. Woythaler JN, Singer SL, Kwan OL, Meltzer RS, Reulner B, Bommer W, DeMaria AN: Accuracy of echocardiography versus electrocardiography in detecting left ventricular hypertrophy: comparison with post-mortem mass measurement. J Am Coll Cardiol 1983; 2: 305.

35. Lewis JF, Kuo LC, Nelson JG, Limacher MC, Quinones MA: Pulsed Doppler echocardiographic determination of stroke volume and cardiac output: clinical validation of two new methods using the apical window. Circulation 1984; 70: 425.

36. Rokey R, Kio LC, Zoghbi WA, Limacher MC, Quinones MA: Determination of parameters of left ventricular diastolic filling with pulsed Doppler echocardiography: comparison with cinéangiography. Circulation 1985; 71: 543.

37. Gardin JM, Tobis JT, Dabestani A, Smith C, Elkayam U, Castleman E, White D, Allfie A, Henry W: Superiority of two-dimensional echocardiographic measurement of aortic vessel diameter in Doppler echocardiographic estimations of left ventricular stroke volume. J Am Coll Cardiol 1985; 6: 66.

38. Daley P, Sagar KB, Wann LS: Doppler echocardiographic measurement of flow velocity in the ascending aorta during supine and upright exercise. Br Heart J 1985; 54: 562.

39. Devereux RB, Alonso DR, Lutas EM, Gottlieb GJ, Campo E, Sachs I, Reichek N: Echocardiographic assessment of left ventricular hypertrophy: comparison to necropsy findings. Am J Cardiol 1986; 57: 450.

40. Gardin JM, Dabestani A, Takenaka K, Rohan MK, Knoll M, Russell D, Henry WL: Effect of imaging view and sample volume location on evaluation of mitral flow velocity by pulsed Doppler echocardiography. Am J Cardiol 1986; 57: 1335.

41. Bryg RJ, Labovitz AJ, Mehdirad AA, Williams GA, Chaitman BR: Effect of coronary artery disease on Doppler-derived parameter of aortic flow during upright exercise. Am J Cardiol 1986; 58: 14.

42. Wallmer K, Wann LS, Sagar KB, Kalbfleisch J, Klopfenstein HS: The influence of preload and heart rate on Doppler echocardiographic indexes of left ventricular performance: comparison with invasive indexes in an experimental preparation. Circulation 1986; 74: 181.

43. Sabbah HN, Khaja F, Brymer JF, McFarland TM, Albert DE, Snyder JE, Goldstein S, Stein P: Noninvasive evaluation of ventricular performance based on peak aortic blood accelation measured with a continuous-wave Doppler velocity meter. Circulation 1986; 74: 323.

44. Higginbotham MB, Morris KG, Williams S, Mchale PA, Coleman RE, Cobb FR: Regulation of stroke volume during submaximal and maximal upright exercise in normal man. Circ Res 1986; 58: 281.

45. Spirito P, Maron BJ, Bellotti P, Chiarella F, Vecchio C: Noninvasive assessment of left ventricular diastolic function: Comparative analysis of pulsed Doppler ultrasound and digitized M-mode echocardiography. Am J Cardiol 1986; 58: 837.

46. Mehdirad AA, Williams GA, Labovitz AJ, Bryg RJ, Chaitman BR: Evaluation of left ventricular function during upright exercise: correlation of exercise Doppler with postexercise two-dimensional echocardiographic results. Circulation 1987; 75: 413.

47. Sabbah HN, Przybylski J, Albert DE, Stein PD: Peak aortic blood acceleration reflects the extent of left ventricular ischemic mass at risk. Am Heart J 1987; 113: 885.

48. Iwase M, Sotobata I, Takagi S, Miyaguchi K, Jing HX, Yokota M: Effects of diltiazem on left ventricular diastolic behavior in patients with hypertrophic cardiomyopathy: evaluation with exercise pulsed Doppler echocardiography. J Am Coll Cardiol 1987; 9: 1099.

49. Labovitz AJ, Pearson AC: Evaluation of left ventricular diastolic function: Clinical relevance and recent Doppler echocardiographic insights. Am Heart J 1987; 114: 836.

50. Maron BJ, Spirito P, Green KJ, Wesley YE, Bonow RO, Arce J: Noninvasive assessment of left ventricular diastolic function by pulsed Doppler echocardiography in patients with hypertrophic cardiomyopathy. J Am Coll Cardiol 1987; 10: 733.

51. Choong CY, Herrmann HC, Weyman AE, Fifer MA: Preload dependance of Doppler-derived indexes of left ventricular diastolic function in humans. J Am Coll Cardiol 1987; 10: 800.

52. Christie J, Sheldahl LM, Tristani FE, Sagar KB, Ptacin MJ, Wann S: Determination of stroke volume and cardiac output during exercise: Comparison of two-dimensional and Doppler echocardiography, Fick oximetry, and thermodilution. Circulation 1987; 76: 539.

53. Ihren H, Endrsesn K, Golf S, Nitter-Hauge S: Cardiac stroke volume during exercise measured by Doppler echocardiography: Comparison with the thermodilution technique and evaluation of reproducibility. Br Heart J 1987; 58: 455.

8. Pulmonary hypertension

1. Gramiak R, Nanda NC, Shah PM: Echocardiographic detection of the pulmonary valve. Radiology 1972; 102: 153.

2. Sakamote T, Matsuhisa M, Hayashi T, Ichiyasu H: Echocardiogram of the pulmonary valve. Jpn Heart J 1974; 15: 360.

3. Weyman AE, Dillon JC, Feigenbaum H, Chag S: Echocardiographic patterns of pulmonic valve motion with pulmonary hypertension. Circulation 1974; 50: 905.

4. Lew W, Karliner JS: Assessment of pulmonary valve echogram in normal subjects and in patients with pulmonary arterial hypertension. Br Heart J 1979; 42: 147.

5. Aquatella H, Schiller NB, Sharpe DN, Chatterjee K: Lack of correlation between echocardiographic pulmonary valve morphology and simultaneous pulmonary arterial pressure. Am J Cardiol 1979; 43: 946.

6. Shiina A, Kondo K, Nakasone Y, Tsuchiya M, Yaginuma T, Hosoda S: Contrast echocardiographic evaluation of change in flow velocity in the right side of the heart. Circulation 1981; 63: 1408.

7. Tahara M, Tanaka H, Nakao S, Yoshimura H, Sakurai S, Tei C, Kashima T: Hemodynamic determinants of pulmonary valve motion during systole in experimental pulmonary hypertension. Circulation 1981; 64: 1249.

8. Hatle L, Angelsen BAJ, Tromsdal A: Noninvasive estimation of pulmonary artery systolic pressure with Doppler ultrasound. Br Heart J 1981; 45: 157.

9. Kitabatake A, Inoue M, Asao M, Masuyama T, Tanouchi J, Morita T, Mishima M, Uematsu M, Shimazu T, Hori M, Abe H: Noninvasive evaluation of pulmonary hypertension by a pulsed Doppler technique. Circulation 1983; 68: 302.

10. Okamoto M, Miyatake K, Kinoshita N, Sakakibara H, Nimura Y: Analysis of blood flow in pulmonary hypertension with the pulsed Doppler flowmeter combined with cross sectional echocardiography. Br Heart J 1984; 51: 407.

11. Kosturakis D, Goldberg SJ, Allen HD, Loeber C: Doppler echocardiographic prediction of pulmonary arterial hypertension in congenital heart disease. Am J Cardiol 1984; 53: 1110.

12. Serwer GA, Cougle AG, Eckerd JM, Armstrong BE: Factors affecting use of the Doppler-determined time from flow onset to maximal pulmonary artery velocity for measurement of pulmonary artery pressure in children. Am J Cardiol 1986; 58: 352.

13. Dabestani A, Mahan G, Gardin JM, Takenaka K, Burn C, Allfie A, Henry WL: Evaluation of pulmonary artery pressure and resistance by pulsed Doppler echocardiography. Am J Cardiol 1987; 59: 662.
14. Chan KL, Currie PJ, Seward JB, Hagler DJ, Mair DD, Tajik J: Comparison of three Doppler ultrasound methods in the prediction of pulmonary artery pressure. J Am Coll Cardiol 1987; 9: 549.

9. Arrhythmia

1. Benchimol A, Desser KB: Clinical application of the Doppler ultrasonic flowmeter. Am J Cardiol 1972; 29: 540.
2. Benchimol A, Desser KB, Wang TF, Morik: Left ventricular blood flow velocity during atrial arrhythmias in man. Am J Cardiol 1974; 34: 271.
3. DeMaria AN, Vera Z, Neumann A, Mason DT: Alterations in ventricular contraction pattern in the Wolff-Parkinson-White syndrome. Circulation 1976; 53: 249.
4. Hishida H, Sotobata I, Koike Y, Okumura M, Mizuno Y: Echocardiographic patterns of ventricular contraction in the Wolff-Parkinson-White syndrome. Circulation 1976; 54: 567.
5. DeMaria AN, Mason DT: Echocardiographic evaluation of disturbances of cardiac rhythm and conduction. Chest 1977; 71: 439.
6. Gomes JAC, Damato AN, Akhtar M, Dhatt MS, Calon AH, Reddy CP, Moran HE: Ventricular septal motion and left ventricular dimensions during abnormal ventricular activation. Am J Cardiol 1977; 39: 641.
7. D'Cruz IA, Prabhu R, Cohen HC, Glock G: Echocardiographic features of second degree atrioventricular block. Chest 1977; 72: 459.
8. Fujii J, Foster JR, Mills PG, Moos S, Graige E: Dual echocardiographic determination of atrial contraction sequence in atrial flutter and other related atrial arrhythmias. Circulation 1978; 58: 314.
9. Fujii J, Watanabe H, Watanabe T, Takahashi N, Ohta A, Kato K: M-mode and cross-sectional echocardiographic study of the left ventricular wall motions in complete left bundle branch block. Br Heart J 1979; 42: 255.
10. Uchiyama T, Corday E, Meerbaum S, Lang T, Gueret P, Povzhitkov M, Peter T: Characterization of left ventricular mechanical function during arrhythmias with two-dimensional echocardiography. 1. Premature ventricular contractions. Am J Cardiol 1981; 48: 679.
11. Cohn K, Kryda W: The influence of ectopic beats and tachy-arrhythmias on stroke volume and cardiac output. J Electrocardiol 1981; 14: 207.
12. Iwase M, Sotobata I, Yokota M, Takagi S, HuXiano Jung, Noda S, Kawai N, Hayashi H, Miyaguchi K, Tsuzuki J: Evaluation of left atrial rhythm with pulsed Doppler echocardiography. Int J Cardiac Imaging 1985; 1: 159.
13. Iwase M, Sotobata I, Yokota M, Takagi S, Hu XJ, Kawai N, Hayashi H, Murase M: Evaluation by pulsed Doppler echocardiography of the atrial contribution to left ventricular filling in patients with DDD pacemakers. Am J Cardiol 1986; 58: 104.
14. David D, Michelson EL, Naito M, Chen CC, Schaffenburg M, Dreifus LS: Diastolic 'locking' of the mitral valve: possible importance of diastolic myocardial properties. Circulation 1986; 73: 997.
15. Penidis IP, Ross J, Munley B, Nestico P, Mintz GS: Diastolic mitral regurgitation in patients with atrioventricular conduction abnormalities: a common finding by Doppler echocardiography. J Am Coll Cardiol 1986; 7: 768.
16. Rokey R, Murphy DJ, Nielsen AP, Abinader EG, Huhta JC, Quinones MA: Detection of diastolic atrioventricular valvular regurgitation by pulsed Doppler echocardiography and its association with complete heart block. Am J Cardiol 1986; 57: 692.

Additional references

The headings here correspond to those found between pages 282–296.

1. Basics and methodology of echocardiography

33. Sahn DJ, Yoganathan AP: Seminar on in vitro studies of cardiac flow and their applications for clinical Doppler echocardiography-I. J Am Coll Cardiol 1988; 12: 1343.

2. Valvular heart disease

92. Peller OG, Wallerson DC, Devereux RB: Role of Doppler and imaging echocardiography in selection of patients for cardiac valvular surgery. Am Heart J 1987; 114: 1445.
93. Carabello BA: Advances in the hemodynamic assessment of stenotic cardiac valves. J Am Coll Cardiol 1987; 10: 912.
94. Gorlin R: Calculation of cardiac valve stenosis: restoring an old concept for advanced applications. J Am Coll Cardiol 1987; 10: 920.
95. Fan PH, Kapur KK, Nanda NC: Color-guided Doppler echocardiographic assessment of aortic valve stenosis. J Am Coll Cardiol 1988; 12: 441.
96. Beard JT, Byrd BF: Saline contrast enhancement of trivial Doppler tricuspid regurgitation signals for estimating pulmonary artery pressure. Am J Cardiol 1988; 62: 486.
97. Jaffe WM, Roche AHG, Coverdale HA, McAlister HF, Ormiston JA, Green ER: Clinical evaluation versus Doppler echocardiography in the quantitative assessment of valvular heart disease. Circulation 1988; 78: 267.
98. Yoshida K, Yoshikawa J, Shakudo M, et al.: Color Doppler evaluation of valvular regurgitation in normal subjects. Circulation 1988; 78: 840.
99. Thomas JD, Wilkins GT, Choong CYP, et al.: Inaccuracy of mitral pressure half-time immediately after percutaneous mitral valvotomy: dependence on transmitral gradient and left atrial and ventricular compliance. Circulation 1988; 78: 980.

4. Coronary artery disease

42. Griffin B, Timmis AD, Sowton E: Contrast echocardiography: distribution and reproducibility of myocardial contrast enhancement in coronary heart disease. Am J Cardiol 1987; 60: 538.
43. Feinstein SB, Lang RN, Dick C, et al.: Contrast echocardiography during coronary arteriography in humans: perfusion and anatomic studies. J Am Coll Cardiol 1988; 11: 59.
44. Keller MW, Glasheen W, Smucker ML, et al.: Myocardial contrast echocardiography in humans. II. Assessment of coronary blood flow reserve. J Am Coll Cardiol 1988; 12: 925.

5. Myocardial diseases

27. McIntosh CL, Maron BJ: Current operative treatment of obstructive hypertrophic cardiomyopathy. Circulation 1988; 78: 487.
28. Come PC, Riley MF, Carl LV, Lorell B: Doppler evidence that true left ventricular-to-aortic pressure gradients exist in hypertrophic cardiomyopathy. Am Heart J 1988; 116: 1253.
29. Zoghbi WA, Haichin RN, Quinones MA: Mid-cavity obstruction in apical hypertrophy: Doppler evidence of diastolic intraventricular gradient with higher apical pressure. Am Heart J 1988; 116: 1469.

6. Other cardiac diseases

47. Erbel R, Borner N, Steller D, Brunier, Thelen M, Pfeiffer C, Moth-Kahaly S, Iversen S, Oelert H, Meyer J: Detection of aortic dissection by transesophageal echocardiography. Br Heart J 1987; 58: 45.
48. Rifkin RD, Pandian NG, Funai JT, et al.: Sensitivity of right atrial collapse and right ventricular diastolic collapse in the diagnosis of graded cardiac tamponade. Am J Noninvas Cardiol 1987; 1: 73.
49. Boyd MT, Seward JB, Tajik AJ, et al.: Frequency and location of prominent LV trabeculations at autopsy in 474 normal human hearts: Implications for evaluation of mural thrombi by two-dimensional echocardiography. J Am Coll Cardiol 1987; 9: 323.
50. Appleton CP, Hatle LK, Popp RL: Demonstration of restrictive ventricular physiology by Doppler echocardiography. J Am Coll Cardiol 1988; 11: 757
51. Fukumitsu T, Tsunekawa A, Watanabe M, Iwase M, Takeuchi E, Abe T: Primary malignant fibrous histiocytoma of the left atrium with acute mitral regurgitation. Am Heart J 1988; 115: 691.
52. Sahasakul Y, Edwards WD, Naessens JM, Tajik AJ: Age-related changes in aortic and mitral valve thickness: Implications for two-dimensional echocardiography based on an autopsy study of 200 normal human hearts. Am J Cardiol 1988; 62: 424.

53. Pollick C, Cujec B, Parker S, Tator C: Left ventricular wall motion abnormalities in subarachnoid hemorrhage: an echocardiographic study. J Am Coll Cardiol 1988; 12: 600.

54. Himelman RB, Kircher B, Rockey DC, Schiller NB. Inferior vena cava plethora with blunted respiratory response: A sensitive echocardiographic sign of cardiac tamponade. J Am Coll Cardiol 1988; 12: 1470.

55. Iwase M, Maeda M, Aoki T, Yokota M, Hayashi H, Tanaka M: Evaluation by Doppler echocardiography of transmitral flow disturbance in patients with left atrial myxoma. Am J Noninvas Cardiol 1988; 2: 264.

56. Hendel R, Silver K, Cuenoud H, Pape L: Giant anomalous left ventricular band: An echocardiographic diagnosis. Am J Noninvas Cardiol 1988; 2: 310.

7. Left ventricular function

54. Picano E, Lattanzi F, Masini M, Distante A, l'Abbate A: Comparison of the high-dose dipyridamole-echocardiography test and exercise two-dimensional echocardiography for diagnosis of coronary artery disease. Am J Cardiol 1987; 59: 225.

55. Held AC, Lavine SJ: Effect of upright exercise on left ventricular diastolic filling in normal subjects. Am J Cardiol 1988; 62: 488.

56. Labovitz AJ, Pearson AC, Chaitman BR: Doppler and two-dimensional echocardiographic assessment of left ventricular function before and after intravenous dipyridamole stress testing for detection of coronary artery disease. Am J Cardiol 1988; 62: 1180.

57. Fujii H, Yasue H, Okumura K, et al.: Hyperventilation-induced simultaneous multivessel coronary spasm in patients with variant angina: an echocardiographic and arteriographic study. J Am Coll Cardiol 1988; 12: 1184.

58. Ferrara N, Vigorito C, Leosco D, et al.: Regional left ventricular mechanical function during isometric exercise in patients with coronary artery disease: correlation with regional coronary blood flow changes. J Am Coll Cardiol 1988; 12: 1215.

59. Maeda M, Yokota M, Iwase M, Miyahara T, Hayashi H, Sotabata I: Accuracy of cardiac output measured by continuous wave Doppler echocardiography during dynamic exercise testing in the supine position in patients with coronary heart disease. J Am Coll Cardiol 1989; 13: 76.

60. Stoddard MF, Pearson A, Kern MJ, Ratcliff J, Mrosek DG, Labovitz AJ: Left ventricular diastolic function: comparison of pulsed Doppler echocardiographic and hemodynamic indexes in subjects with and without coronary heart disease. J Am Coll Cardiol 1988; 13: 327.

61. Iwase M, Hatano K, Saito F, Kato K, Maeda M, Miyaguchi K, Aoki T, Yokota M, Hayashi H, Saito H, Murase M: Evaluation by exercise Doppler echocardiography of maintenance of cardiac output during ventricular pacing with or without chronotropic response. Am J Cardiol 1989; in press.

8. Pulmonary hypertension

15. Graettinger WF, Greene ER, Voyles WF: Doppler predictions of pulmonary artery pressure, flow, and resistance in adults. Am Heart J 1987; 113: 1426.

9. Arrhythmia

17. Iwase M, Takagi S, Maeda M, Aoki T, Yokota M, Hayashi H: Evaluation of the left ventricular hemodynamic derangements due to ventricular premature contractions by pulsed Doppler echocardiography. Am J Noninvas Cardiol 1988; 2: in-press.

18. Iwase M, Aoki T, Maeda M, Yokota M, Hayashi H: Relationships between beat to beat interval and the left ventricular function in patients with atrial fibrillation. Int J Cardiac Imaging 1988; in press.

Index of subjects

Abnormal atrio-ventricular conduction 249
Abscess formation 52, 264
Acoustic shadowing 80
Acoustic window 11
A-dip 88
Age-related changes 213
Aliasing 7, 281
Ambiguous sample volume 25
A-mode 2
Amyloidosis 159
Aneurysm of the aorta 188
Annuloaortic ectasia 121
Anomalous origin of the left main coronary artery
    from pulmonary trunk 121
Aortic regurgitation 46, 83, 261–64, 271–72
Aortic stenosis 37, 262
Aortic valve perforation 52, 263
Aortic valve prolapse 46, 83, 271–72
Aortitis syndrome 46
Apical 11
Area–length method 189
Arrhythmia 219
Arrhythmogenic right ventricular dysplasia 140
Asymmetric septal hypertrophy 138
Atrial contraction 19, 196
Atrial fibrillation 223
Atrial flutter 223
Atrial septal aneurysm 187
Atrial septal defect 81, 268
Atriogenic diastolic reflux 248, 281
Attenuation 1
Autocorrelation 250
AV interval 248
Azimuth plane 18

B–B' step 140
Bernoulli equation 24, 79, 88, 138
Bicuspid aortic valve 105
Blood flow stasis 32
B-mode 2
Bowing 37
Buckling 37
Bundle branch block 218

Cardiac output 190
Cardiac pacing 190, 249

Chamber stiffness 196
Chiari network 187
Color Coded Doppler flow mapping 250
Congenital Heart Disease 81
Constrictive pericarditis 169
Continuous wave (CW) Doppler 7, 21, 190, 266
Contrast echocardiography 15, 101
Coronary artery fistula 106, 277
Coronary artery disease 122
Corrected transposition of great arteries 99
Cor triatriatum 103
Coupling interval 237

DDD pacing 248
Deceleration half-time 196
Diastolic behavior 195, 243
Diastolic filling 138
Dilated cardiomyopathy 140
Dissecting aortic aneurysm 121, 188, 280
Doppler effect 2
Doppler equation 3
Double outlet of the right ventricle 99

Echo-free space 168
Ebstein's anomaly 93, 276
Echocardiographic examination 11
Ectopic atrial rhythm 237
Eisenmenger complex 82, 273
Endocardial cushion defect 81
Exercise testing 197

Fabry's disease 159
False tendon 169
Fd_{max} 5, 282
Filling volume 223
Floating thrombi 31
Four-chamber view 12
Flailing mitral valve 37
Flow mapping technique 52
Flow velocity integral 190

Gain 18
Giant left atrium 32
Granular sparkling texture 159

Hepatic veins 79, 267

High PRF Doppler   7
Hypertrophic cardiomyopathy   138, 278

Infective endocarditis   52, 256, 264, 265
Intrapericardial hemorrhage   169
Ischemic cardiomyopathy   137

Kawasaki's disease   137

Laminar   5
Left atrial myxoma   160, 279
Left atrial rhythm   237
Left atrial thrombus   31
Left ventricular fibroma   168
Left ventricular filling   195
Left ventricular function   189
Left ventricular inflow   19
Left ventricular long axis view   11
Left ventricular outflow   19
Left ventricular short axis view   12
Left ventricular thrombus   123, 140

Malignant primary cardiac tumor   168
Marfan's syndrome   121
Mitral annular calcification   188
Mitral regurgitation   32, 81, 136, 138, 159, 160, 255,
   256, 257, 259
Mitral stenosis   28, 255, 260, 261, 262
Mitral valve area   31
Mitral valve cleft   81
Mitral valve fluttering   46
Mitral valve prolapse   33, 81, 121, 258
M-mode   2, 14, 189, 195, 214, 218
M-mode scan   14
Moving target   250
Multi-gated Doppler   8
Mural thrombus   123
Myocardial Diseases   138
Myocardial abnormality due to toxic agents   159
Myocardial inflammation   159
Myxomatous degeneration   37

Nyquist   5

Packet size   250
Parasternal   11
Paravalvular leak   259
Patent ductus arteriosus   88, 277
Peak velocity   190
Pericardial effusion   168
Pericardial defect   169
Persistent left superior vena cava   82
Phased array   2
Placement of the transducer   11
Pleural effusion   169
Pressure half-time   31, 52, 213
Presystolic mitral regurgitation   248

Prosthetic valve   80, 261
Pulmonary hypertension   188, 214
Pulmonary regurgitation   79, 268
Pulmonary stenosis   88
Pulmonary valve   15
Pulmonary wedge pressure (PWP)   197
Pulsed Doppler   5, 192, 196, 217
Pulsed Doppler examination   17

Qp/Qs assessment   81

Rapid filling   19, 196
Ratio of peak velocity in the rapid filling phase to that
   in the atrial contraction phase (A/R)   196, 213
Retrograde P wave   249, 281
Rhabdomyoma   160
Right atrial myxoma   160
Right ventricular collapse   168
Right ventricular infarction   136
Right ventricular inflow   21
Right ventricular outflow   21
Ruptured chordae tendineae   37

Secondary cardiomyopathy   159
Secondary tumors of the heart   168
Shaggy echoes   52
Shoulder formation   248
Sigmoid septum   188
Single ventricle   99
Sinus of Valsalva aneurysm   84, 273
Smoke-like echoes   40
Stroke volume   190
Subcostal   11
Suprasternal   11
Supravalvular aortic stenosis   106
Supraventricular premature contraction   237
Supraventricular tachycardia   248
Systolic anterior movement (SAM)   47, 138
Systolic Function   192
Systolic pressure gradient   46, 79, 88, 266

Tetralogy of Fallot   93, 275
Tissue characterization   122
Transesophagial echocardiography   188
Transmitral flow   160
Transvalvular regurgitation   260
Treadmill exercise   190
Tricuspid atresia   102, 270
Tricuspid regurgitation   79, 93, 266, 267
Tricuspid stenosis   73
Tricuspid valve   15
Tricuspid valve prolapse   37
Turbulent   5
Two-dimensional echocardiography   189
Two-dimensional examination   11

Ultrasound   1

Valvular perforation   52
Variance   251, 282
Vegetations   52, 256
Ventricular aneurysm   123, 278
Ventricular premature contraction   237
Ventricular septal aneurysm   83
Ventricular septal defect   82, 270, 272, 274
Ventricular septal rupture   136
Ventricular tachycardia   248

Wall-Parkinson-While (WPW) syndrome   218
Wall motion filter   18
Wall motion abnormalities   122
Wall thickening   122
Wall thinning   122
Wavelength   1

Zero shift   7

Developments in cardiovascular medicine

Recent volumes

Perry, H.M., ed.: Lifelong management of hypertension. 1983. ISBN 0-89838-582-2.

Jaffe, E.A., ed.: Biology of endothelial cells. 1984. ISBN 0-89838-587-3.

Surawicz, B., Reddy, C.P., Prystowisky, E.N., eds.: Tachycardias. 1984. ISBN 0-89838-588-1.

Spencer, M.P., ed.: Cardiac Doppler diagnosis. 1983. ISBN 0-89838-591-1.

Villarreal, H., Sambhi, M.P., eds.: Topics in pathophysiology of hypertension. 1984. ISBN 0-89838-595-4.

Messerli, F.H., ed.: Cardiovascular disease in the elderly. 1984. ISBN 0-89838-596-2.

Simoons, M.L., Reiber, J.H.C., eds.: Nuclear imaging in clinical cardiology. 1984. ISBN 0-89838-599-7.

Ter Keurs, H.E.D.J., Schipperheyn, J.J., eds.: Cardiac left ventricular hypertrophy. 1983. ISBN 0-89838-612-8.

Sperelakis, N., ed.: Physiology and pathophysiology of the heart. 1984. ISBN 0-89838-615-2.

Messerli, F.H., ed.: Kidney in essential hypertension. 1984. ISBN 0-89838-616-0.

Sambhi, M.P., ed.: Fundamental fault in hypertension. 1984. ISBN 0-89838-638-1.

Marchesi, C., ed.: Ambulatory monitoring: Cardiovascular system and allied applications. 1984. ISBN 0-89838-642-X.

Kupper, W., MacAlpin, R.N., Bleifeld, W., eds.: Coronary tone in ischemic heart disease. 1984. ISBN 0-89838-646-2.

Sperelakis, N., Caulfield, J.B., eds.: Calcium antagonists: Mechanisms of action on cardiac muscle and vascular smooth muscle. 1984. ISBN 0-89838-655-1.

Godfraind, T., Herman, A.S., Wellens, D., eds.: Calcium entry blockers in cardiovascular and cerebral dysfunctions. 1984. ISBN 0-89838-658-6.

Morganroth, J., Moore, E.N., eds.: Interventions in the acute phase of myocardial infarction. 1984. ISBN 0-89838-659-4.

Abel, F.L., Newman, W.H., eds.: Functional aspects of the normal, hypertrophied, and failing heart. 1984. ISBN 0-89838-665-9.

Sideman, S., Beyar, R., eds.: Simulation and imaging of the cardiac system. 1985. ISBN 0-89838-687-X.

Van der Wall, E., Lie, K.I., eds.: Recent views on hypertrophic cardiomyopathy. 1985. ISBN 0-89838-694-2.

Beamish, R.E., Singal, P.K., Dhalla, N.S., eds.: Stress and heart disease. 1985. ISBN 0-89838-709-4.

Beamish, R.E. Panagio, V., Dhalla, N.S., eds.: Pathogenesis of stress-induced heart disease. 1985. ISBN 0-89838-710-8.

Morganroth, J., Moore, E.N., eds.: Cardiac arrhythmias. 1985. ISBN 0-89838-716-7.

Mathes, E., ed.: Secondary prevention in coronary artery disease and myocardial infarction. 1985. ISBN 0-89838-736-1.

Lowell Stone, H., Weglicki, W.B., eds.: Pathology of cardiovascular injury. 1985. ISBN 0-89838-743-4.

Meyer, J., Erberl, R., Rupprecht, H.J., eds.: Improvement of myocardial perfusion. 1985. ISBN 0-89838-748-5.

Reiber, J.H.C., Serruys, P.W., Slager, C.J.: Quantitative coronary and left ventricular cineangiography. 1986. ISBN 0-89838-760-4.

Fagard, R.H., Bekaert, I.E., eds.: Sports cardiology. 1986. ISBN 0-89838-782-5.

Reiber, J.H.C., Serruys, P.W., eds.: State of the art in quantitative coronary arteriography. 1986. ISBN 0-89838-804-X.

Roelandt, J., ed.: Color Doppler Flow Imaging. 1986. ISBN 0-89838-806-6.

Van der Wall, E.E., ed.: Noninvasive imaging of cardiac metabolism. 1986. ISBN 0-89838-812-0.

Liebman, J., Plonsey, R., Rudy, Y., eds.: Pediatric and fundamental electrocardiography. 1986. ISBN 0-89838-815-5.

Hilger, H.H., Hombach, V., Rashkind, W.J., eds.: Invasive cardiovascular therapy. 1987. ISBN 0-89838-818-X.

Serruys, P.W., Meester, G.T., eds.: Coronary angioplasty: a controlled model for ischemia. 1986. ISBN 0-89838-819-8.

Tooke, J.E., Smaje, L.H.: Clinical investigation of the microcirculation. 1986. ISBN 0-89838-819-8.

Van Dam, R. Th., Van Oosterom, A., eds.: Electrocardiographic body surface mapping. 1986. ISBN 0-89838-834-1.

Spencer, M.P., ed.: Ultrasonic diagnosis of cerebrovascular disease. 1987. ISBN 0-89838-836-8.

Legato, M.J., ed.: The stressed heart. 1987. ISBN 0-89838-849-X.

Safar, M.E., ed.: Arterial and venow systems in essential hypertension. 1987. ISBN 0-89838-857-0.

Roelandt, J., ed.: Digital techniques in echocardiography. 1987. ISBN 0-89838-861-9.

Dhalla, N.S. et al., eds.: Pathophysiology of heart disease. 1987. ISBN 0-89838-864-3.

Dhalla, N.S. et al., eds.: Heart function and metabolism. 1987. ISBN 0-89838-865-1.

Dhalla, N.S. et al., eds.: Myocardial Ischemia. 1987. ISBN 0-89838-866-X.

Beamish, R.E. et al., eds.: Pharmacological aspects of heart disease. 1987. ISBN 0-89838-867-8.

Ter Keurs, H.E.D.J., Tyberg, J.V., eds.: Mechanics of the circulation. 1987. ISBN 0-89838-870-8.

Sideman, S., Beyar, R., eds.: Activation, metabolism and perfusion of the heart. 1987. ISBN 0-89838-871-6.

Aliot, E., Lazzara, R., eds.: Ventricular tachycardias. 1987. ISBN 0-89838-881-3.

Schneeweiss, A. et al., eds.: Cardiovascular drug therapy in the elderly. 1987. ISBN 0-89838-883-X.

Chapman, J.V., Sgalambro, A., eds.: Basic concepts in Doppler echocardiography. 1987. ISBN 0-89838-888-0.

Chien, S. et al., eds.: Clinical hemocheology. 1987. ISBN 0-89838-807-4.

Morganroth, J., ed.: Congestive heart failure. 1987. ISBN 0-89838-955-0.

Messerli, F.H., ed.: Cardiovascular disease in the elderly. 2nd ed. 1988. ISBN 0-89838-962-3.

Heintzen, P.H., Bürsch, J.H., eds.: Progress in digital angiocardiography. 1988. ISBN 0-89838-965-8.

Scheinman, M.A., ed.: Catheter ablation of cardiac arrhythmias. 1988. ISBN 0-89838-967-4.

Spaan, J.A.E., Bruschke, A.V.G., Gittenberger-de Groot, A.C., eds.: Coronary circulation. 1987. ISBN 0-89838-978-X.

Visser, C., Kan, G., Meltzer, R., eds.: Echocardiography in coronary artery disease. 1988. ISBN 0-89838-979-8.

Bayés de Luna, A., Betriu, A., Permanyer, G., eds.: Therapeutics in cardiology. 1988. ISBN 0-89838-981-X.

Mirvis, D.M., ed.: Body surface electrocardiographic mapping. 1988. ISBN 0-89838-983-6.

Konstam, M.A., Isner, J.M., eds.: The right ventricle. 1988. ISBN 0-89838-987-9.

Kappagoda, C.T., Greenwood, P.V., eds.: Long-term management of patients after myocardial infarction. 1988. ISBN 0-89838-352-8.

Gaasch, W.H., Levine, H.J., eds.: Chronic aortic regurgitation. 1988. ISBN 0-89838-364-1.

Singal, P.K., ed.: Oxygen radicals in the pathophysiology of heart disease. 1988. ISBN 0-89838-375-7.

Reiber, J.H.C., Serruys, P.W., eds.: New developments in quantitative coronary arteriography. 1988. ISBN 0-89838-377-3.

Morganroth, J., Moore, E.N., eds.: Silent myocardial ischemia. 1988. ISBN 0-89838-380-3.
Ter Keurs, H.E.D.J., Noble, M.I.M., eds.: Starling's law of the heart revisited. 1988. ISBN 0-89838-382-X.